EVIDENCE-BASED TREATMENT WITH OLDER ADULTS

EVIDENCE-BASED PRACTICES

Family Psychoeducation for Serious Mental Illness
Harriet P. Lefley

School Social Work
An Evidence-Informed Framework for Practice
Michael S. Kelly, James C. Raines, Susan Stone, and Andy Frey

Mental Health Treatment for Children and Adolescents
Jacqueline Corcoran

Individual Placement and Support
An Evidence-Based Approach to Supported Employment
Robert E. Drake, Gary R. Bond, and Deborah R. Becker

Preventing Child and Adolescent Problem Behavior
Evidence-Based Strategies in Schools, Families, and Communities
Jeffrey M. Jenson and Kimberly A. Bender

School Social Work
An Evidence-Informed Framework for Practice
Michael Kelly, James Raines, Susan Stone, and Andy Frey

Supporting Families of Children with Developmental Disabilities
Evidence-Based and Emerging Practices
Mian Wang and George H. S. Singer

Evidence-Based Treatment with Older Adults
Theory, Practice, and Research
Nancy P. Kropf and Sherry M. Cummings

The Evidence Based Practices Series is published in collaboration with the Jack, Joseph and Morton Mandel School of Applied Social Sciences at Case Western Reserve University.

EVIDENCE-BASED TREATMENT WITH OLDER ADULTS

THEORY, PRACTICE, AND RESEARCH

Nancy P. Kropf
Sherry M. Cummings

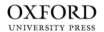

OXFORD
UNIVERSITY PRESS

Oxford University Press is a department of the University of Oxford. It furthers
the University's objective of excellence in research, scholarship, and education
by publishing worldwide. Oxford is a registered trade mark of Oxford University
Press in the UK and certain other countries.

Published in the United States of America by Oxford University Press
198 Madison Avenue, New York, NY 10016, United States of America.

© Oxford University Press 2017

CIP data is on file at the Library of Congress
ISBN 978–0–19–021462–3

CONTENTS

Part III   Challenges in Implementating Evidence-Based Treatment

EVIDENCE-BASED TREATMENT WITH OLDER ADULTS

I

OVERVIEW OF LATER LIFE ISSUES

1

INTRODUCTION TO THE AGING
POPULATION

I have discovered that there is a crucial difference between society's image of old people and "us" as we know and feel ourselves to be. . . . To break through that image, we must first understand why, how, and by whom it is perpetrated. We must also glimpse some new possibilities and new directions, both as individuals and as a society, that belie that image . . . there are choices we can make along the journey we all, sooner or later, must take that truly open surprising new possibilities.

—B. Friedan, *The Fountain of Age*, p. 31

As the baby boom generation enters their later years, significant changes are taking place within the older population and US society. The increase in the aging population is not limited to the United States, however; it is a global issue that is reshaping family life and social policy throughout the world. Why are these changes expected?

There are several reasons that the older population is increasing and changing. First, the sheer number of older adults is altering social and economic trends, including family life and responsibilities. Second, the older population is becoming more diverse in significant ways that impact health and social welfare. Additionally, the variation within the older population is increasing as greater life expectancy results in multiple cohorts within later life. Taken together, these are significant issues for professionals who practice with older adults in health, mental health, and social welfare contexts.

In recent decades, numerous biomedical advances have extended the life span and have increased life expectancy rates. Previously, later adulthood was viewed as a period of disengagement and decline (Cummings & Henry, 1961). Currently, there are many examples of adults of advanced age who are expanding the boundaries of functioning during later life. In fact, a snapshot of contemporary society reveals individuals in families, workplaces, and cultural venues who are thriving well into later adulthood.

Although the population of older adults is experiencing higher levels of health and well-being than in previous generations, the probability still exists that health and social changes will accompany advancing years. These challenges may test the functioning and resilience of older adults. In addition, many in later life are managing chronic illnesses and require additional supports in the activities of daily living (ADLs) or the instrumental activities of daily living (IADLs). As a result, families and other informal supports often assume caregiving roles and provide assistance to older adults. The demands and stress of caregiving can take a toll on their own levels of health and well-being.

The aging of society has important implications for health and human service professions. Sadly, many professions are woefully behind in preparing practitioners to work with older adults. Decades ago, Elaine Brody, a pioneer in geriatric social work, admonished social work for being unprepared for the coming advent of older adults (Brody, 1970). Since then, numerous efforts have been involved to increase the level of gerontological and geriatric care, including interprofessional education, upgrading labor force capacity, and developing pipelines into geriatric care (Heise, Johnsen, Himes, & Wing, 2012; Hooyman, 2009; Kropf, Idler, Flacker, Clevenger, & Rothschild, 2015; Sisco, Volland, & Gorin, 2005). Clearly, the aging of the population has created an awareness that clinicians, service providers, and health-care workers need to understand the issues of later life if they are to be effective in their practice.

While "experts in aging" are needed, such as geriatric social workers, nurses, and geriatricians, aging issues will be part of health, mental health, and social welfare practice regardless of settings. As a result, *all professionals* need to have a basic understanding of aging, as there will certainly be issues that are included in their scope of practice. Several examples can help illustrate this point:

- Professionals within school systems (school social workers, teachers, school nurses, and psychologists) are working with custodial grandparents who are raising their grandchildren. Census data indicate that about 10% of all US grandchildren live with a grandparent (Ellis & Simmons, 2014).
- The population of prisoners is aging. By the year 2019, prisoners over age 50 are projected to comprise about 28% of the total incarcerated population. This estimated percentage is a 10% increase since 2011 (Kim & Peterson, 2014). Those who work in criminal justice will work with these individuals who are "aging in place" within correctional facilities.
- As the baby boomers grow older, addiction patterns are increasing and changing. Alcoholism and marijuana use are two areas where there are increases in addictions within older adults (Cooper, 2012).

- Although the percentage of older adults who are homeless is lower than other age groups, these numbers are rising. One estimate indicates that the number of older adults who are homeless will double between 2010 and 2050, resulting in over 95,000 in this population (Sermons & Henry, 2010).

These examples are but a few illustrations of non-geriatric service areas that will require knowledge and skills in aging. Chapter 2 will discuss more traditional service settings in aging, such as community-based and long-term care settings.

OLDER ADULTHOOD: A BIOPSYCHOSOCIAL OVERVIEW

Before proceeding to an analysis of evidence-based practice approaches, we present information about the older population. To understand practice with older adults, it is important to have a good foundation to understand the breadth and diversity of issues during later life. In addition, health and functioning information is critical, as often these are issues that precipitate involvement with health-care providers.

INCREASES IN THE AGING POPULATION

Currently, more individuals are living past infancy, childhood, and young adulthood into later life. Illnesses that claimed the lives of young people, such as polio, smallpox, and flu epidemics, have been eradicated or controlled by public health practices, vaccines, and medical advances. In addition, changes in our economy have brought about new (and safer) occupations that have decreased accidental deaths in the labor force.

As a result, there are fewer deaths earlier in the life course. Early detection, advances in pharmaceuticals, surgical procedures, and preventive approaches allow individuals to live with conditions that previously would have claimed their lives; notable examples include cancer, hypertension, pneumonia, cardiac conditions, and diabetes, among others. However, these advances also result in more chronic conditions in the older population. Although older adults account for about 14% of the US population, this group consumes 34% of all prescription and 30% of over-the-counter drugs (Albert et al., 2014).

Life expectancy rates have increased; people are staying alive longer, with increased rates at both age 65 and 85 years. Currently, people who reach age 65 can expect to live an additional 19.2 years (Federal Interagency Forum, 2012). This period is 5 years longer than life expectancy rates at the same age in 1960. Yet within the older population, there is variation in these rates. In all racial and ethnic groups, women's life expectancy is greater than that of men (Arias, 2014). There are also differences in life expectancy by racial/ethnic background. Asian Americans have the longest life expectancy at 86.5 years. Latinos (82.8) have the second longest life space, outliving Whites (78.9) by nearly 4 years. African Americans (74.6) have the shortest life span, and Native Americans are expected to live to be 76.9 years old (The Social Science Research Council, 2014).

An additional reason that there are greater numbers of older adults today is the large number of baby boomers who are aging. As already stated, the baby boom generation consists of those individuals who were born between 1946 and 1964. This cohort was born after World War II during a time of prosperity in the United States, when families could afford children. This period also preceded the advent of widely available and convenient contraception, and thus family sizes were larger. These baby boomers are now in their fifties, sixties, and seventies and are reaching their later years.

Aging trends are significant when growth is viewed as a proportion of the population. In 1900, 5% of the population was over 65 years of age. As stated earlier, this group currently accounts for about 14% of the overall population. By 2050, when all the baby boom generation is in later life, 20.2% of the population is expected to be 65 years or older (US Census Bureau, 2015). That is, in 1900 *one in 20* people was over 65 years. By 2050, the proportion of older adults will increase to *one in four* individuals.

As stated previously, the population of the oldest old is growing most rapidly. The greatest growth is in the over-85-year-old group, with the population of centenarians (those 100 years or older) having the overall greatest increase (US Department of Health and Human Services, 2013). While living a century or more was once a major feat, centenarians are now found in societies across the world (United Nations, 2013). In addition, supercentenarians are those individuals who live past 110 years of age. The Gerontology Research Group compiles an updated list of validated supercentenarians worldwide (http://supercentenarian-research-foundation.org/TableE.aspx). Currently, these 47 individuals are found across the globe, with almost half living in Japan ($n = 23$).

DIVERSITY IN LATER ADULTHOOD

During later life, there is greater heterogeneity than there is during any other period of life. This situation is attributed to both individual factors, such as one's personality and unique history, as well as the social era in which one lived (e.g., Vietnam War and Watergate). These lived experiences, both as an individual and a member of a cohort group, have shaped worldview and behavior in unique ways. As a result, there is substantial behavioral and attitudinal variation among older adults.

Race and Ethnicity

The older population is diverse by race and ethnicity. While White older adults still comprise the majority of the population, this trend is changing. By 2050, the older population is expected to be made up of 12% African American, 20% Hispanic, and 9% Asian. Native Americans and Alaskan Natives can expect to see large growth relative to their small populations (US Census Bureau, 2010b).

Immigration trends are important in understanding the later life experiences of those who are aging. Within the United States, the number of older adults who were born in other countries has been increasing (see Figure 1.1). In 2010, more than one in eight US adults ages 65 and older were foreign-born, a share that is expected to continue to grow.

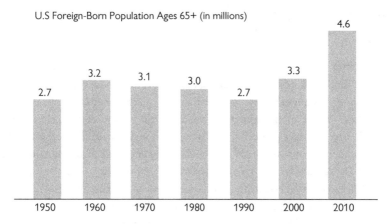

U.S Foreign-Born Population Ages 65+ (in millions)

FIGURE 1.1 Foreign-born older adults in the United States. *Source:* US Census Bureau, historical census data, 1950–2000; and Current Population Survey, 2010.

As an example, the US elderly immigrant population rose from 2.7 million in 1990 to 4.6 million in 2010, a 70% increase in 20 years (US Census Bureau, Historical Census Data, 1950–2000; and Current Population Survey, 2010a).

The changing racial/ethnic composition is significant for health and social service providers. The concept of *double jeopardy* defines the later life experiences of older persons of color who bring a lifetime of cumulative social disadvantage to their later years. Racism, combined with ageism, results in marginalized social experiences for many within these groups. Within the Hispanic and Asian groups, this condition is further complicated by language barriers, as many immigrate later in life to help support their families. As a result, they have low levels of language skills, and lack social connections and assimilation into society, which results in isolation and depression (Kim, Park, & Heo, 2010).

Gender Differences

There are also significant gender issues within the older population. Women's life expectancy is greater than that of men in all racial and ethnic groups (Arias, 2014). As a result, widowhood is a normative social role for women. Because of the pool of available women, men who lose a spouse in later life are more likely to re-partner (US Department of Health and Human Services, 2013). However, the lack of available men results in women living alone or with their adult children.

Poverty is another late-life gender issue. While programs such as Social Security and Medicare have reduced the overall poverty rate in the older population, segments within the population continue to struggle with adequate resources. For example, there are substantial differences in poverty rates by race and gender. White males had the lowest poverty rate, while older Black and Hispanic women had the highest (Federal Interagency Forum, 2012):

- The poverty rate for White men over 65 years was 5%, as compared to 14% for older Black, Hispanic, and Asian men.

- White women over age 65 years had an 8% poverty rate. This percentage compares to 15% for Asian women, and 21% for both Black and Hispanic women.

Cohort Variations

The older adult years span several decades, from age 60 to 100+ years, and includes different cohorts. As a result, there are variations and differences within the older adult population, which is another aspect of diversity. Birth cohorts are defined as a "group of people born during a particular period or year" (*Segen's Medical Dictionary*, 2011). Older adulthood includes multiple generations, including those who have experienced the Great Depression (born between 1901 and 1924), World War II (born between 1925 and 1945), and the baby boom generation (born between 1946 and 1964).

The social era in which an individual develops will impact and shape behavior and responses. For example, the baby boom generation experienced the Vietnam War, Watergate, and the rise of the civil rights movement. As a result, this generation has been more questioning of authority, with the expectation that baby boomers will be more "consumer-oriented" in their approach to health and social welfare services. That is, they will be less apt than the previous generation to take information from health and service providers at face value, and they may investigate alternatives or seek multiple options more often than their parents and grandparents (Olson & Wiley, 2006).

HEALTH AND FUNCTIONING

Although older adults are living longer than previously, advancing age often includes health-related declines and decreases in functional ability. There are examples of exceptional individuals who maintain high levels of fitness into very late life. For example, Olga Kotelko successfully competed in track and field events until her death at age 95 (Grierson, 2014). However, most individuals are not at this peak level of capacity at this point in the life course. Approximately 91% of older adults have at least one chronic health issue; 75% of older adults have at least two chronic conditions, such as diabetes, arthritis, or hypertension (National Council on Aging, 2014), and often these conditions have a negative impact on their functioning and well-being.

Within a health-care context, acute health problems were previously associated with high death rates. For example, the Spanish flu of 1918 had a dramatic impact on the population worldwide, especially on young adults. Estimates of death range between 50–100 million people (Taubenberger & Morens, 2006), which is about one of every five individuals in the world. These global pandemics now are quite rare as vaccines, technology, and advanced public health practices have become more sophisticated and have decreased the prevalence of outbreaks.

As a result, the more typical pattern is for an older individual to manage a chronic health problem. All but one of the leading causes of death of older adults are chronic conditions. Although heart disease has declined since the 1980s, this remains the leading cause of death for people over age 65. The other leading causes of death in the older population are (in order): cancer, chronic lower respiratory disease, stroke, and Alzheimer's disease, diabetes, and pneumonia/influenza (Federal Interagency Forum, 2012). While these chronic conditions are serious, many can be managed by appropriate treatment. However, there is also a probability that individuals with these health conditions will require other types of support to manage these conditions, such as care provision, modification of their household, or a move to a more supportive residential situation, such as a long-term care facility.

Differences exist in health conditions by sociodemographic variables. Women have higher rates of asthma, hypertension, and arthritis than men. However, men have more cancer, heart disease, and diabetes than women (Centers for Disease Control & Prevention, 2014). Different health patterns are also reported by race and ethnicity. Older African Americans and Hispanics had higher rates of diabetes than Whites of similar ages. In addition, older African Americans also had higher rates of hypertension than Whites. However, older Hispanics had lower levels of arthritis as compared to similar age Whites (Federal Interagency Forum, 2012).

One of the most challenging conditions of older life is Alzheimer's disease, the most common type of dementia, which is characterized by memory impairment, personality changes such as agitation and hostility, and decreased judgment and orientation. Alzheimer's disease can last for years, and requires increasing support, which is mainly provided by family (US Department of Health and Human Services, 2014). As a result, those who are in care provider roles (mainly spouses, partners, adult children) benefit from interventions and resources to help them cope with the multiple and complex tasks of care associated with dementia. Dementia is a serious concern, both as a health and public policy issue, because of the nature of the disease process. With the advancing growth of older adults who are 85 years and older, the rates of Alzheimer's disease and other dementias are expected to double for every 5-year interval beyond age 65 (US Department of Health and Human Services, 2014).

MENTAL HEALTH ISSUES IN LATER LIFE

In addition to health conditions, later life may include mental health issues for older adults. For example, the multiple changes that are experienced during this part of the life course—such as role shifts (e.g., retirement, widowhood) and functional limitations (e.g., no longer driving)—can be precipitating factors in geriatric depression. However, other conditions are lifelong experiences that older adults bring to their later years. For example, people with severe mental illness (SMI) are living longer lives than previously (Cummings & Kropf, 2011). In later life, people with SMI may exhibit different symptoms, and require care and support to deal with the interaction of aging with their mental health condition.

Therefore, the mental health conditions of older adults may emerge during this period of life, or might be a long-standing issue that is carried into their later years.

Geriatric Depression

The most prevalent mental health conditions of later life are geriatric depression and anxiety. The Geriatric Mental Health Foundation (2015) references the following statistics about geriatric depression:

- Depression affects 15 out of every 100 adults over age 65.
- Rates of depression in the community range from 1% to 13%.
  - The prevalence rate of major depressive disorders (MDD) is 1.8% in the over-65 population.
  - 13.5% of depressive syndromes are considered clinically relevant in this population.
  - During the first year, over half of the residents of long-term care facilities experience depression (54.1%).

Depression can have grave consequences for older adults. Those older adults who suffer from geriatric depression have poor physical and cognitive functioning, poorer perceptions of their own health status, lower health utilization rates, and increased health-care costs (Cole & Dendukuri, 2003).

A particularly devastating outcome of geriatric depression is elder suicide. In many countries in the world, including the United States, older adults have high suicide rates, especially older men (Conwell & Thompson, 2008). In the United States, suicide rates for males are highest among those aged 75 and older, with a rate 36 per 100,000 individuals (CDC, 2010). Suicide is a significant public health concern during later life, and this trend is continuing as the baby boom generation ages. Between 1999 and 2010, the suicide rate among men aged 45–64 years increased 43%. For adult women, the largest percentage increase in suicide rate was in the 45–64-year age group, a (Curtin, Warner, & Hedegaard, 2016).

Substance Abuse and Addiction

Addiction is another serious concern in later life, and rates and patterns of addictions are changing as baby boomers enter their later years. Currently, the annual number of older adults with substance abuse disorders is about 2.8 million. This number is expected to double by 2020, when it is expected to increase to 5.7 million (Han, Gfoerer, Colliver, & Penne, 2009).

Nicotine is the most common addiction and impacts 18%–22% of the older adult population. The next most prevalent addiction is alcohol, which impacts up to 18% of older adults (Blazer & Wu, 2009a). Currently, illegal drug rates remain low (less than 1% of the over-65 population). However, marijuana use is increasing as the baby boom generation ages. Marijuana dependency accounted for .12% of the over-65 age group, but was about 4% in the 50–64-year group (Blazer & Wu, 2009b; Han, Gfoere, & Colliver, 2009). With changing patterns and types of addiction, additional research is needed on effective treatment approaches, as well as interactions with other medication.

Older adults are an over-prescribed population, and medication can create several problems with this population. First, the interaction of prescription drugs and alcohol can be dangerous or lethal. An estimate is that 19% of older Americans may be impacted by using both medications and alcohol (Blow, 2013). Additionally, age-related changes create more health-related problems when older adults use alcohol. Decreases in the percentage of water in the body means that alcohol impacts older adults more quickly (especially older women) and absorbs more slowly. Therefore, alcohol is cleared less efficiently and stays within the system, risking drug reactions and health problems (e.g., ulcers, risk of falls). Additionally, those who are long-term drinkers are at risk for psychiatric illness. Older adults are three times more likely to develop depression, cognitive losses, or anxiety disorders if they have a lifetime diagnosis of alcohol abuse (Blow, 2013).

Severe Mental Illness

As the general aging population is increasing, so is the population that is aging with a severe mental illness (SMI). The typical diagnoses that are classified as SMI are schizophrenia and schizophrenia-related disorders, bipolar disorder, major recurrent depressive disorder, and personality disorders (Cummings & Kropf, 2011). Current estimates suggest that about 1.4% of the US population have a severe mental illness and are over age 65 (Hudson, 2012). As the baby boom generation ages, challenges in meeting the increased mental health needs of the older population are also expected to increase. Unfortunately, the mental health needs of older adults continue to be overlooked in treatment and policy arenas (Friedman, Williams, Kidder, & Furst, 2013).

The intersection of aging and SMI creates particular challenges in treatment and care provision. Compared to their counterparts without psychiatric disorders, older adults with SMI have more health-related challenges. In addition, older adults with SMI or addictions are more likely to have multiple chronic illnesses (Lin, Zhang, Leung, & Clark, 2011). Due to the nature of certain psychiatric conditions, persons with SMI may also have compromised social, financial, and emotional resources that are needed in later life (Shepherd, Depp, Harris, Halpain, Palinkas, & Jeste, 2012). These combined factors can create challenges for the care of older adults who age with a severe psychiatric condition.

SOCIAL CONDITIONS

Several social conditions have also created changes that impact the experience of later life for older individuals, families, and societies. Family structures have changed, with greater diversity in the family forms of today. In addition to diversity in race and ethnicity, as already discussed in this chapter, family structures are shifting by sexual orientation and identity. These trends are changing the dynamics of later life and have an impact on caregiving and support for older adults.

Shifting Family Structures

Since the baby boom years were a time of high birth rates and lower life expectancy rates, the population had a greater number of younger individuals than older adults. Since then, birth and pregnancy rates have changed, which has resulted in different generational configurations within families. During the baby boom years, families had a pyramidal shape; that is, there were many children, two parents, and perhaps a grandparent or two. Families of today have a "beanpole" shape; that is, there are fewer children and multiple generations in later life. On a population level, the pyramids are shifting and becoming more of a rectangle than an actual pyramid. In Figure 1.2, two population pyramids are displayed, and the change in the shape over the 45-year time period is dramatic. Corresponding changes in family structure result in greater numbers of older adults (e.g., older parents, grandparents, and possibly great-grandparents) with fewer in younger generations to provide care and assistance.

Families are changing in other ways as well. For example, the United States has recently experienced a transformation in marriages. In 2004, San Francisco became the first location in the United States to legalize same-sex marriage (although the ruling was later overturned). The first couple wed was Del Martin and Phyllis Lyon, who were in their eighties when they married, after having been together for decades. Later that year, Massachusetts legalized same-sex marriage, and subsequently, states had the ability to allow same-sex marriage, although these unions were not recognized at the federal level. In June 2015, the Supreme Court overturned the ban on same-sex marriage, thus allowing gay and lesbian couples to legally marry in all states within the United States (http://www.supremecourt.gov/opinions/14pdf/14-556_3204.pdf).

Since the 1960s, when advances in civil rights opened up new opportunities for gay and lesbian populations, significant advancements in social and political responses to LGBT issues have been dramatic. Although there continue to be discrimination and backlash, LGBT individuals have rights to bear and adopt children and openly serve in the armed forces (with benefits to their spouses), as just two examples. In addition, specialized services to LGBT older adults also exist, which is imperative, as an estimated 2 million Americans aged 50 or older identify as LGBT, with that number expected to double by 2030 (Fredriksen-Goldsen et al., 2011). For example, research on Area Agencies on Aging (AAA) indicate that four-fifths of the agencies surveyed were willing to provide training on sexual identity and aging to agency staff to be a more inclusive and welcoming organization for older LGBT individuals (Knochel, Croghan, Moone, & Quam, 2012).

Caregiving Issues

As the older population increases, families are dealing with issues related to support for older adults. The majority of care for older adults is provided by informal support such as family, friends, or other close relationships. As a result, interventions, support, and resources for the care provider are part of aging services. The "average" US care provider is "a 49-year-old woman who works outside the home and spends nearly 20 hours per week providing unpaid care to her mother for nearly five years. Almost two-thirds

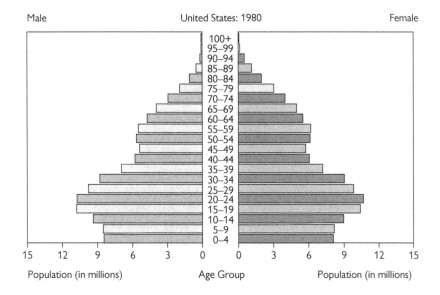

Male   United States: 1980   Female

Population (in millions)   Age Group   Population (in millions)

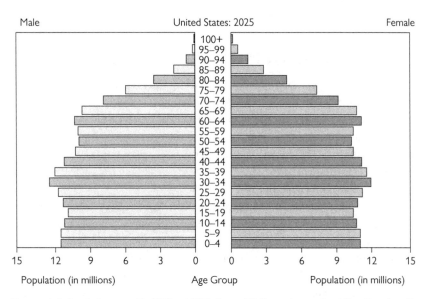

Male   United States: 2025   Female

Population (in millions)   Age Group   Population (in millions)

FIGURE 1.2 Population pyramids: 1980 and 2025. *Source:* US Census International Data Base, http://www.census.gov/population/international/data.

of family caregivers are female (65%). More than eight in ten are caring for a relative or friend age 50 or older" (Feinberg, Reinhard, Houser, & Choula, 2011, p. 1). As this description suggests, caregiving is another "job" for many in this role. Additionally, care provision is frequently assumed in addition to other role responsibilities, such as being a parent, employee, and spouse or partner.

Caregiving is associated with significant costs for families. One estimate is that unpaid family caregiving equals about $450 billion per year (Family Caregiving Alliance, 2012). However, there is great variability in the cost of care by different conditions. The average out-of-pocket costs for someone with dementia was 81% higher than caring for patients with other health conditions (Kelley, McGarry, Gorges, & Skinner, 2015).

However, not all caregiving is provided *to older adults*, as substantial numbers provide care to younger generations. Parents who remain in care-provision roles for adult children with cognitive, physical, or psychiatric conditions have unique support needs. Typically, these caregivers provide physical, economic, and/or emotional support long past the usual time period of parenting. Often, they are managing their own age-related changes and challenges in conjunction with the care needs of their adult child (Greene & Kropf, 2014). In addition, other family members may assume caregiving roles, such as grandparents who are raising grandchildren. Currently, approximately 2.5 million grandparents are responsible for raising one or more of their grandchildren, with 59 years being the average age of the caregiver (Ellis & Simmons, 2014). Clearly, late-life caregiving needs to include attention and support for older adults who are in caregiving roles for their children and grandchildren.

ELEMENTS OF EFFECTIVE PRACTICE WITH OLDER ADULTS

Although the older population is diverse in terms of functioning and experience, effective practice needs to take into account the age-related changes of later adulthood. While subsequent chapters provide more specific principles, there are some basic and fundamental tenets that are a foundation for practice with the older population. The Gerontological Society of America (GSA) has compiled an evidence-based summary of communication practices with older adults (GSA, 2012). These include both content and method of interactions when communicating with older adults.

Although older adults bring a vast experience from their decades of living, those communicating with them may use a demeaning or infantilizing tone. Younger generations may address older individuals in *elderspeak*—that is, with short, simple sentences, exaggerated intonation such as a sing-song effect, or endearing or diminutive terms such as "dear" or "sweetie" (Balsis & Carpenter, 2006; Williams, Kemper & Hummert, 2004). In interactions with older adults, practitioners should begin by recognizing if they have any preexisting ideas about working with aging individuals (stereotypes about cognitive and physical limitations, for example). In addition, communication needs to be respectful (e.g., "Hello, Mr. Anderson") and convey a sense of dignity for their life circumstances (e.g., a knock on a door before entering a nursing home room).

In order to overcome some of the changes that can make communication more difficult, there are some strategies that need to be in place to maximize interactions with older adults. Hearing and sight changes can make reading, talking, and listening more difficult. As a result, good practices include attending to the environment when interact-ing with older adults (e.g., reduce background noises, reduce glare, face older person when speaking). To be sure that important points are comprehended correctly, a good practice is to distribute critical information in visual form (e.g., handouts, diagrams, bul-let lists).

One strategy that older adults use to help with communication is to bring a family member or close friend to appointments. In a study of physician visits, about 19% of older adults brought someone along to appointments (Wolff, Boyd, Gitlin, Bruce, & Roter, 2012). This strategy is helpful; however, practitioners need to be sensitive to com-munication patterns when another person is involved. In these situations, older adults need to be involved in discussions and addressed within the dialogue. Avoid marginal-izing the older adult by using third-person language with the individual is present (e.g., "How is *he* feeling?").

Much communication is based upon language used, and there are cultural and cohort variations that can compromise understanding by older adults. Practitioners may become entrenched in the jargon of their discipline, and terminology may be unclear to older adults. Additionally, vague language can cause confusion, such as "take two pills twice a day." A clearer statement is to tell an older patient to take two pills after breakfast and two pills after dinner. This provides a clear picture that enhances understanding and adherence. As younger cohorts, we are accustomed to dealing with abstract phrases and language. As adults age, plain and specific language is most helpful in communicating.

ORGANIZATION OF CHAPTERS IN THIS VOLUME

Practitioners across professions need to be knowledgeable about effective interventions in practicing with older adults and their families. The purpose of this book is to examine evidence-based practice with the older population—that is, to analyze which interven-tions have credible, empirical evidence associated with their implementation with the older population. With the significant changes in the older population—including size, life expectancy, health and mental health challenges, and increased diversity—practitioners in multiple practice contexts need to be well versed in intervention approaches that pro-mote functioning and quality of life with older adults and their families.

This book is organized into three major parts to provide an analysis of evidence-based practice. Part I (Chapters 1 and 2) provides an overview of the older population. Content on the diversity of the population, including sociodemographics, health, mental health, and functional abilities, is provided. In addition, the various contexts for treatment and practice are introduced. Settings include community-based, long-term care, and acute-care settings. Integrated health care issues and models will also be presented within this part.

Part II (Chapters 3–12) critically examines evidence-based intervention approaches with older adults. The American Psychological Association (APA) defines evidence-based practice as "the integration of the best available research with clinical expertise in the context of patient characteristics, culture, and preferences" (American Psychological Association, 2006, p. 280). Based upon the standards promulgated by the Division 12 (Clinical Psychology) Task Force of the APA (1995), the following criteria are used to evaluate evidence-based treatment (Chambless & Hollon, 1998):

1. At least two good between-group design experiments must demonstrate efficacy in one or more of the following ways:
   a. Superiority to pill, psychotherapy placebo, or other treatment
   b. Equivalence to already established treatment with adequate sample sizes.
2. Experiments must be conducted with treatment manuals or equivalent clear description of treatment.
3. Characteristics of samples must be specified.
4. Effects must be demonstrated by at least two investigators or teams.

In addition, this book focuses on those interventions that have been implemented with samples that either are specifically older adults, or with a substantial number of adults who are beyond 60 years of age.

Five intervention approaches are included within the chapters. The first type of treatment presented is cognitive behavior therapy (CBT), which is the most commonly used evidence-based practice to treat mental disorders, especially depression (Field, Beeson, & Jones, 2015). An individual's cognitive appraisal (e.g., thoughts, images) shapes the internal landscape, such as the way the person feels about a situation. As a treatment approach, CBT works to modify automatic thoughts (Beck, Rush, Shaw, & Emery, 1979) that trigger maladaptive perceptions such as "I'm a burden," or "I can't do anything." The practitioner works with clients to bring understanding about these thoughts and feelings in an effort to change to more adaptive and functional ones. Since geriatric depression is one of the most common mental health conditions of later life, CBT is a treatment approach that has utility with the older population.

The second treatment approach is problem-solving therapy (PST). This approach assists individuals by enhancing coping abilities to decrease the stresses of negative physical and mental health conditions. The goal of PST is to help clients engage in resolving problems that they are currently experiencing (c.f., Hegel & Areán, 2012). The process involves identifying the particular problems experienced, generating solutions to the problem, implementing selected options, and evaluating the outcome. Since later life often involves stresses resulting from managing health and mental conditions, decreased functional abilities, and residential and social transition, PST is an appropriate treatment choice to assist older clients with these and related issues.

A third approach is motivational interviewing (MI). This is a counseling approach that assists clients in resolving ambivalence in an effort to create behavioral changes. In MI, the process of change involves engaging the client, focusing on a direction for change, evoking the process that the client will undergo to achieve change, and planning strategies to change behavior. This method has been used widely with problems in younger generations, such as addictions and weight loss (c.f., Armstrong et al., 2011; Heckman & Egleston, 2010). Although a relatively new approach with older adults, a growing literature indicates that MI is effective with older adults who have addictions, as well as in promoting behaviors to support health and wellness in this population.

Two of the more typical treatment types with older adults are psychoeducational and social support interventions. These are used with a range of conditions, including situations in which older adults or caregivers need to learn new behaviors (e.g., diet management in diabetes or hypertension), ways of coping (e.g., caregiving for a person with dementia), or providing connection with others (e.g., bereavement group). These approaches are often structured around the unique issues of the individuals, such as a support group where caregivers have a space to discuss whatever they are dealing with in the care situation. As such, few of these interventions employ a manualized approach. However, a robust literature exists around the effectiveness of these two approaches and the breadth of conditions and contexts where these approaches can be implemented. For those reasons, psychoeducational and social support interventions are included in the chapters.

The final intervention approach is unique to aging, as life review and reminiscence are typically used with older adults over other age cohorts. Although these approaches have a different focus, both life review and reminiscence use the process of recall and remembering past situations and experiences to enhance present functioning. These interventions are easily employed in various community-based and residential contexts, and can be used to maintain and preserve functioning and to deal with challenges and functional decline. Unlike some of the other approaches in this book, reminiscence in particular has been used widely in dementia care.

For each of these five approaches, theoretical foundations are presented and discussed. To illustrate implementation, a case example of a practice issue with an older adult client is presented. Additionally, the empirical research on this intervention with older adults will be summarized.

Part III of the book (Chapters 13 and 14) examines implementation and challenges of evidence-based practice in more detail. Factors and conditions that facilitate successful implementation and produce effective results will be highlighted, as well as challenges and barriers to successful implementation. As a brief introduction, treatment fidelity refers to the degree that essential elements of an intervention approach are delivered as intended within the standards and protocols of the approach (Cohen et al., 2008; Gearing et al., 2011; Naleppa & Cagle, 2010; Tucker & Blythe, 2008). Different factors can comprise fidelity, such as lack of training for interventionists, or organizational or structural issues in the setting (e.g., lack of privacy in a nursing home or staff turnover). Within intervention research, studies typically summarize the degree and magnitude of change in the dependent variable, such as a decrease in depression scores after participating in CBT. However, there has been less description of the treatment, or independent variable, including description of the treatment approach and duration, and modifications in using the approach with older clients. Due to the importance of this issue, treatment fidelity will be discussed in greater detail in Chapter 13.

Chapter 14, the final chapter, looks toward the future and includes a summary of "promising interventions" with older adults. In particular, behavioral activation and mindfulness-based stress reduction will be discussed, as a substantive body of literature in practice with younger cohorts exists for these two approaches. Finally, the book will conclude with some thoughts about next steps in geriatric research and practice.

REFERENCES

Albert, S. M., Bix, L., Bridgeman, M. M., Carstensen, L. L., Dyer-Chamberlain, M., Neafsey, P. J., & Wolf, M. S. (2014). Promoting safe and effective use of OTC medications: CHPA-GSA National Summit. *The Gerontologist, 54*(6), 909–918.

American Psychological Association. (2006). Evidence-based practice in psychology. *American Psychologist, 61*(4), 271–285.

American Psychological Association Task Force on Psychological Intervention Guidelines. (1995). *Template for developing guidelines: Interventions for mental disorders and psychological aspects of physical disorders.* Washington, DC: APA.

Arias, E. (2014). *U.S. Department of Health and Human Services: National vital statistics reports.* Vol. 62, no. 7, p. 3. Retrieved June 28, 2014, from http://www.cdc.gov/nchs/data/nvsr62/nvsr62_07.pdf.

Armstrong, M. J., Mottershead, T. A., Ronkley, P. E., Sigal, R. J., Campbell, T. S., & Hemmelgarn, B. R. (2011). Motivational interviewing to improve weight loss in overweight and/or obese patients: a systematic review and meta-analysis of randomized controlled trials. *Obesity Reviews, 12,* 709–723.

Balsis, S., & Carpenter, B. D. (2006). Evaluations of elderspeak in a caregiving context. *Clinical Gerontologist, 29*(1), 79–96.

Beck, A. T., Rush, A. J., Shaw, B. F., & Emery, G. (1979). *Cognitive therapy of depression.* New York: Guilford Press.

Birth cohort. (n.d.). *Segen's Medical Dictionary.* (2011). Retrieved July 12, 2014, from http://medical-dictionary.thefreedictionary.com/birth+cohort.

Blazer, D., & Wu, L. T. (2009a). The epidemiology of at-risk and binge drinking among middle-aged and elderly community adults: National Survey on Drug Use and Health. *American Journal of Psychiatry, 166*(10), 1162–1169.

Blazer, D. G., & Wu, L. T. (2009b). The epidemiology of substance use and disorders among middle aged and elderly community adults: national survey on drug use and health. *The American Journal of Geriatric Psychiatry, 17*(3), 237–245.

Blow, F. C. (2013, September 27). *Overview: Aging substance misuse: background, prevalance and comorbidity.* Presentation, Atlanta Regional Geriatric Education Center Conferece: Building Workforce Competency.

Brody, E. M. (1970). Serving the aged: educational needs as viewed by practice. *Social Work, 15*(4), 42–51.

Centers for Disease Control and Prevention, National Center for Injury Prevention and Control. Web-based Injury Statistics Query and Reporting System (WISQARS) [online]. (2010). Available from www.cdc.gov/injury/wisqars/index.html.

Chambless, D. L., & Hollon, S. D. (1998). Defining empirically supported therapies. *Journal of Consulting and Clinical Psychology, 66*(1), 7–18.

Cohen, D. J., Crabtree, B. F., Etz, R. S., Balasubramanian, B. A., Donahue, K. E., Leviton, L. C., . . . Green, L. W. (2008). Fidelity versus flexibility: translating evidence-based research into practice. *American Journal of Preventive Medicine, 35*(5), S381–S389.

Cole, M. G., & Dendukuri, N. (2003). Risk factors for depression among elderly community subjects: a systematic review and meta-analysis. *American Journal of Psychiatry, 160*(6), 1147–1156.

Conwell, Y., & Thompson, C. (2008). Suicidal behavior in elders. *Psychiatric Clinics of North America, 31*(2), 333–356.

Cooper, L. (2012). Combined motivational interviewing and cognitive-behavioral therapy with older adult drug and alcohol abusers. *Health & Social Work, 37*(3), 173–179. doi:10.1093/hsw/hls023.

Cumming, E., & Henry, W. E. (1961). *Growing old: the process of disengagement.* New York: Basic.

Cummings, S. M., & Kropf, N. P. (2011). Aging with a severe mental illness: challenges and treatments. *Journal of Gerontological Social Work, 54*(2), 175–188.

Curtin, S.C., Warner, M., & Hedegaard, H. (2016). Suicide Rates for Females and Males by Race and Ethnicity: United States, 1999 and 2014. Centers for Disease Control. Retrieved December 17, 2016. https://www.cdc.gov/nchs/data/hestat/suicide/rates_1999_2014.pdf

Ellis, R. R., & Simmons, T. (2014). Coresident grandparents and their grandchildren: 2012. US Bureau of the Census. Retrieved July 16, 2016, from http://www.census.gov/content/dam/Census/library/publications/2014/demo/p20-576.pdf.

Family Caregiving Alliance. (2012). *Fact sheet: selected caregiver statistics.* Retrieved December 17, 2016 from http://www.caregiver.org/caregiver/jsp/content_node.jsp?nodeid=439.

Federal Interagency Forum. (2012). *Older Americans 2012: key indicators of well- being.* Retrieved May 12, 2014, from www.agingstats.gov.

Feinberg, L. F., Reinhard, S. C., Houser, A., & Choula, R. (2011). *Valuing the invaluable: 2011 update—The growing contributions and costs of family caregiving.* Washington, DC: AARP Policy Institute.

Field, T. A., Beeson, E. T., & Jones, L. K. (2015). The new ABCs: a practitioner's guide to neuroscience-informed cognitive-behavior therapy. *Journal of Mental Health Counseling, 37*(3), 206–220.

Fredriksen-Goldsen, K. I., Kim, H.-J., Emlet, C. A., Muraco, A., Erosheva, E. A., Hoy-Ellis, C. P., . . . Petry, H. (2011). *The aging and health report: disparities and resilience among lesbian, gay, bisexual, and transgender older adults.* Seattle, WA: Institute for Multigenerational Health.

Friedan, B. (1993). *The fountain of age.* New York: Simon & Schuster.

Friedman, M. B., Williams, K. A., Kidder, E., & Furst, L. (2013). Meeting the mental health challenges of the elder boom. In J. Rosenberg & S. J. Rosenberg (Eds.), *Community mental health: challenges for the 21st century* (2nd ed.) (pp. 109–132). New York: Routledge/Taylor & Francis Group.

Gearing, R. E., El-Bassel, N., Ghesquiere, A., Baldwin, S., Gillies, J., & Ngeow, E. (2011). Major ingredients of fidelity: a review and scientific guide to improving quality of intervention research implementation. *Clinical Psychology Review, 31*(1), 79–88.

Geriatric Mental Health Foundation. (2015). Depression in late life: not a natural part of aging. Retrieved from July 12, 2015. http://www.gmhfonline.org/gmhf/consumer/factsheets/depression_latelife.html.

Gerontological Society of America. (2012). *Communicating with older adults: an evidence-based review of what really works.* Washington, DC: Author. http://www.agingresources.com/cms/wp-content/uploads/2012/10/GSA_Communicating-with-Older-Adults-low-Final.pdf.

Greene, R. R., & Kropf, N. P. (2014). *Caregiving and caresharing: a life course perspective.* Washington, DC: NASW Press.

Grierson, B. (2014). *What makes Olga run: the mystery of the 90 something track star and what she can teach us about living longer, happier lives.* New York: Henry Holt.

Han, B., Gfroerer, J., & Colliver, J. (2009). *An examination of trends in illicit drug use among adults aged 50 to 59 in the United States.* Washington, DC: Office of Applied Studies, Substance Abuse and Mental Health Service Administration.

Han, B., Gfroerer, J. C., Colliver, J. D., & Penne, M. A. (2009). Substance use disorder among older adults in the United States in 2020. *Addiction, 104*(1), 88–96.

Heckman, C. J., & Egleston, B. L. (2010). Efficacy of motivational interviewing for smoking cessation: a systematic review and meta-analysis. *Top Control, 19,* 410–416.

Hegel, M. T., & Areán, P. A. (2012). Problem-Solving Treatment for Primary Care (PST-PC): a treatment manual for depression. University of Washington Psychiatry and Behavioral Sciences. Retrieved July 15, 2015 from http://impact-uw.org/tools/pst_manual.html.

Heise, B. A., Johnsen, V., Himes, D., & Wing, D. (2012). Developing positive attitudes toward geriatric nursing among millennials and generation Xers. *Nursing Education Perspectives, 33*(3), 156–161.

Hooyman, N. R. (2009). *Transforming social work education: the first decade of the Hartford Geriatric Social Work Initiative.* Alexandria, VA: Council on Social Work Education.

Hudson, C. G. (2012). Declines in mental illness over the adult years: an enduring finding or methodological artifact? *Aging and Mental Health, 16*(6), 735–752.

Kelley, A. S., McGarry, K., Gorges, R., & Skinner, J. S. (2015). The burden of health care costs for patients with dementia in the last 5 years of life. *Annals of Internal Medicine, 163*(10), 729–736.

Kim, J., Park, J., & Heo, J. (2010). What should recreational professionals do when providing services to elderly immigrants? *Physical & Occupational Therapy in Geriatrics, 28*(2), 195–202. doi:10.3109/02703180903438761

Kim, K. & Peterson, B. (2014). Aging behind bars: Trends and implications of graying prisoners in the federal prison system. Urban Institute. Retrieved July 15, 2016, from http://www.urban.org/sites/default/files/alfresco/publication-pdfs/413222-Aging-Behind-Bars-Trends-and-Implications-of-Graying-Prisoners-in-the-Federal-Prison-System.PDF.

Knochel, K. A., Croghan, C. F., Moone, R. P., & Quam, J. K. (2012). Training, geography, and provision of aging services to lesbian, gay, bisexual, and transgender older adults. *Journal of Gerontological Social Work, 55*(5), 426–443.

Kropf, N. P., Idler, E., Flacker, J., Clevenger, C., & Rothschild, E. (2015). Interprofessional dialogues within a senior mentoring program: incorporating gerontology students as facilitation leaders. *Educational Gerontology, 41*(5), 373–383.

Lin, W. C., Zhang, J., Leung, G. Y., & Clark, R. E. (2011). Chronic physical conditions in older adults with mental illness and/or substance use disorders. *Journal of the American Geriatrics Society, 59*(10), 1913–1921.

Naleppa, M. J., & Cagle, J. G. (2010). Treatment fidelity in social work intervention research: a review of published studies. *Research on Social Work Practice, 20*(6), 674–681.

National Council on Aging. (2014) *Center for health aging*. Retrieved April 22, 2015 from http://www.ncoa.org/improve-health/center-for-healthy-aging/chronic-disease/.

Olson, D. L., & Wiley, P. (2006). Benefits, consumerism and an "Ownership Society." *Benefits Quarterly*, 22(2), 7–14.

Sermons, M. W., & Henry, M. (2010). Demographics of the homeless: the rising elderly population. Homelessness Research Institute, National Alliance to End Homelessness. Retrieved July 15, 2016, from http://www.endhomelessness.org/page/-/files/2698_file_Aging_Report.pdf.

Shepherd, S., Depp, C. A., Harris, G., Halpain, M., Palinkas, L. A., & Jeste, D. V. (2012). Perspectives on schizophrenia over the lifespan: a qualitative study. *Schizophrenia Bulletin*, 38(2), 295–303.

Sisco, S., Volland, P., & Gorin, S. (2005). Social work leadership and aging: meeting the demographic imperative. *Health & Social Work*, 30(4), 344.

The Social Science Research Council (2014). *Measure of America 2013–2014, American human development report*. Retrieved June 20, 2014, from http://www.measureofamerica.org/docs/MOA-III-June-18-FINAL.pdf

Taubenberger, J. K., & Morens, D. M. (2006, Jan.). 1918 influenza: the mother of all pandemics. *Emerging Infectious Diseases*, 17, 69–79. Retrieved May 15, 2014, from http://dx.doi.org/10.3201/eid1209.050979

Tucker, A., & Blythe, B. (2008). Attention to treatment fidelity in social work outcomes: a review of the literature from the 1990s. *Social Work Research*, 32(3), 185–190.

United Nations, Department of Economic and Social Affairs, Population Division (2013). *World population ageing 2013*. ST/ESA/SER.A/348. Retrieved February 12, 2015 from http://www.un.org/en/development/desa/population/publications/pdf/ageing/WorldPopulationAgeing2013.pdf.

US Census Bureau. (2010a). *Current population survey*. Washington, DC: US Government Printing Office.

US Census Bureau. (2010b). *The next four decades: The older population in the United States: 2010 to 2050*. Retrieved June 22, 2014, from http://www.census.gov/prod/2010pubs/p25-1138.pdf.

US Census Bureau. (2015). *Older Americans month: May 2015*. Retrieved July 16, 2016, from http://www.census.gov/content/dam/Census/newsroom/facts-for-features/2015/cb15-ff09_older_american_month.pdf.

US Department of Health and Human Services. (2013). *A profile of older Americans: 2013*. Retrieved June 20, 2014, from http://www.aoa.gov/Aging_Statistics/Profile/2013/docs/2013_Profile.pdf.

US Department of Health and Human Services. (2014). *About Alzheimer's disease: Alzheimer's basics*. Retrieved October 15, 2015 http://www.nia.nih.gov/alzheimers/topics/alzheimers-basics#howmany.

Williams, K., Kemper, S., & Hummert, M. L. (2004). Enhancing communication with older adults: overcoming elderspeak. *Journal of Gerontological Nursing*, 30(10), 17–25.

Wolff, J. L., Boyd, C. M., Gitlin, L. N., Bruce, M. L., & Roter, D. L. (2012). Going it together: persistence of older adults' accompaniment to physician visits by a family companion. *Journal of the American Geriatrics Society*, 60(1), 106–112.

2

SETTINGS AND CONTEXTS FOR GERIATRIC PRACTICE

Just as the population of older adults is diverse, geriatric practice settings are also wide ranging. One of the myths of later life is that the majority of older adults live in nursing homes, yet currently only a small percentage (3.8%) of people over age 65 live in some type of institutional setting (Administration on Aging, 2013). However, this number increases with advanced age, with 10% of the population over the age of 85 residing in a long-term care setting. In the older population overall, the majority live in community-based settings and reside in their own homes. For example, 12.53% of the 65–75-year-old population are head of their household, which means that the individual had primary responsibility for support of the home and co-residential family members. An additional 10% of householders are over the age of 75 (US Census, 2013).

The residential context is important in understanding geriatric practice, intervention, and practitioner/clinician roles. In community settings, there are a number of different residential situations. Some older adults who live alone may require assistance with activities of daily living (ADLs) or instrumental activities of daily living (IADLs). In addition, their health and functioning may create incongruence with their abilities and the demands of their environment (e.g., going up stairs, reaching items in cupboards). Psychosocial issues are also present, such as feeling isolated, lonely, or depressed. These examples are all important considerations in assessment and intervention.

This chapter examines several contexts for geriatric practice with older adults and their families. The first section analyzes community-based practice with older adults, evaluating some of the living arrangements and service needs for older individuals who reside in their own homes or with others. The second section focuses on residential settings such as assisted living, long-term care, and medical settings. Practice issues that are specific to various contexts will be presented. Taken together, Chapters 1 and 2 provide an overview of the older population and the experience of aging settings for practice, and present a framework for understanding the various interventions that constitute evidence-based practice with older adults and their families.

COMMUNITY-BASED RESIDENTIAL ARRANGEMENTS

The preferred residence for most older adults is their own home, and this trend is expected to increase as the baby boomers make decisions about residential options. A report by AARP (2005) indicated that about 9 of every 10 adults aged 50 and older expressed a desire to live in their own homes as they age. In order to remain in the home, older adults often require supports, services, and environmental modifications that promote safety and functioning. This section describes various community-based residential situations for older adults. In addition, implications for practice at the individual, family, and community levels are highlighted.

OLDER HOUSEHOLDS

As stated, the majority of older adults reside within community-based, not long-term care residential settings. However, there are various configurations within the community, including living with a spouse/partner, living alone, and living within intergenerational families. Community models have been developed to promote supports and services within community settings, and to foster relationships among older adults themselves. This section explores the various residential options within the community, and discusses how residential transitions impact older adults in situations when a move is necessary.

Shared Household Arrangements

Older adults' living arrangements differ by gender (US Department of Health and Human Services, 2012). Most older men share a household with their spouse (72%), while less than half of older women live with a spouse (42%). In looking at males only, Asian men were most likely to live with a spouse (79%), while Black men (55%) were least likely to have this type of arrangement. For women, non-Hispanic White women (45%) were most likely to live with a spouse, while Black women were least likely to live with one (23%).

Besides living with a spouse or partner, older adults share a household with other family members. In general, women were much more likely than men to live in a household with other relatives (18% compared to 6%). Hispanic men (17%) and women (36%) had the highest rate of co-residence with other family, while non-Hispanic White men (4%) and women (13%) had the lowest rate (US Department of Health and Human Services, 2012).

These co-residential situations may include some type of caregiving arrangement. Approximately 43.5 million caregivers, aged 18 and up, provide care to family members or friends over the age of 50, with 20% of caregivers residing in the same house as the care recipient (National Alliance of Caregiving, AARP, 2009). Not all of these arrangements entail caregiving for older adults, however, as older adults also hold caregiving roles for younger generations. For example, older parents may remain in caregiving roles for adult sons and daughters with intellectual or psychiatric disabilities (Cummings & Kropf, 2011; Heller & Caldwell, 2006; Song, Mailick, & Greenberg, 2014). In addition, older adults may assume care of their grandchildren, as an estimated 10% of children are in the care of their grandparents (Ellis & Simmon, 2014).

Living Alone

A sizable number of older adults, especially older women, live alone. Almost twice as many women (36%) live by themselves as compared to older men (19%) (US Department of Health and Human Services, 2012). Both older Black and non-Hispanic White women are the most typical single-person household, with 39% in each of these groups living along.

Individuals who live by themselves in later life face some unique challenges. Portacolone (2013) describes single-person households as experiencing a sense of "precariousness," as some struggle to maintain their household with challenges in physical and mental functioning, along with navigating complex services and programs with limited or no assistance. In fact, older adults who live alone, especially those who are 80 years and older and who have limited levels of social support, have significant health and mortality risks (Gopinath, Rochtchina, Anstey, & Mitchell, 2013).

Living alone may also contribute to older adults' feelings of isolation and loneliness. For women, however, these conditions may be associated with the loss of a spouse or significant partner (Chan, Malhotra, Malhotra, & Østbye, 2011; Greenfield & Russell, 2011). Unfortunately, living alone may be a significant risk factor for older men. The highest suicide rate in the older population is for White men over the age of 80 who live alone. At this age, the suicide rate is six times higher than the average (Mental Health America, n.d).

Supportive Community Models

Since older adults have a strong preference for remaining in their own homes, community models have been created to promote functioning and provide support. Naturally occurring retirement communities (NORC) are "housing developments that are not planned or designed for older people, but which over time come to house largely older people" (Hunt & Guner-Hunt, 1986, p. 4). In 2006, the Older Americans Act defined a NORC as a community that has a concentrated population of at least 40% of heads of households over the age of 60, or where the location includes a critical mass of older adults, which makes delivery of services to this location an efficient method of service provision (Older American Act Amendments of 2006). The goal of NORCs is to provide high concentration areas of older adults access to coordinated services, and opportunities for developing social networks through activities and social engagement (Bedney, Goldberg, & Josephson, 2010). Some areas have high rates of NORC residency. For example, approximately 50,000 residents in New York City reside within a NORC (Stone, 2013).

The limited literature on the outcomes of NORCs for older residents suggests that a major benefit is the positive social relationships that develop. Older adults who participate in NORCs report positive relationships with other older adults as well as with staff (Cohen-Mansfield, Dakheel-Ali, & Frank, 2010; Greenfield, 2016; Ivery, Akstein-Kahan & Murphy, 2010). Residents also report trusting relationships with service providers (e.g., household repair, lawn maintenance) since NORCs may serve as a clearinghouse for reputable and quality services (Bronstein, Gellis, & Kenaley, 2009).

A second type of community-based initiative is the Village model. Compared to NORCs, Villages tend to include more middle-income residents and have greater volunteer (versus paid) staff, which creates a more consumer-driven environment (McDonough & Davitt, 2011; Scharlach, Graham, & Lehning, 2012). Since the majority of Villages have about half of their operating budgets from membership fees (Greenfield, Scharlach, Graham, Davitt, & Lehning, 2012), this model is more appropriate for those older adults who have secure financial resources.

Although there are differences between the Village and NORC models, they share important similarities. Both of these community-support models promote civic engagement, social relationships, and healthy functioning so that older adults can remain in their own homes (Greenfield, Scharlach, Lehning, & Davitt, 2012). Clearly, there are some positive aspects of these models, and additional research on the outcomes, cost, and sustainability will be necessary as greater numbers of baby boomers make decisions about residential arrangements.

PRACTICE ISSUES WITH COMMUNITY-BASED OLDER ADULTS

There are several practice issues that emerge when older adults are residing within the community. For some, decisions about continued residence in their homes and families can be emotional and complex. For example, social workers often become involved with families when crises arise that impact older adults' abilities to remain in their home and community (Greene, 2008). At these junctures, older adults and their families may need assistance with decision-making about residential changes (e.g., moving to a more supportive environment) or involvement with support services (e.g., community or in-home services).

Because most care for older adults is performed by informal sources of supports, practice issues also involve support for the care providers. Assisting the care providers to use available services, or to become associated with others in care roles, can help decrease adverse health and mental health outcomes of care. In addition, more macro-level approaches, such as the establishment of community partnerships and social policies to support caregiving families, are needed (Kropf, 2006). Additionally, greater emphasis on community-level planning is required, as few locations are ready for the increased number of older adults (National Association of Area Agencies on Aging, 2011). Additional resources within communities, such as accessible and affordable transportation options, will benefit older adults and their families.

Residential Transitions

One of the most difficult decisions for older adults and their families is whether the older individuals have the capacity to live in their current situation. At this point, the decision to relocate to a more structured or restricted environment (e.g., nursing home) can be one of the most difficult questions of later life. Even when there is clear evidence that older adults require greater support, the move to a different residential setting is a major transition (Lee, Simpson, & Froggatt, 2013; Rossen & Knafl, 2003). While positive outcomes include greater safety, opportunities for social contact, and health and medical care, there are also potential difficulties for the older adult. Residential transitions are a major life event at any age; however, there are unique issues with older adults that contribute to the stressful nature of moving. These include grief and the loss of their familiar surroundings, fear of an unknown future, less choice and flexibility in the new environment, and changes in their social network (Jungers, 2010).

Residential relocations in later life differ significantly from moves during early periods. For older adults, residential changes are associated other life-course transitions, such as changing role status (e.g., retirement, widowhood) or health/functioning abilities (Sergeant, Ekerdt, & Chapin, 2010). The practice dilemma is often balancing the risks between the current (preferred) living arrangement and a move to a more restrictive and unfamiliar environment.

Social Integration and Access to Services

Practitioners also are involved in both micro- and macro-practice efforts to facilitate the social integration of older adults within their communities, and to ensure access to health care and social welfare services. Unfortunately, the majority of local communities are unprepared for the increased number of older adults who will reside in their homes and neighborhoods. In an analysis of community readiness, the National Association of Area Agencies on Aging (2011) issued a reported titled "The Maturing of America: Communities Moving Forward for An Aging Population." Several major challenges were identified that local communities experience in planning for greater numbers of older residents. These include identifying sources of funding to support specialized initiatives, increasing appropriate and affordable housing for older adults, increasing transportation and mobility access, and increasing access to health resources. These issues are critical, as the functioning and well-being of older adults are associated with environmental factors that support their continued engagement within communities (Landorf, Brewer, & Sheppard, 2008; Rosso, Auchincloss, & Michael, 2011).

From a micro-practice level, geriatric case management plays an important role in various contexts. As *geriatric* case managers, practitioners manage a smaller caseload to respond more individually to clients, work with families who might reside in different locations, and construct individualized service plans to promote and preserve functioning of the older individual (Cress, 2015). Geriatric case managers are frequently involved in working with crisis and transition issues (e.g., medical issues), as well as maintaining functioning for older adults who experience challenging situations (e.g., transitioning into retirement or widowhood) (Greene, Cohen, Galambos, & Kropf, 2007).

Community development and social action are macro-practice roles to create more aging-friendly environments. As Scharlach (2012) states, "Communities throughout the United States are ill equipped for dealing with the dramatic demographic changes they will experiences as their residents age. Existing physical infrastructures were not designed for an aging population, and fewer than one-half of America's cities and towns have even begun to make the types of changes that an aging society will require" (p. 26). Older adults need to be involved within the planning process to provide guidance on the course that community development can take (Austin, Des Camp, Flux, McClelland, & Sieppert, 2005). Some strategies to involve older residents in particular initiatives include outreach to diverse groups of older adults, and the addition of social components that make the planning process an enjoyable experience. When individuals are involved in these ways, a higher level of collective efficacy develops, which promotes a greater sense of community and network (Ohmer & Beck, 2006).

SUPPORT FOR CAREGIVERS

The long-term care system is based upon the involvement of the informal support systems of older adults. Informal caregivers—family, partners, close friends—are the "backbone of long term services and supports" (Redfoot, Feinberg, & Houser, 2013). As such, providing assistance to those in caregiving roles is an important dimension of geriatric practice.

Caregivers benefit from support in various ways. First, their own physical and mental health may suffer as a result of their responsibilities. Caregivers of older adults report higher levels of both physical and mental health symptoms than non–care providers (c.f., Etters, Goodall, & Harrison, 2008; Schulz & Sherwood, 2008). As a result, interventions to help caregivers maintain optimal health and functioning status are necessary. Second, care providers need support in their roles, as caregiving may require new skills or knowledge. Support and psychoeducational groups provide caregivers with information and skill-building opportunities, as well as connection to others who are in similar situations (Savundranayagam, Montgomery, Kosloski, & Little, 2011). Additionally, the financial toll can be dramatic, as increased expenditures are often combined with decreased wages and employment opportunities (National Alliance for Caregiving, 2009). Connection to resources to assist with these costs (e.g., home remodeling, medical care) help caregivers with these resources.

LONG-TERM CARE

Even though the majority of older adults prefer to age in their homes and communities, there are health-related and social reasons that they relocate to more supportive environments. The long-term care system includes options that provide various levels of support for older adults (cf., longtermcare.gov). Some older adults require assistance with instrumental activities of daily living (IADLs), such as managing their household, taking medications, shopping and meal preparation, or caring for self in emergency situations. Other long-term care services have a greater medical focus and assist older adults with their activities of daily living (ADLs), which includes bathing, dressing, feeding, and hygiene needs. Typically, assistance in these areas require a higher level of, or more skilled, care.

ASSISTED LIVING

An assisted living facility (ALF) is a type of residential option for individuals who have some limitations in functioning and require a greater level of support than they have within their own home. Mostly commonly, ALF residents require assistance in their ADLs and/or IADLs, and typically are living with dementia, functional impairments, and one or more chronic illnesses such as heart disease and diabetes (Golant, 2004; McNabney et al., 2014). These facilities vary greatly in type, with about half being residences of 4–10 beds. The remaining properties were medium facilities with 11–25 beds (16%), large facilities with 26–100 beds (28%), and extra large facilities with more than 100 beds (7%) (Park-Lee et al., 2011). An estimate is that almost one million older adults reside within an ALF at any point in time (National Center for Assisted Living, 2013).

Because residents of ALFs are in a congregate living arrangement, social challenges emerge that impact the experiences for the older adults. Although ALFs provide activities, residents may not be involved with these events, especially those who have lower functional abilities (Jang, Park, Dominguez, & Molinari, 2013). However, engagement with other residents is a primary factor in reports of satisfaction and quality of life at the ALF (Cummings & Cockerham, 2004; Street et al., 2007).

Geriatric depression is a factor in both assisted living and nursing home residence. In one study of ALF residents, 27% scored within the range of probable depression (Park, Jang, Lee, Schonfeld, & Molinari, 2012). In spite of this high proportion, very few residents were receiving any mental health services. Transitions, such as relocations or medical changes, are risk junctures when residents need to be assessed for depression.

NURSING HOMES

A second type of residence is nursing homes, and there are two ways that these facilities are used. Short-term stays in nursing homes are used as sites for rehabilitation after hospitalization, for example, after a hip fracture or stroke. After discharge from a hospital setting, older patients may not be ready to return to their home or prior residence. In this way, nursing homes provide specialized care that allows patients to regain levels of functioning prior to their return home.

For other older adults, nursing homes become their permanent residence. In a national study of nursing home residents, the average age of the typical resident was

84 years, with women being slightly older (M = 85) than men (M = 81). The major medical conditions associated with nursing home admission are dementia, stroke, cognitive impairment, and depression (Moore, Boscardin, Steinman, & Schwartz, 2012). Social factors are also associated with nursing home admissions. These include unavailability of social support, lack of a potential care provider, multiple and severe care needs, and inability to adapt to a major life change (Gaugler, Duval, Anderson, & Kane, 2007; Luppa et al., 2009).

Alzheimer's disease (AD) and other dementias are additional conditions of residents in nursing homes. Almost half (49%) of residents have AD or another form of dementia (Harris-Kojetin, Sengupta, Park-Lee, & Valverde, 2013). The clinical symptomology associated with this disease process includes memory loss, decreased capacity in judgment, disorientation, and personality changes, among other conditions. Nursing homes are often the safest environment for persons with AD, as they require round-the-clock supervision and care.

Geriatric depression is present within nursing homes in higher rates as well. Similar to the incidence of dementia, almost half of nursing home residents are depressed (Drageset, Eide, & Ranhoff, 2011). In spite of the high level of depression and other mental health conditions, residents may not receive adequate treatment. In fact, disparities exist, with Black residents and those with lower levels of education receiving lower levels of treatment (Siegel et al., 2012). In the two-tier system of nursing home funding, these residents are frequently the ones who live in Medicaid-accepting facilities, which provide fewer mental health interventions (Feng, Fennell, Tyler, Clark, & Mor, 2011).

The environment in some nursing homes is far from tranquil. Larger facilities and those with high levels of residents with dementia and other psychiatric conditions can create turmoil and disorder that are disrupting for some residents and can lead to hostility and aggression. Research suggests that both individual factors (e.g., psychiatric conditions, being male, being older, having lower levels of functional impairments) and organizational context (e.g., larger facilities, stricter facility policies) are associated with higher levels of aggressive behaviors in residents (Cassie, 2012).

As many nursing home residents are physically and cognitively impaired, they can be vulnerable to abuses. In 1987, the Nursing Home Reform Act was passed to protect the rights of residents and establish standards for nursing homes to receive federal funding (Medicare or Medicaid). As part of this legislation, the Patients' Bill of Rights was promulgated (see Box 2.1). These rights promote dignity and respect for all residents, and those who feel that their rights are violated have access to an ombudsman, as mandated by federal law.

In 2013, nursing home ombudsmen provided 335,088 consultations to individuals, and worked to resolve 190,592 complaints. Ombudsmen resolved or partially resolved 73% of all complaints to the satisfaction of the resident or complainant (US Department of Health and Human Services, Administration on Aging, 2015; http://www.aoa.gov/aoa_programs/elder_rights/Ombudsman/index.aspx).

BOX 2.1 NURSING HOME PATIENTS' BILL OF RIGHTS

The 1987 Nursing Home Reform Law protects the following rights of nursing home residents:

THE RIGHT TO BE FULLY INFORMED OF

- Available services and the charges for each service
- Facility rules and regulations, including a written copy of resident rights
- Address and telephone number of the state ombudsman and state survey agency
- State survey reports and the nursing home's plan of correction
- Advance plans of a change in rooms or roommates
- Assistance if a sensory impairment exists
- Residents have a right to receive information in a language they understand (Spanish, Braille, etc.)

THE RIGHT TO COMPLAIN

- Present grievances to staff or any other person, without fear of reprisal and with prompt efforts by the facility to resolve those grievances
- To complain to the ombudsman program
- To file a complaint with the state survey and certification agency

THE RIGHT TO PARTICIPATE IN ONE'S OWN CARE

- Receive adequate and appropriate care
- Be informed of all changes in medical condition
- Participate in their own assessment, care planning, treatment, and discharge
- Refuse medication and treatment
- Refuse chemical and physical restraints
- Review one's medical record
- Be free from charge for services covered by Medicaid or Medicare

THE RIGHT TO PRIVACY AND CONFIDENTIALITY

- Private and unrestricted communication with any person of their choice
- Residents have right to privacy and confidentiality during treatment and care of one's personal needs
- Regarding medical, personal, or financial affairs

RIGHTS DURING TRANSFERS AND DISCHARGES

- Remain in the nursing facility unless a transfer or discharge

(a) is necessary to meet the resident's welfare;

(b) is appropriate because the resident's health has improved and she or he no longer requires nursing home care;

(c) is needed to protect the health and safety of other residents or staff;

(d) is required because the resident has failed, after reasonable notice, to pay the facility charge for an item or service provided at the resident's request

- Receive 30-day notice of transfer or discharge, which includes the reason, effective date, location to which the resident is transferred or discharged, the right to appeal, and the name, address, and telephone number of the state long-term care ombudsman
- Safe transfer or discharge through sufficient preparation by the nursing home

THE RIGHT TO DIGNITY, RESPECT, AND FREEDOM

- To be treated with consideration, respect, and dignity
- To be free from mental and physical abuse, corporal punishment, involuntary seclusion, and physical and chemical restraints
- To self-determination
- Security of possessions

THE RIGHT TO VISITS

- By a resident's personal physician and representatives from the state survey agency and ombudsman programs
- By relatives, friends, and others of the residents' choosing
- By organizations or individuals providing health, social, legal, or other services
- Residents have the right to refuse visitors

THE RIGHT TO MAKE INDEPENDENT CHOICES

- Make personal decisions, such as what to wear and how to spend free time
- Reasonable accommodation of one's needs and preferences
- Choose a physician
- Participate in community activities, both inside and outside the nursing home
- Organize and participate in a resident council
- Manage one's own financial affairs.

Once an older adult is in a long-term care setting, multilevel practice issues emerge. One area is working with families to help them remain connected to the older resident and to define their role in care. When there is a care-sharing experience, such when an older adult resides in a long-term care facility, difficulties can develop between families and formal service providers (Greene & Kropf, 2014). Assistance in setting expectations and establishing roles (and boundaries) might be needed.

Practice issues also may emerge with the residents, especially around transition points. These include entering a facility, when there is a change in health/functioning status that requires relocation, or changes in social conditions (e.g., death of a friend or companion). Practitioners can help residents establish new supports and relationships, or become engaged in other social enterprises.

Long-term residences include others besides the family and the individual, as staff have an integral place in the residents' lives. In a classic anthropological study of long-term care, Joel Savishinsky (1991) analyzed the different experiences that exist within the nursing home context. Human service professionals have crucial administrative roles to make the facility an attractive workplace for the staff. Currently, this is not the case, as turnover rates are high and staff development opportunities are low (Harahan, 2010). Since these individuals provide direct care provision to frail and vulnerable older adults, this aspect of long-term care needs to change.

Work with Families

When a family member moves into a residential facility, there are practice issues that still require attention and involvement by a practitioner. Contrary to a common myth, families do not abandon or disengagement from their loved one when he or she is admitted to a long-term care facility. The majority of families remain engaged, and these connections result in positive outcomes in quality of life and care for the residents (Gaugler, 2005). Practitioners can help families with the emotional experiences that often accompany a residential placement, such as feelings of guilt or overcompensation.

There are also ways to help foster positive relationships between staff at the facility and residents' families. One is to help set expectations between family and staff, and to help set an organizational culture within the facility that fosters positive communications and relationships (Abrahamson, Pillemer, Sechrist, & Suitor, 2011). Families may need information about the conditions of their family member, and what to expect as changes occur. This is especially true with dementia patients, with increased memory loss, personality changes, and agitation.

However, families also need to be vigilant about the care that their loved one is receiving. Too frequently, residents in long-term care settings are over-prescribed medications that increase their risk of injury or drug interaction (Beloosesky, Nenaydenko, Nevo, Adunsky, & Weiss, 2013). For example, the average number of prescribed medications per resident is 6.7, with 27% of residents taking 9 or more medications (Allen,

2010). Medication rates for residents with dementia were even higher (Vetrano et al., 2013). Although families are not experts in this area, practitioners need to encourage and empower families to review medications and to request justification for each one prescribed. In addition, families can monitor functioning of an older resident after prescriptions are altered and can alert staff in the event of significant changes. Families may be reluctant to interfere, yet they often know the behavior and functioning of their loved one better than staff.

Social Engagement and Transitions

Although the majority of older adults state preferences for remaining in the community, a move to a residential option that has greater services and support may be necessary. Additionally, some older adults report that this type of move improved their quality of life, and offered additional security and relief to them (Jungers, 2010; Newson, 2011). However, a move involves a number of transitions, and practitioners need to be sensitive to the degree of change that individuals experience when they enter an ALF or nursing home.

There are ways to make this transition less traumatic for new residents. Sussman and Dupuis (2014) identify practices that can aid in the transition for new residents. One is to welcome new residents into the facility. While these efforts provide a type of ritual for beginnings, new residents are also reassured, as their presence in the facility is acknowledged. Families and new residents want additional information during this transition. Discussion about the structure and schedule at the facility, and how the facility functions, is helpful in setting expectations. Additionally, new residents need to make decisions about their space and experience to the greatest degree possible. To non-residents, some of these choices may seem trivial (e.g., picture or bed placements), but to a resident, even small decision-making can be empowering.

Staff and Organizational Issues

Although staff in long-term care settings work with frail and vulnerable populations, there are often high turnover rates. In one national study, the 3-month turnover rate for registered nurses was 10.2%, for licensed practice nurses 14.3%, for home health aides 12.5%, and for certified nursing assistants 10.2% (Luo, Lin, & Castle, 2013). This research suggests that facilities are in a constant situation of hiring and training staff, with potential disruptions in continuity of care for the residents. Facility administration needs to consider ways to retain staff by creating conditions that are associated with work satisfaction. Even if there cannot be pay adjustments, administrators can work to enhance job conditions that will result in higher retention rates.

While working in a long-term care facility can be rewarding for staff, conditions exist that make this environment difficult. In one study on the incidence of aggression, for example, staff reported that 15% of the residents in their care had exhibited verbal or physical aggression within the past 2 weeks (Lachs et al., 2013). Cassie (2012) found that higher levels of aggressive behaviors were found in those facilities that had more rigid policies surrounding care. Instead of trying to prevent and manage these behaviors by strict guidelines, investing in training and skill development of staff is optimal. Facility administrators can promote training programs for staff that will enable them to innovative and to be effective in dealing with aggression in residents.

HEALTH AND MENTAL HEALTH CONTEXTS

Other practice contexts are in medical and psychiatric facilities that have older adults as patients. In hospital settings, for example, 15.9% of the patients that had one or more hospital admissions in 2012 were aged 65 years and older. Additionally, the risk of hospitalization increases with advancing age (US Department of Health and Human Services, 2013). The older population with psychiatric conditions and/or addictions is also increasing. Settings for treatment of these conditions include both inpatient and outpatient facilities. Additionally, end-of-life care includes palliative interventions for comfort and pain management. Interventions in end-of-life settings include work with the older patient, as well as the family who is preparing for the death of their loved one.

ACUTE MEDICAL CARE

In hospital settings, practice issues include helping the patient and family deal with medical conditions, as well as decisions about discharge placement. Inadequate preparation for discharge, lack of transition in care, and absence of resources post-discharge result in readmission and rehospitalization rates that range between 20% and 30% (Jencks, Williams, & Coleman, 2009; Mor & Besdine, 2011; Wolff, Meadows, Weiss, Boyd, & Leff, 2008). With proper protocols established, many of these readmissions could be avoided. One estimate is that 75% of readmissions of older adults are preventable (Medicare Advisory Commission, 2009).

Interventions to bring down rehospitalizations are critical. An example of an effective program is the Enhanced Discharge Planning Program that included post-discharge assessment and individualized treatment by social workers (Altfeld et al., 2013). Two days after discharge, the patient or caregiver is contacted to determine adjustment, and referrals to resources are made as necessary. In addition, adherence to the aftercare plan (e.g., follow up with physician, medication) is assessed. This type of individualized aftercare results in better care outcomes, including connection to health-care providers, support for caregivers, and early intervention with unmet needs. The program is an example of aftercare that can help decrease financial and emotional costs of hospital readmissions.

Hospitalizations are particularly complex for older adults with dementia. In addition, hospital rates and costs are as much as five times as high as the population without dementia and last up to three times longer (Rudolph et al., 2010; Zhao, Kuo, Weir, Kramer, & Ash, 2008). Care providers of patients with Alzheimer's disease indicate that many feel unprepared to manage the complex set of issues related to dementia and the health diagnoses (Bauer, Fitzgerald, Koch, & King, 2011). Especially with these patients, aftercare and support for the care providers is critical.

PSYCHIATRIC AND ADDICTION SERVICES

Within the coming years, the expectation is that increases in both psychiatric and addiction rates will occur with the advancing age of the baby boomers. Anxiety and depression are the most typical psychiatric conditions of late life, yet often these conditions are untreated within the older population. Adults over the age of 65 are more likely to underutilize mental health services compared to the general population (Karel, Gatz, & Smyer, 2012).

For those with the onset of a psychiatric condition in later life, there is evidence that patient preference is for psychotherapy over psychopharmacology. In a study with older adults who were not experiencing emotional distress currently, participants were asked to choose various interventions and treatment modalities should a psychiatric need arise (Mohlman, 2012). Interestingly, all cohorts in the older population chose psychotherapy instead of psychopharmacology. While the youngest members of the study, aged 65–75, reported a preference for individual psychotherapy, older cohorts had a stated preference for group modalities. This difference is significant, as it suggests that fostering relationships with others is important for those in the older cohorts of later life.

Addiction rates in the older population are expected to increase with the aging of the baby boomers as well. In a national study of alcohol use, 13% of men aged 50–64 were classified as at risk and 14% were considered binge drinkers, which means that over one-quarter had significant issues with their use of alcohol (Blazer & Wu, 2009). Additionally, marijuana use is on the rise in the older population, with chronic users also more likely to have other forms of addiction, such as alcohol and nicotine (DiNitto & Choi, 2011). Since addiction in the older population may be overlooked or unsuspected by family and service providers, efforts to raise awareness about this growing issue are needed. Additionally, intervention approaches that have demonstrated efficacy with the older population must be instituted.

HOSPICE AND PALLIATIVE CARE

Although patients of all ages use hospice and palliative care programs at the end of life, these services are disproportionately used by older adults. Close to 85% of patients in hospice care are aged 65 or older, and one-third are aged 85 or older (National Hospice and Palliative Care Organization, 2013). Once a patient is in hospice or receives palliative care, the goal of treatment is focused on pain management, symptom relief, and support to the family and caregivers. The most typical type of care is within the family home (66%), and the current average stay in hospice care is about 19 days (NHPCO, 2013).

Hospice care is delivered within the context of an interdisciplinary team approach. Typical staff includes physicians, nurses, health aides, and psychosocial/spiritual personnel including social workers, clergy, and bereavement counselors. Often, volunteers are part of the team and provide support to the family. Hospices have different organizational structures, with some being freestanding, and others being part of a hospital or health-care agency.

In general, attitudes about hospice services are positive in the older population. Research indicates that older adults are open to involvement with hospice, if necessary, and would desire to have treatment reduce pain and suffering associated with terminal conditions (June, Segal, Klebe, & Watts, 2012; Manu, et al., 2013). Since the hospice involves support for caregivers, practice with the family must include sensitivity to and awareness of the configuration of care that exists. Caregiving differs by racial/ethnic group, and families have different patterns of care provision and decision-making that need to be considered with end-of-life practice (Carrion, Park, & Lee, 2011). Understanding various cultural, religious, and spiritual experiences in end-of-life care and planning is crucial for medical and hospice personnel.

Palliative and hospice care are critical practice approaches for patients who are at the end of their life. In a report, *Dying in America*, a consensus group of experts promulgated recommendations for professionals across disciplines to increase the scope and quality of end-of-life care (Institute of Medicine, 2014). In particular, recommendations include expanded coverage for costs of care, additional education and training for health-care professionals in end-of-life interventions, and increased attention to end-of-life planning by patients and families. In addition, quality standards for end-of-life care were articulated that promote dignity, compassion, comfort, and support for patients who are in terminal stages and their families (see Table 2.1).

CONCLUSION

As this chapter indicates, practice with older adults and their families takes place in various contexts and settings. Most older adults live within the community, so safety, caregiving, and psychosocial functioning are important issues within practice. With the onset of chronic conditions or health changes, a relocation to a more supportive setting may be necessary. Assisted living and nursing homes are examples of residential options. In these situations, practice issues involve the integration of the resident into the facility, the connection between the formal and informal supports, and working with facility staff to provide the most effective level of care for older adults. Other practice contexts include those related to acute health or mental health issues, and end-of-life care.

Taken together, Chapters 1 and 2 provide a context for practice as a foundation for the remainder of the book. In the following chapters, various interventions that have

TABLE 2.1 IOM COMMITTEE'S PROPOSED CORE COMPONENTS OF QUALITY END-OF-LIFE CARE

Component	Rationale
Frequent assessment of the patient's physical, emotional, social, and spiritual well-being	Interventions and assistance must be based on accurately identified needs.
Management of emotional distress	All clinicians should be able to identify distress and direct its initial and basic management. This is part of the definition of palliative care, a basic component of hospice, and clearly of fundamental importance.
Offer referral to expert-level palliative care	People with palliative needs beyond those that can be provided by non-specialist-level clinicians deserve access to appropriate expert-level care.
Offer referral to hospice if the patient has a prognosis of 6 months or less	People who meet the hospice eligibility criteria deserve access to services designed to meet their end-of-life needs.
Management of care and direct contact with patient and family for complex situations by a specialist-level palliative care physician	Care of people with serious illness may require specialist-level palliative care physician management, and effective physician management requires direct examination, contact, and communication.
Round-the-clock access to coordinated care and services	Patients in advanced stages of serious illness often require assistance, such as with activities of daily living, medication management, wound care, physical comfort, and psychosocial needs. Round-the-clock access to a consistent point of contact that can coordinate care obviates the need to dial 911 and engage emergency medical services.
Management of pain and other symptoms	All clinicians should be able to identify and direct the initial and basic management of pain and other symptoms. This is part of the definition of palliative care, a basic component of hospice, and clearly of fundamental importance.
Counseling of patient and family	Even patients who are not emotionally distressed face problems in areas such as loss of functioning, prognosis, coping with diverse symptoms, finances, and family dynamics, and family members experience these problems as well, both directly and indirectly.
Family caregiver support	A focus on the family is part of the definition of palliative care; family members and caregivers both participate in the patient's care and require assistance themselves.
Attention to the patient's social and cultural context and social needs	Person-centered care requires awareness of patients' perspectives on their social environment and of their needs for social support, including at the time of death. Companionship at the bedside at time of death may be an important part of the psychological, social, and spiritual aspects of end-of-life care for some individuals.

(continued)

TABLE 2.1 (CONTINUED)

Component	Rationale
Attention to the patient's spiritual and religious needs	The final phase of life often has a spiritual and religious component, and research shows that spiritual assistance is associated with quality of care.
Regular personalized revision of the care plan and access to services based on the changing needs of the patient and family	Care must be person-centered and fit current circumstances, which may mean that not all of the preceding components will be important or desirable in all cases.

Source: Institute of Medicine, *Dying in America*. www.iom.edu/endoflife.

evidence of effectiveness with the older population are presented. As readers, there are several important questions to consider as these interventions are analyzed:

- How does the intervention assist older adults and their families with the challenges that are faced?
- Does the intervention have specific utility for subpopulations of older adults (e.g., those with dementia, those who live alone, LGBT seniors, diversity by race and ethnicity, etc.)?
- Does the intervention approach differ across practice settings or contexts (e.g., nursing home residents vs. those living community settings)?
- How might the interventions change as the baby boomers reach advanced ages?

In order to address these issues, the book will highlight some promising interventions in the final chapter. The goal of the book is not only to analyze the intervention approaches that currently have evidence of effectiveness, but also to consider some practice approaches that may yield additional ways to address challenges and issues with the coming generation of older adults.

REFERENCES

AARP. (2005). *State of 50+ America 2005*. Retrieved May 31, 2015 from http://assets.aarp.org/rgcenter/econ/fifty_plus_2005.pdf.

Abrahamson, K., Pillemer, K., Sechrist, J., & Suitor, J. (2011). Does race influence conflict between nursing home staff and family members of residents? *The Journals of Gerontology Series B: Psychological Sciences and Social Sciences, 66*(6), 750–755.

Administration on Aging. (2013). *Profile of older Americans*. Retrieved May 31, 2015 from http://www.aoa.gov/Aging_Statistics/Profile/2013/Index.aspx.

Allen, J. E. (2010). *Nursing home federal requirements: Guidelines to surveyors and survey protocols* (7th ed.). New York: Springer.

Altfeld, S. J., Shier, G. E., Rooney, M., Johnson, T. J., Golden, R. L., Karavolos, K., . . . Perry, A. J. (2013). Effects of an enhanced discharge planning intervention for hospitalized older adults: a randomized trial. *Gerontologist, 53*(3), 430–440.

Austin, C. D., Des Camp, E., Flux, D., McClelland, R. W., & Sieppert, J. (2005). Community development with older adults in their neighborhoods: the elder friendly communities program. *Families in Society: The Journal of Contemporary Social Services, 86*(3), 401–409.

Bauer, M., Fitzgerald, L., Koch, S., & King, S. (2011). How family carers view hospital discharge planning for the older person with a dementia. *Dementia, 10*(3), 317–323.

Bedney, B. J., Goldberg, R. B., & Josephson, K. (2010). Aging in place in naturally occurring retirement communities: transforming aging through supportive service programs. *Journal of Housing for the Elderly, 24*(3–4), 304–321.

Beloosesky, Y., Nenaydenko, O., Nevo, R. F. G., Adunsky, A., & Weiss, A. (2013). Rates, variability, and associated factors of polypharmacy in nursing home patients. *Clinical Interventions in Aging, 8*, 1585.

Blazer, D., & Wu, L. T. (2009). The epidemiology of at-risk and binge drinking among middle-aged and elderly community adults: National Survey on Drug Use and Health. *American Journal of Psychiatry, 166*(10), 1162–1169.

Bronstein, L., Gellis, Z. D., & Kenaley, B. L. (2009). A neighborhood naturally occurring retirement community: views from providers and residents. *Journal of Applied Gerontology, 30*(1), 104–112.

Carrion, I. V., Park, N. S., & Lee, B. S. (2011). Hospice use among African Americans, Asians, Hispanics, and Whites: implications for practice. *American Journal of Hospice and Palliative Medicine, 29*(2), 116–121. doi:1049909111410559.

Cassie, K. M. (2012). A multilevel analysis of aggressive behaviors among nursing home residents. *Journal of Gerontological Social Work, 55*(8), 708–720.

Chan, A., Malhotra, C., Malhotra, R., & Østbye, T. (2011). Living arrangements, social networks and depressive symptoms among older men and women in Singapore. *International Journal of Geriatric Psychiatry, 26*(6), 630–639.

Cohen, C. I. (2003). Introduction. In C. I. Cohen (Ed.), *Schizophrenia into later life* (pp. xiii–xx). Washington, DC: American Psychiatric Publishing.

Cohen-Mansfield, J., Dakheel-Ali, M., & Frank, J. K. (2010). The impact of a naturally occurring retirement communities service program in Maryland, USA. *Health Promotion International, 25*(2), 210–220.

Cress, C. (2015). *Handbook of geriatric care management.* Gaithersburg, MD: Aspen Publishers.

Cummings, S. M., & Cockerham, C. (2004). Depression and life satisfaction in assisted living residents: impact of health and social support. *Clinical Gerontologist, 27*, 25–42

Cummings, S. M., & Kropf, N. P. (2011). Aging with a severe mental illness: challenges and treatments. *Journal of Gerontological Social Work, 54*, 175–188.

DiNitto, D. M., & Choi, N. G. (2011). Marijuana use among older adults in the U.S.A.: user characteristics, patterns of use, and implications for intervention. *International Psychogeriatrics, 23*(5), 732–741.

Drageset, J., Eide, G. E., & Ranhoff, A. H. (2011). Depression is associated with poor functioning in activities of daily living among nursing home residents without cognitive impairment. *Journal of Clinical Nursing, 20*(21–22), 3111–3118. doi:10.1111/j.1365-2702.2010.03663.x.

Ellis, R. R., & Simmons, T. (2014). Coresident grandparents and their grandchildren: 2012 population characteristics. P20-576U.S. Department of Commerce Economics and Statistics Administration U.S. CENSUS BUREAU. Retrieved December 17, 2016 from https://www.census.gov/content/dam/Census/library/publications/2014/demo/p20-576.pdf.

Etters, L., Goodall, D., & Harrison, B. E. (2008). Caregiver burden among dementia patient caregivers: a review of the literature. *Journal of the American Academy of Nurse Practitioners, 20*(8), 423–428.

Feng, Z., Fennell, M. L., Tyler, D. A., Clark, M., & Mor, V. (2011). Growth of racial and ethnic minorities in US nursing homes driven by demographics and possible disparities in options. *Health Affairs, 30*(7), 1358–1365.

Gaugler, J. E. (2005). Family involvement in residential long-term care: a synthesis and critical review. *Aging and Mental Health, 9*(2), 105–118.

Gaugler, J. E., Duval, S., Anderson, K. A., & Kane, R. L. (2007). Predicting nursing home admission in the US: a meta-analysis. *BMC Geriatrics, 7*(1), 13.

Golant, S. M. (2004). Do impaired older persons with health care needs occupy U.S. assisted living facilities? An analysis of six national studies. *Journals of Gerontology: Series B: Psychological Sciences and Social Sciences, 59B*(2), S68–S79.

Gopinath, B., Rochtchina, E., Anstey, K. J., & Mitchell, P. (2013). Living alone and risk of mortality in older, community-dwelling adults. *JAMA Internal Medicine, 173*(4), 320–321.

Greene, R. R. (2008). *Social work with the aged and their families* (3rd ed.). New Brunswick, NJ: Transaction.

Greene, R. R., Cohen, H., Galambos, C. & Kropf, N. P. (2007). *Foundations of social work practice in the field of aging: a competency-based approach.* Washington, DC: NASW Press.

Greene, R. R. & Kropf, N. P. (2014). *Caregiving and caresharing: a life course perspective.* Washington, DC: NASW Press.

Greenfield, E. A. (2016) Support from neighbors and aging in place: can NORC programs make a difference? *The Gerontologist, 54*(4), 651–659.

Greenfield, E. A., Scharlach, A. E., Graham, C., Davitt, J., & Lehning, A. (2012). *A national overview of villages: results from a 2012 organizational survey.* New Brunswick, NJ: Rutgers University.

Greenfield, E. A., Scharlach, A., Lehning, A. J., & Davitt, J. K. (2012). A conceptual framework for examining the promise of the NORC program and Village models to promote aging in place. *Journal of Aging Studies, 26*(3), 273–284.

Greenfield, E. A., & Russell, D. (2011). Identifying living arrangements that heighten risk for loneliness in later life: evidence from the US National Social Life, Health, and Aging Project. *Journal of Applied Gerontology, 30*(4), 524–534.

Harahan, M. F. (2010). A critical look at the looming long-term-care workforce crisis. *Generations, 34*(4), 20–26.

Harris-Kojetin, L., Sengupta, M., Park-Lee, E., & Valverde, R. (2013). *Long-term care services in the United States: 2013 overview.* Hyattsville, MD: National Center for Health Statistics.

Heller, T., & Caldwell, J. (2006). Supporting aging caregivers and adults with developmental disabilities in future planning. *Mental Retardation, 44*(3), 189–202.

Hunt, M. E., & Gunter-Hunt, G. (1986). Naturally occurring retirement communities. *Journal of Housing for the Elderly, 3*(3–4), 3–22.

Institute of Medicine. 2014. *Dying in America.* Retrieved May 15, 2016 from http://www.iom.edu/~/media/Files/Report%20Files/2014/EOL/Key%20Findings%20and%20Recommendations.pdf.

Ivery, J. M., Akstein-Kahan, D., & Murphy, K. C. (2010). NORC supportive services model implementation and community capacity. *Journal of Gerontological Social Work, 53*(1), 21–42.

Jang, Y., Park, N. S., Dominguez, D. D., & Molinari, V. (2013). Social engagement in older residents of assisted living facilities. *Aging & Mental Health, 18*(5), 642–647.

Jencks, S. F., Williams, M. V., & Coleman, E. A. (2009). Rehospitalizations among patients in the Medicare fee-for-service program. *New England Journal of Medicine, 360*(14), 1418–1428.

June, A., Segal, D. L., Klebe, K., & Watts, L. K. (2012). Views of hospice and palliative care among younger and older sexually diverse women. *American Journal of Hospice and Palliative Medicine, 29*(6), 455–461.

Jungers, C. M. (2010). Leaving home: an examination of late-life relocation among older adults. *Journal of Counseling & Development, 88*(4), 416–423.

Karel, M. J., Gatz, M., & Smyer, M. A. (2012). Aging and mental health in the decade ahead: what psychologists need to know. *American Psychologist, 67*(3), 184–198. doi:10.1037/a0025393.

Kropf, N. P. (2006). Community caregiving partnerships in aging: promoting alliances to support care providers. In R. R. Greene (Ed.), *Contemporary issues in caregiving* (pp. 327–340). New York: Haworth Press.

Lachs, M. S., Rosen, T., Teresi, J. A., Eimicke, J. P., Ramirez, M., Silver, S., & Pillemer, K. (2013). Verbal and physical aggression directed at nursing home staff by residents. *Journal of General Internal Medicine, 28*(5), 660–667.

Landorf, C., Brewer, G., & Sheppard, L. A. (2008). The urban environment and sustainable ageing: critical issues and assessment indicators. *Local Environment, 13*(6), 497–514.

Lee, V. P., Simpson, J., & Froggatt, K. (2013). A narrative exploration of older people's transitions into residential care. *Aging and Mental Health, 17*(1), 48–56.

Luo, H., Lin, M., & Castle, N. G. (2013). The correlates of nursing staff turnover in home and hospice agencies: 2007 national home and hospice care survey. *Research on Aging, 35*(4), 375–392.

Luppa, M., Luck, T., Weyerer, S., König, H. H., Brähler, E., & Riedel-Heller, S. G. (2009). Prediction of institutionalization in the elderly: a systematic review. *Age and Ageing, 39*(1), 31–38.

Manu, E., Mack-Biggs, T. L., Vitale, C. A., Galecki, A., Moore, T., & Montagnini, M. (2013). Perceptions and attitudes about hospice and palliative care among community-dwelling older adults. *American Journal of Hospice and Palliative Medicine, 30*(2), 153–161.

McDonough, K. E., & Davitt, J. K. (2011). It takes a village: community practice, social work, and aging-in-place. *Journal of Gerontological Social Work, 54*(5), 528–541. doi:10.1080/01634372.2011.581744.

McNabney, M. K., Onyike, C., Johnston, D., Mayer, L., Lyketsos, C., Brandt, J., & Samus, Q. (2014). The impact of complex chronic diseases on care utilization among assisted living residents. *Geriatric Nursing, 35*, 26–30. doi:10.1016/j.gerinurse.2013.09.003.

Medicare Payment Advisory Commission. (2009). *Report to Congress: Improving incentives in the Medicare program*. Washington, DC: MedPAC. Retrieved June 21, 2012, from http://www.medpac.gov/documents/Jun09_EntireReport.pdf.

Mental Health America. (n.d.). *Suicide statistics*. Retrieved June 30, 2015 from http://www.mentalhealthamerica.net/suicide.

Mohlman, J. (2012). A community based survey of older adults' preferences for treatment of anxiety. *Psychology and Aging, 27*(4), 1182–1190.

Moore, K. L., Boscardin, W. J., Steinman, M. A., & Schwartz, J. B. (2012). Age and sex variation in prevalence of chronic medical conditions in older residents of US nursing homes. *Journal of the American Geriatrics Society, 60*(4), 756–764.

Mor, V., & Besdine, R. W. (2011). Policy options to improve discharge planning and reduce rehospitalization. *JAMA, 305*(3), 302–303.

National Alliance of Caregiving in Collaboration with AARP (2009). *Caregiving in the U.S.: a focused look at caring for the 50+*. Retrieved June 30, 2015 from http://assets.aarp.org/rgcenter/il/caregiving_09.pdf.

National Alliance on Caregiving. (2009). *Caregiving in the U.S. 2009*. Retrieved June 30, 2015 from http://www.caregiving.org/data/Caregiving_in_the_US_2009_full_report.pdf.

National Association of Area Agencies on Aging. (2011). *Maturing of America: communities moving forward for an aging population*. Retrieved from January 18, 2013 http://www.n4a.org/files/MOA_FINAL_Rpt.pdf.

National Center for Assisted Living. (2013). *Assisted living state regulatory review*. Washington, DC: Author.

Newson, P. (2011). At home then away: supporting new residents as they settle in. *Nursing and Residential Care, 13*(1), 32.

Ohmer, M., & Beck, E. (2006). Citizen participation in neighborhood organizations in poor communities and its relationship to neighborhood and organizational collective efficacy. *Journal of Sociology and Social Welfare, 33*, 179.

Older Americans Act Amendments of 2006, Title IV: Activities for health, independence and longevity. Sec. 409, Community innovations for aging in place (Public Law 109-365).

Park, N. S., Jang, Y., Lee, B. S., Schonfeld, L., & Molinari, V. (2012). Willingness to use mental health services among older residents in assisted living. *Journal of Applied Gerontology, 31*(4), 562–579.

Park-Lee, E., Caffrey, C., Sengupta, M., Moss, A. J., Rosenoff, E., Harris-Kojetin, L. D. (2011). *Residential care facilities: a key sector in the spectrum of long-term care providers in the United States*. NCHS data brief no. 78. Hyattsville, MD: National Center for Health Statistics.

Portacolone, E. (2013). The notion of precariousness among older adults living alone in the US. *Journal of Aging Studies, 27*(2), 166–174.

Redfoot, D., Feinberg, L., & Houser, A. (2013, August). *The aging of the baby boom and the growing care gap: a look at future declines in the availability of family caregivers*. Washington, DC: AARP Public Policy Institute.

Rossen, E. K., & Knafl, K. A. (2003). Older women's response to residential relocation: description of transition styles. *Qualitative Health Research, 13*(1), 20–36.

Rosso, A. L., Auchincloss, A. H., & Michael, Y. L. (2011). The urban built environment and mobility in older adults: a comprehensive review. *Journal of Aging Research*, 1–10. doi:10.4061/2011/816106.

Rudolph, J. L., Zanin, N. M., Jones, R. N., Marcantonio, E. R., Fong, T. G., Yang, F. M., . . . & Inouye, S. K. (2010). Hospitalization in community-dwelling persons with Alzheimer's disease: frequency and causes. *Journal of the American Geriatrics Society, 58*(8), 1542–1548.

Savishinsky, J. (1991). *The ends of time: Life & work in a nursing home*. NY: Bergin & Garvey.

Savundranayagam, M. Y., Montgomery, R. V., Kosloski, K., & Little, T. D. (2011). Impact of a pscyhoeducational program on three types of caregiver burden among spouses. *International Journal Of Geriatric Psychiatry, 26*(4), 388–396. doi:10.1002/gps.2538

Scharlach, A. (2012). Creating aging-friendly communities in the United States. *Ageing International, 37*(1), 25–38.

Scharlach, A., Graham, C., & Lehning, A. (2012). The 'Village' model: A consumer-driven approach for aging in place. *The Gerontologist, 52*(3), 418–427. doi:10.1093/geront/gnr083

Schulz, R., & Sherwood, P. R. (2008). Physical and mental health effects of family caregiving. *The American Journal of Nursing, 108*(9 Suppl), 23.

Sergeant, J. F., Ekerdt, D. J., & Chapin, R. K. (2010). Older adults' expectations to move: Do they predict actual community-based or nursing facility moves within 2 years?. *Journal of Aging and Health, 22*(7), 1029–1053.

Siegel, M. J., Lucas, J. A., Akincigil, A., Gaboda, D., Hoover, D. R., Kalay, E., & Crystal, S. (2012). Race, education, and the treatment of depression in nursing homes. *Journal of Aging and Health*, 24(5), 752–778.

Song, J., Mailick, M. R., & Greenberg, J. S. (2014). Work and health of parents of adult children with serious mental illness. *Family Relations*, 63(1), 122–134.

Stone, R. (2013). What are the realistic options for aging in community? *Generations*, 37(4), 65–71.

Street, D., Burge, S., Quadagno, J., & Barrett, A. (2007). The salience of social relationships for resident well being in assisted living. *Journal of Gerontology: Social Sciences*, 62B, S129–S134.

Sussman, T., & Dupuis, S (2014). Supporting residents moving into long-term care: multiple layers shape residents' experiences. *Journal of Gerontological Social Work*, 57, 438–459.

US Census Bureau. (2013). *American families and living arrangements 2013: Table H2*. Retrieved April 17, 2015 from http://www.census.gov/hhes/families/data/cps2013H.html.

US Census Bureau. (2013). *American community survey (2013)*. Retrieved April 17, 2015 from http://factfinder2.census.gov/faces/tableservices/jsf/pages/productview.xhtml?pid=ACS_13_1YR_B10050&prodType=table.

US Department of Health and Human Services. (2012). *A profile of older Americans: 2012*. Retrieved April 18, 2015 from http://www.aoa.gov/Aging_Statistics/Profile/2012/docs/2012profile.pdf.

US Department of Health and Human Services (2013). *Health, United States, 2013: with special feature on prescription drugs* (p. 294). Retrieved April 21, 2015 from http://www.cdc.gov/nchs/data/hus/hus13.pdf#094.

US Department of Health and Human Services, Administration on Aging. (2015). *Long-Term Care Ombudsman Program (OAA, Title VII, Chapter 2, Sections 711/712)*. Retrieved from http://www.aoa.gov/aoa_programs/elder_rights/Ombudsman/index.aspx.

Vetrano, D. L., Tosato, M., Colloca, G., Topinkova, E., Fialova, D., Gindin, J., . . . Onder, G. (2013). Polypharmacy in nursing home residents with severe cognitive impairment: results from the SHELTER Study. *Alzheimer's & Dementia*, 9(5), 587–593.

Wolff, J. L., Meadow, A., Weiss, C. O., Boyd, C. M., & Leff, B. (2008). Medicare home health patients' transitions through acute and post-acute care settings. *Medical Care*, 46(11), 1188–1193.

Zhao, Y., Kuo, T. C., Weir, S., Kramer, M. S., & Ash, A. S. (2008). Healthcare costs and utilization for Medicare beneficiaries with Alzheimer's. *BMC Health Services Research*, 8(1), 108.

II

EVIDENCE-BASED INTERVENTIONS WITH THE OLDER POPULATION

3

COGNITIVE BEHAVIORAL THERAPY
THEORY AND PRACTICE

As addressed in Chapters 1 and 2, later life may include challenges that can create negative and dysfunctional thoughts and feelings about a person's experience and well-being. According to cognitive behavioral theory, negative psychological states are not a result of undesirable situations or events that befall an individual. Rather, psychological disorders stem from faulty thinking patterns in response to a situation.

Individuals' thoughts influence their emotions and behaviors (Beck, 2011). For example, the day following retirement, a person may wake up and think, "Now I can finally relax!" then gets up, has a leisurely breakfast while reading the paper, and feels happy. Another person may think, "Now I have the time to explore new activities," then gets up, calls a volunteer agency, and feels excited. Yet another person could think, "Now there's nothing for me to do. I am useless," then turns over, stays in bed, and feels depressed. It is our thoughts or beliefs about events, instead of the events themselves, that impact how we feel and behave.

As individuals go through the day, thoughts constantly run through their minds and, without their awareness, help to interpret and give meaning to the experienced events. This inner dialogue can be understood as a stream of consciousness, and an ongoing commentary in reaction to the events encountered. Because these arise spontaneously, they have been termed "automatic thoughts" (Beck et al., 1979) and are typically not subject to scrutiny. They are accepted by the individual without examination, regardless of their accuracy.

The following is an example of faulty assumptions of an older woman about the unresponsiveness of her daughter. Mrs. Boone, age 74, calls her daughter, whom she hasn't heard from in several days. Her daughter doesn't answer the phone and so she leaves a message. Mrs. Boone waits all day but doesn't hear back from her daughter. She begins to think, "My daughter must have something more important to do than talk to me. Why can't she just take a few minutes to give me a call? I'm just not that important to her." A mental image flashes through her mind of her daughter off enjoying time with friends. Mrs. Boone begins to feel rejected and sad.

The next day her daughter calls and explains that she had misplaced her cell phone and so hadn't received her mother's message. Although Mrs. Boone's interpretation of the events was inaccurate, and may not reflect the reality of her relationship with her daughter, the feelings that she experienced in response to her thoughts were very real and had a powerful impact on her. As is evident from this example, at times our thoughts do not accurately reflect reality. The cognitive behavioral therapy (CBT) practitioner would work with clients to replace these faulty assumptions and distorted thoughts, which cause very real pain and suffering.

HISTORY AND BACKGROUND

After World War II, with the return of thousands of veterans who were facing psychological distress, many therapists recognized the need for effective brief treatment. Concomitantly, behavioral therapy arose in reaction to psychodynamic therapy, which was the prevailing model of therapy at that time. Psychodynamic treatment focused on the unconscious, involved lengthy treatment often spanning years, and lacked empirical evidence to support its effectiveness (Westbrook, Kennerley, & Kirk, 2011). Attention turned to the work of behavioral scientists such as John Watson (1913), the founder of the psychological school of behaviorism, who argued that unconscious and mental constructs are not publicly observable and that only behaviors can be measured. Observation of events in the environment (stimuli) and the individual's reaction (responses) to these events, which can be observed and measured, became the point of focus. Behavioral science posited that it is possible to eliminate or "extinguish" problematic behaviors, and to learn new, more adaptive behaviors, and by this means decrease negative outcomes and emotions (Martin & Pear, 2007). With the development of social learning theory, Albert Bandura (1969) asserted that learning is not only a behavioral activity, but also a cognitive process in which individuals learn by observing behaviors and the consequences of behaviors. Based upon behavioral science and social learning theory, behavioral therapy focused on modifying unwanted behavior using time-limited methods endorsed by scientific research. This approach has been termed the "first wave" of behavioral therapy (Miller, 2003).

The "cognitive revolution" began in the 1960s due to dissatisfaction with the limitations of a purely behavioral approach. Psychologists and others began the empirical study of thoughts and how these affect emotions and behavior. This revolution became known as the "second wave" (Miller, 2003). Practicing therapists began to integrate concepts from cognitive science into therapy with the goal of addressing problematic psychological states by helping clients identify and change inaccurate and unhelpful thoughts. The publication of John Beck's (1979) book, *Cognitive Therapy of Depression*, helped to popularize this approach. While thoughts influence behaviors, behaviors can reinforce or help modify thoughts. Therapists began to examine clients' observable behaviors and, also, to assess their conscious thoughts to further understand and treat the presenting problem. Over time, the behavioral and cognitive approaches influenced one another and grew together.

THEORETICAL FOUNDATION

According to cognitive behavioral therapy, an individual's affect and behavior are largely determined by the way in which he or she structures the world. A person is not directly affected by stimuli, but rather by the way these stimuli are interpreted by the individual. The combination of events and the person's particular cognitions leads to a person's feelings. Cognitions (e.g., thoughts, visual images) represent a person's appraisal of his or her situation (see Figure 3.1). How we think or interpret events influences how we feel and behave (Westbrook et al., 2011).

Thoughts that negatively skew reality are known as "cognitive distortions" and act as a warped filter through which we perceive, interpret, and react to events and situations (Sorocco & Lauderdale, 2011). Distorted thoughts influence feelings and subsequent behaviors, which, in turn, can reinforce the distortions. All individuals may engage in some thoughts that do not accurately reflect reality. If mild and sporadic, these thoughts do not cause psychological distress. However, ongoing patterns of distorted cognitions pave the way for the development of psychological disorders such as depression and anxiety (see Table 3.1). Certain patterns of cognitive distortions are more prevalent in the general population and are more commonly present in those experiencing psychological distress (Cully & Teten, 2008; Gallagher-Thompson & Thompson, 2010).

Cognitions, whether positive or negative, are rooted in individuals' underlying assumptions about themselves, the world, and the future. Because we believe that these thoughts are true, we don't question them. Underlying assumptions, also called "intermediate beliefs," are basic themes or formulas about life that help each person make sense of and interpret the world (Beck, 2011). They can be viewed as conditional beliefs or rules of life, such as "Without my looks I am nothing" or "Most people are trustworthy." Underlying assumptions often also take the form of "if . . . then" propositions, such as "If I always go along with others then they will like me, but if I assert myself, they'll reject me"; or "If I don't achieve success, then I am nothing." Underlying assumptions are

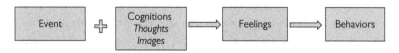

Figure 3.1 Relationship between cognitions, thoughts, and behaviors.

TABLE 3.1 COMMON COGNITIVE DISTORTIONS

Cognitive Distortion	Description	Example
All-or-nothing thinking	Tendency to evaluate personal qualities in extreme black or white categories	I can't drive any longer; I've lost all independence.
Overgeneralization	Seeing a single event as a never-ending pattern of defeat	My daughter said she couldn't come over for dinner on Sunday. My children never make time for me.
Minimizing	Downplaying or discounting the significance of events	My photograph was chosen to be part of the art exhibit at the senior center. But it's not as good as some of the other entries.
Mind reading	Concluding that someone is reacting negatively toward you without bothering to check it out	She didn't stop and talk to me because she doesn't like me.
Emotional reasoning	Assuming that your negative feelings reflect the way things really are	I feel overwhelmed. My problems are impossible to solve.
Should statements	Assuming there is only one truth or way of looking at things	I should be able to care for my husband without getting frustrated or mad.
Labeling	Generalizing one or two qualities, or an error, into a negative global judgment	I get so frustrated at times with having to stay home constantly to care for my wife. I'm a horrible husband.
Comparative thinking	Comparing yourself to someone and finding that you don't measure up	My sister bounced back so quickly after her husband's death and I've been struggling for months since my husband died. I'm not as competent as my sister.
Personalization	Assuming responsibility for a negative event when there is no basis for doing so	When I went over to my son's house for dinner, his wife snapped at me. I don't know what I did wrong.
Fortune telling	Assuming that things will turn out negatively with little or no evidence	If I move into a new living situation, I won't be able to make any friends there.

often such a part of us that we typically do not realize we hold these beliefs. Underlying assumptions can be functional or dysfunctional. Dysfunctional assumptions differ from functional ones in that they are maladaptive, disproportionate, and rigid.

Underlying assumptions are rooted in *schema*, which are core beliefs that are fundamental to the person's understanding of self, others, and the world. Schema are foundational and global, and additionally, most often they are also unexamined and

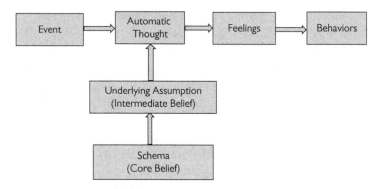

FIGURE 3.2 Influence of schema and underlying assumptions.

unquestioned. Schema develop from early, usually childhood, experiences. The nature of an individual's schema depend upon the child's interactions with the world and how the child interprets these experiences (Westbook, Kennerley, & Kirk, 2011). Core beliefs can be positive or negative, and people generally possess a combination of both. Healthier functioning people, however, have more positive schema. Core beliefs are generally expressed as general and absolute beliefs, such as "I am lovable" or "I have no value."

In addition to being positive or negative, schema may be operational or latent. *Operational schema* are the active core beliefs that typically guide our behaviors and responses to interactions. A *latent schema* is a core belief an individual possess that is currently inactive. A latent schema can be activated by a series of minor stressful events or by a single negative experience. Once a schema is activated, the person tries to fit his or her perceptions and interpretations of events into that particular schema. Schema is the basis for screening in or out stimuli that confront the person (see Figure 3.2).

Returning to the original examples of this chapter can illustrate how schema and underlying assumptions influence recent retirees' thoughts and behaviors. The first retiree has a core belief "I am of value" and an underlying assumption based on that core belief of "I deserve good things in my life." Upon waking up the first day after retirement, she thinks, "Now I can finally relax" (automatic thought). She feels positive, gets up, and enjoys morning coffee and the paper. The last retiree has a core belief of "I have no value" and the underlying assumption "to be of value I must be productive" rooted in this core belief. The morning following his retirement, he awakes and thinks, "Now there's nothing for me to do. I am useless" (automatic thought). He feels depressed and chooses to stay in bed.

PRACTICE APPROACHES AND APPLICATION

CBT is an active, structured, and time-limited therapy for treating a wide range of psychological disorders by helping clients identify and modify maladaptive thoughts, beliefs, and related behaviors. At the core, CBT helps clients understand the relationship between thoughts, feelings, and behaviors; identify the distorted cognitions they possess that negatively influence their feelings and behaviors; and change their disruptive thought patterns to ones that are healthier and more adaptive. CBT is a problem-oriented therapy focused on helping clients deal with a specific problem in the here and now and learn how to handle troublesome future symptoms (Butler & Beck, 1995).

The process of treatment is a collaborative approach in which the client and therapist work together to investigate and discover automatic thoughts and test the truthfulness or reality of these thoughts. Through a process of "guided discovery," the therapist helps the client recognize dysfunctional thoughts and consider alternative interpretations (Cully & Teten, 2008). Based on the Socratic method, the therapist asks the client questions to assist in the investigative process. The therapist does not try to persuade or convince the client, or engage in interpretations. Rather, the clinician or practitioner asks questions to help the client gather evidence from his or her own life that either supports or disputes the disruptive thought. If there is limited evidence to support the distorted thought, the therapist will ask the client what other possible interpretations might exist.

In the following case, the therapist works with a woman to challenge her thoughts about her marital relationship. Mrs. Johnson, age 68, reports that she has been feeling anxious and stressed about her marriage. She notes that her husband has been irritable and distant of late, and she can't figure out what she is doing that is causing him to behave this way. Mrs. Johnson may be engaging in the cognitive distortion of *personalization*: assuming responsibility for a negative event when there may be no reason to do so. After educating Mrs. Johnson about CBT and the relationship between thoughts and feelings, the therapist asks Mrs. Johnson to consider her thought that she is doing something to cause her husband to be irritable and distant, and inquires as to the evidence Mrs. Johnson has that indicates something she has done has led to her husband's current behavior. Mrs. Johnson replies that her inability to identify what she has done wrong is the source of the anxiety she is experiencing. The therapist then asks Mrs. Johnson to consider other possible reasons, outside of herself, that may be causing her husband's behavior. Through this process the therapist helps the client understand the relationship between thoughts and feelings, to observe and critically analyze his or her thoughts, and to develop alternate hypotheses or interpretations about the event. To further engage the client in this process, both cognitive and behavioral techniques are employed (Karlin, 2011).

COGNITIVE STRATEGIES IN CBT

Cognitive strategies are designed to help clients understand the relationship between events, thoughts and feeling, observe their own cognitions, and recognize and modify cognitive distortions. The targeting of underlying assumptions and core beliefs may be necessary for symptom resolution, and for these, cognitive strategies are also employed. Cognitive and behavioral techniques are often used in tandem to reinforce discovery and learning. To actively engage in cognitive strategies, a client must be functioning at a reasonable level. If a client is severely depressed, anxious, or suffers from another serious psychological disorder, behavioral techniques will form the cornerstone of the treatment until the client has regained moderate functioning. Behavioral, rather than cognitive, strategies are more often used with cognitively impaired clients (Gallagher-Thompson & Thompson, 2010).

As part of the orientation process to CBT, the therapist explains the association between events, thoughts, feelings, and behaviors. With the therapist's help, the client initially learns how to recognize and record automatic interpretations of his or her experience. A Brief Automatic Thought Record may be used to help a client recognize the link between events, thoughts, feelings, and behaviors. For example, a client is asked to think about a time when negative feelings were particularly troublesome, to describe the circumstance in which the feelings occurred, and then to identify cognitions (thoughts or mental representations) that he or she experienced during this event. The therapist gently guides the client through this process and elicits information by asking questions. The event, thoughts, feelings, and consequent behaviors are then recorded on the Brief Automatic Thought Record.

In the following example a therapist uses the Brief Automatic Thought Record to help an older client explore the relationship between her thoughts and feelings. Agnes Henley is an 87-year-old widow who has just moved from the home she shared with her husband until his death 6 months ago into an apartment in a continuous care retirement community. She complains of experiencing anxiety and depression since her relocation. She spends most of her time in her apartment alone. The worker asks Mrs. Henley to think of a time within the past couple of days when she felt particularly anxious or depressed, and together they talk through the scenario and complete the Brief Automatic Thought Record (see Table 3.2).

The therapist helps the client to examine the veracity of his or her thoughts, and to determine if alternative explanations of the event are possible. In the example in Table 3.2, Mrs. Henley states that it is possible that some residents would have been open to having her at their table. After exploring this possibility with the therapist, Mrs. Henley concludes that if she had approached a table with an open seat she would likely have been welcomed to join the group. When asked what she could say to herself if she faces this same scenario in the future, she replies, "I'll say to myself, someone will want me at their table, I just need to ask." Having the client write down the new adaptive thought(s) on an Automatic Thought Record (ATR) gives the client a concrete visual of the outcome of examining and disputing cognitive distortion and developing concrete adaptive responses (see Table 3.3).

An important strategy in CBT is to have a client engage in homework. Clients are asked to use an ATR while at home to record problematic feelings and related thoughts and behaviors. The client brings the ATR to the next session for further discussion with the therapist. As patients learn to identify cognitive distortions and to develop adaptive

TABLE 3.2 BRIEF AUTOMATIC THOUGHT RECORD

Event	Automatic Thoughts	Feelings	Behavior
Walking into the dining room of the new retirement community for dinner two nights ago.	1) I don't know anyone. 2) Everyone already has friends. 3) No one wants me at their table.	1) Anxious 2) Depressed	1) Took my plate and went back to my apartment to eat.

responses, these can be added to the ATR homework. Homework enables clients to practice, utilize, and reinforce cognitive strategies between sessions, and teaches the clients strategies to use on their own in the future should the need arise.

At times, clients may have difficulty coming up with alternate thoughts that they can believe or which will endure in the presence of their cognitive distortions. Such cognitive distortions may be rooted in underlying assumptions or core beliefs that must be addressed. One technique for uncovering an underlying assumption or belief is to ask the client about the meaning of the thought to him or her (Beck, 2011), as demonstrated in the following example. Harvey Westen, a retired manager at an auto repair shop, has been seeing a counselor due to depression and anger issues. At his wife's suggestion, Mr.

TABLE 3.3 AUTOMATIC THOUGHT RECORD

Event	Automatic Thoughts and Ratings of Belief in These (%)	Feelings and Ratings of Strength of Feelings (%)	Adaptive Response and Ratings of Belief in These (%)	Outcomes (%) Re-rate Belief in ATs; Re-rate Feelings and Probability of New Behavior
Walking into the dining room of the new retirement community for dinner two nights ago.	1) I don't know anyone. (100%) 2) Everyone already has friends. (80%) 3) No one wants me at their table. (80%)	1) Anxious (75%) 2) Depressed (70%)	1) Some people will be open to meeting new folks. (70%) 2) If I see an empty seat at a table and ask, others will probably welcome me. (90%)	Automatic Thoughts 1) 100% 2) 70% 3) 40% Resultant Feelings 1) 50% 2) 40% Planned New Behavior Ask if I see an empty seat (95%)

Westen decides to volunteer at the local Lion's Club. He is asked to work on a project with three other volunteers. While brainstorming with the group, Mr. Westen brings up an idea that one of the group members quickly shoots down. Mr. Westen becomes very angry and verbally aggressive with the other volunteer, who eventually backs down. When recounting this incident to his counselor, Mr. Westen is able to state that he reacted so strongly because he believed the other volunteer was disrespecting him. When asked what it means if someone does act disrespectfully toward him, Mr. Westen states, "I can't allow it. If I allow it, I'm weak" (underlying assumption). After further discussion, the counselor asks, "What it would mean if you were weak?" Mr. Westen responds, "If a man is weak, what is he worth? Nothing, he's worthless" (core belief).

BEHAVIORAL STRATEGIES IN CBT

Behavioral strategies are useful for clients with low activity levels, decreased motivation, greater passivity, difficulty initiating action, and those who complain of limited pleasure and productivity (Dobson & Dobson, 2009). Increased activity can help motivate a client and pave the way for cognitive change. Helping a client to modify or increase behaviors can also serve to demonstrate an error in the client's generalized negative beliefs. Behavioral techniques such as activity rehearsal and problem-solving can also be beneficial for higher functioning clients (Cully & Teten, 2008). Severely depressed patients may engage in very few activities throughout the day, and are often pessimistic about their ability to carry out and derive any pleasure from activities. Through behavioral monitoring, the practitioner helps clients to focus on activities in which they are currently engaged, regardless of how limited or beneficial. The Weekly Activity Schedule (WAS) is used for this purpose. The practitioner asks the client to name all activities in which he or she engaged during the last week; these may include things as small as having a cup of coffee in the morning, reading the paper, or watching a game show on television. All activities are listed on the WAS form, and the client is asked to rate his or her mastery in accomplishing this activity as well as the pleasure he or she derived.

The case of Charley Donovan demonstrates the use of the WAS form with a depressed client experiencing low motivation. Charley Donovan is a 79-year-old widower whose wife died 9 months ago. Since that time, he has become increasingly depressed. He lives alone in the house they shared. He states that he is depressed and bored. When asked to recount what he's done the previous few days he states, "Nothing, just stared out the window." With some guiding questions from the therapist, Mr. Donovan describes a few activities he did engage in during the past few days, which the therapist records on the WAS (see Table 3.4).

The therapist asks Mr. Donovan to rate the activities on the chart to indicate how much pleasure he received and the degree of accomplishment he derived from each activity. For example, the therapist queries, "On a scale of 0–10 with 10 being the greatest accomplishment and 0 being no accomplishment at all, how much of an

TABLE 3.4 WEEKLY ACTIVITY SCHEDULE

Weekly Activities Schedule Rate—Accomplishment (A) and Pleasure (P)

	Monday	Tuesday	Wednesday	Thursday	Friday
9–10	Got up, dressed Breakfast A = 4, P = 3				
10–11	Drove to doctor appointment A = 5, P = 5	Got up Breakfast A = 3, P = 2	Got up and dressed A = 4, P = 3		
11–12	Doctor appointment A = 4, P = 3	Sat in chair A = 1, P = 0	Breakfast A = 4, P = 3		
12–1	Doctor apt A = 4, P = 3	Nap A = 0, P = 1	Read paper A = 4, P = 4		
1–2	Drove home A = 5, P = 5	Nap A = 0, P = 1	Daughter called A = 3, P = 6		
2–3	Lunch A = 4, P = 4	Nap A = 0, P = 1	Drove to therapist appointment A = 5, P = 5		
3–4	Read mail A = 3, P = 3	Read mail A = 3, P = 3	Therapist appointment		
4–5	Nap A = 0, P = 1	Sat in chair A = 1, P = 1			
5–6	Watched News A = 3, P = 3	Dinner A = 3, P = 2			
6–7	Jeopardy A = 6, P = 5	Jeopardy A = 5, P = 4			
7–8	Dinner A = 4, P = 4	Bed			
9–12	Bed				

accomplishment do you feel it was for you to get up, get dressed, and have breakfast?" The therapist also asks Mr. Donovan to rate the degree of pleasure he received from this activity. Mr. Donovan responds, "Well, since I didn't feel like getting out of bed or getting dressed at all, I guess I'll give it a 4 for accomplishment and a 3 for pleasure since I didn't enjoy it all that much, but it was better than just lying around in bed in my pajamas." By reviewing the remaining ratings together, the worker and client are able to pinpoint those activities that do bring Mr. Donovan the greatest, and least, feelings of accomplishment and pleasure. As can be seen from the WAS in Table 3.4, Mr. Donovan derives the most pleasure and sense of accomplishment from driving (an activity he has always enjoyed), watching *Jeopardy* (a game at which he is very good), and speaking with his daughter (whom he loves). At the opposite end of the pleasure and accomplishment spectrum are napping and sitting in a chair. The therapist then asks Mr. Donovan to reconsider the accuracy of his earlier statement that he does nothing all day but stare out the window. Mr. Donovan admits that this statement was not accurate, that he has engaged in some activities, and that realizing this makes him feel a little less hopeless. The information gained from constructing and discussing the WAS with the client can then be used for activity scheduling.

With activity scheduling, the client constructs a plan of activities for the coming days or week. In this case, using the information gleaned from the WAS, Mr. Donovan agrees to get up and get dressed every morning. He realizes that the day he stayed in his pajamas was the day he napped the most and felt the least pleasure and accomplishment. He is concerned, however, that he has nothing to do and will just end up sitting in his chair and feeling bad. When the therapist suggests that he take a drive, Mr. Donovan complains that he has nowhere he needs to go in the next couple of days. He finally states that he is getting low on a few groceries. He agrees to drive the following day to a grocery store that is farther away but that has a better selection of produce and that requires him to drive though an interesting area of town. When working with clients to construct an activity schedule, it is important to help them work through problems that may prevent them from accomplishing their tasks. Asking questions such as "How likely do you think it is that you'll be able to do the things you planned?" "What could get in the way of your doing the things you planned?" "What might you be able to do to prevent this from happening?" are critical in assisting clients to recognize and prevent barriers to success.

Problem-solving is a useful strategy in work with clients such as Mr. Donovan and also with higher functioning clients, especially those whom the therapist wishes to engage in behavioral experiments. Behavioral experiments are used to help clients test the accuracy of their thoughts and assumptions (Beck, 2011). In the following example, behavioral experiments are used to assist a woman struggling with anxiety related to public speaking.

Ms. Julie Hedrick, a 64-year-old librarian, has reduced her work schedule to part-time and wishes to engage in volunteer work with children. She always loved reading out loud to her own children and would like to read books to children at the local bookstore, but she has always hated any type of public speaking. She is fearful that she will become nervous, stumble over her words, and look like a fool in front of all the children and their mothers. When asked to rate her belief in the likelihood that she will stumble over her words, she indicates 80%, and 90% that people would think she's a fool if this did occur. As homework the therapist asks Ms. Hedrick to pick out a children's book and read it out loud to herself until she is very comfortable with the story, and then to bring the book to their next session. During their next session, Ms. Hedrick is able to read the story out loud in front of the therapist with few errors. She reports feeling more confident about her ability, but still concerned about reading to a group.

The therapist and Ms. Hedrick engage in problem-solving to see if they can identify a less threatening group setting in which Ms. Hedrick could practice her speaking skills. Ms. Hedrick decides on a kindergarten class at local elementary school where she believes that, in addition to the children, only a teacher and, perhaps, a teacher's assistant would be present. While in the therapist's office she calls the school principal and arranges the reading session. She agrees with the therapist that she will pick a book and thoroughly practice reading it aloud for several days before going to the school. When asked to rate her belief that she will have problems reading to the kindergarten class and be judged a fool, she reports 50% and 55%, respectively.

At their next session, Ms. Hedrick reported that she did read to the kindergarteners and that the principal had unexpectedly sat in during this time. Although this initially made her very nervous, she had practiced so much she was able to complete the story. Although she did stumble over the words once while reading, the children didn't seem to notice, and afterward both the principal and teacher thanked her for taking the time to be with the class. Ms. Hedrick now believes that she is ready to call the bookstore and volunteer to read there. She will thoroughly practice again and will remind herself that no one minded when she got a few words mixed up the last time. The schoolchildren just seemed grateful she was there. After developing this new adaptive response based upon her own experience, Ms. Hedrick stated that she feels more confident, less anxious, and even a little excited about reading at the bookstore.

When working with a client to set up behavioral experiments, the counselor and the client need to consider and determine the strength of the client's thoughts and beliefs. Initial behavioral experiments should consist of small achievable tasks that are thoroughly planned, including specifics about the exact activity the client will engage in and where and when the task will be accomplished (Beck, 2011). Prior to the experiment, the worker and client consider problems that may occur and develop coping strategies. Another beneficial strategy is engaging the client in behavioral rehearsal while in the worker's office. While planning the execution of the behavioral experiment is critical for success, review of the client's experience after the experiment is of equal import. Through post-experiment review, the therapist helps the client evaluate what was learned, what thoughts have or have not changed, and the strengths of these thoughts. If necessary, graduated behavioral experiments can be devised to help a client slowly engage in new behaviors, test out disruptive thoughts, and develop more adaptive beliefs.

CBT WITH OLDER CLIENTS

CBT interventions are effective with clients of various ages. Although frequently spoken of as one consistent age group, those defined as "older adults" comprise separate, often distinct, age cohorts who have lived through specific historical events that shape their assumptions and beliefs. For those who lived through the Great Depression, for example, maintaining physical possessions as a means to ensure basic security may be a core value, while for baby boomers the link between independence and self-worth may be funda-mental. Once again, it is necessary that the worker be cognizant of these issues when employing CBT with the older population.

When employing CBT with older clients, it is necessary to pay special attention to age-related events and contextual factors. Older adults may face the challenges of depres-sion, anxiety, substance misuse, and other psychological disorders for a variety of reasons. A growing number of individuals with ongoing mental health disorders are living longer, and in late life find that they must manage not only the symptoms of these disorders, but also the medical, functional, financial, and social challenges that become more com-mon in later years. Others may develop mental health concerns later in life. Events that occur as one ages, such as loss of loved ones, transitions in employment status and living environment, and the emergence of medical and functional difficulties, may not only rep-resent current challenges, but also trigger the operation of dormant schema, especially those involving self-worth, competence, and security (Chand & Grossberg, 2013). Such assaults can hamper the individual's ability to effectively perceive and respond to events, and may manifest as dysfunctional behaviors such as withdrawal, excess dependence, and substance misuse. CBT actively engages older adults in a non-threatening process that seeks to address and reformulate problematic thoughts and behaviors.

As indicated in one of the basic tenets of CBT, the meaning of the events is what mat-ters, not the actual event itself. Many events that occur in later life do require practical and, at times, complex responses. In the midst of this assessment, however, the worker needs to investigate older clients' thoughts and beliefs about the situations they are confront-ing. For example, the loss of the ability to drive results in the need to secure alternative transportation. However, older adults also experience a loss of independence and a threat to perceived competence. Likewise, the death of a spouse may usher in both feelings of grief and a debilitating fear of never being loved again. The much-documented associa-tion between chronic illness, functional impairment, and psychological distress also war-rants special attention (Clarke & Currie, 2009). The therapist must be knowledgeable of and have the ability to discuss these issues with the client (Satre, Knight, & David, 2006).

Research and reports of expert panels indicate that CBT is effective when used with older adults (Steinman et al., 2007); however, adaptations to the CBT process may be necessary due to age-related cognitive and sensory changes. Normal cognitive changes do occur as part of the aging process. Older adults experience a decline in cognitive speed, spontaneous recall of newly learned material, selective attention, and fluid intelligence (Chand & Grossberg, 2013). Cognitive changes in older adults may require that mate-rial be presented more slowly, with more frequent repetition and summaries, and the use of aids to help retention of information from session to session. Sensory changes, such as decreased hearing and vision loss, may also impact the older client's ability to grasp the information presented and may necessitate the use of special aids. Although modifications may be required for some older clients, it is important not to assume that adaptations must be made just because of the client's age (Gallagher-Thompson & Thompson, 2010). Adjustments should be made based upon client assessment and learning about the client's needs and abilities. The following adaptations are often useful when conducting CBT with older adults.

1. *Socialize the older client into CBT*. Older clients, especially those from earlier cohorts, are typically unfamiliar with therapy and may be suspicious or hesitant to engage in the process. As with all work with older adults, establishing rapport and trust is essential. CBT uses a collaborative model in which the therapist and client jointly investigate the client's thoughts and beliefs. This approach may run counter to the older clients' experience with other practitioners, such as medical doctors, who are seen as experts who inform clients as to the nature of their problems and the needed solutions (Satre et al., 2006).

2. *Provide the necessary structure for the older client to stay on track*. Older adults often appreciate the opportunity to "tell their story" and may digress or get off topic. In such cases the therapist should gently redirect the client back to the topic. If the client continues to digress, the therapist should discuss the time-limited nature of therapy with the client and the importance of using time well in order to accomplish the client's goals.

3. *Slow the pace of therapy*. The worker should speak more slowly, check frequently for comprehension, and periodically ask the client to summarize what has been discussed throughout the session. Also, taking the time to have the client make notes of key points in a notebook can help reinforce important points in the client's mind, as well as ensure that the client has a record of this information after the session is over.

4. *Present materials in different modes*. Combining verbal information with written resources reinforces the information and provides the older client with a physical reference for future use. Written materials should be provided in larger type.

5. *Use teaching aids during the session*. Flip charts can be used to write down a summary of key points, note the progress of the session, document thoughts and assumptions, and record brainstorming outcomes. A notebook, note cards, and folders or binders to organize materials are also often employed. A tape recorder to capture important information and conclusions from cognitive restructuring, which the client can use between sessions for review, often helps to reinforce and strengthen learning.

6. *Reinforce the use of homework*. Research indicates that older adults' completion of homework between sessions significantly improves therapy outcomes (Coon & Thompson, 2003). However, older clients may find the term "homework" demeaning or burdensome. The term "home practice" is often more agreeable to older clients. Techniques for home practice should first be demonstrated and practiced in session. It is important to begin with small steps to support early success. Brief between-session calls to the client to discuss progress with home practice can help remind

clients of the home-practice task, and provide a time for needed clarification and/or troubleshooting.

7. *Use a bridge from the previous to the current session.* Bridge use is a standard part of CBT, but may be especially helpful for the older client. At the beginning of a session, the practitioner asks the client to recount what she found to be the most important or helpful from the previous session. If the client has trouble responding, the therapist suggests a couple of key points from the prior session.

8. *Consider the use of a longer treatment period.* Longer duration in treatment has been associated with better treatment outcomes for older adults (Pinquart & Sörensen, 2001). A slower pace in therapy may necessitate an elongation of the treatment period.

9. *Carefully plan termination.* Because of the role that loss may have played in an older clients' life, it is important to explore the meaning of loss of the therapeutic relationship with the client, to deal with any related distorted cognitions, and to develop a plan for the maintenance of therapy gains (Karlin, 2011). Tapering of sessions and decreasing their frequency toward the end of therapy from weekly to biweekly, for example, and planning for a "booster" session or two following the official end of therapy are useful strategies for successful termination.

CONTEXTS AND IMPLEMENTATION

Cognitive behavioral therapy is a flexible psychosocial intervention that can be used in a variety of contexts and with diverse older populations. Individual and group-based cognitive behavioral treatments with older adults most frequently occur in community-based settings such as out-patient clinics, private practice offices, and community mental health centers. Treatment duration commonly extends from 12 to 16 weeks. With the emergence of integrated health care, however, the use of CBT with older patients in primary care settings is also becoming more common (Serfaty, Haworth, Blanchard, Buszewicz, Murad, & King, 2009). Older adults confront medical issues that heighten stress and negatively impact quality of life and psychological well-being. Increased psychological stress, in turn, may exacerbate health conditions. Research demonstrates the efficacy of cognitive behavioral approaches to address depression, anxiety, pain, and insomnia in various medical patient populations (Mitchell, Gehrman, Perlis, & Umscheid, 2012; Veehor, Oskam, Schreus, & Bohlmeijer, 2011). CBT in primary care settings in which blended medical and behavioral health treatment occur is typically brief (e.g., 1–8 sessions) in duration and focuses on lifestyle issues, such as diet, exercise, and smoking cessation, and on negative psychological states, such as depression and anxiety, that interfere with medical treatment and/or exacerbate health conditions (Jameson & Cully, 2011). Because of the condensed format and treatment focus, goals are limited and measurable. Patients with long-standing mental health disorders such as bipolar disorder, major recurrent depressive disorder, and post-traumatic stress disorder that require further attention are referred to community-based mental health services.

CBT is also effectively employed in the hospice setting. Cognitive behavioral interventions help mitigate grief, depression, guilt, and anxiety experienced by patients and family members in the palliative care environment, as well enable individuals to more effectively deal with the sleep disturbances and pain that often accompany life-limiting illnesses. The interdisciplinary team, patient, and family work together to develop CBT treatment goals focused on the alleviation of physical and emotional distress. Treatment goals are realistic, achievable, and focused on the immediate circumstance. Treatment duration is typically very brief and may span one to four sessions. A characteristic scenario may include an initial session for assessment, two sessions for cognitive or behavioral strategies, and a final session to summarize work that had been accomplished and to develop a plan for maintaining gains (Anderson, Watson, & Davison, 2008). Cognitive strategies are used to assist patients and families in dealing with maladaptive thoughts surrounding death and loss. Behavioral techniques, such as scheduling meaningful pleasant events that can be achieved by the patient either alone or with assistance, and relaxation techniques, such as deep breathing and guided imagery, serve to help relieve stress and anxiety, distract from negative thoughts, and provide periods of enjoyment (Freeman, 2011).

As stated in Chapter 2, nursing home residents suffer from high rates of depression. Up to 48% experience major depressive disorder or significant depressive symptomatology (Zarit & Zarit, 2007). Although not as common as other psychosocial interventions, such as reminiscence therapy (see Chapters 11 and 12), CBT is employed in nursing homes. Cognitive behavioral approaches in nursing homes are most typically conducted in group settings and focus on alleviating stress, depression, and anxiety, and on enhancing socialization. Group sessions in nursing homes frequently occur twice a week and last 30–60 minutes. Although non-completion of treatment is not uncommon due to illness or death, research has shown significant decrease in depressive symptoms among residents participating in CBT group therapy (Konnert, Dobson, & Stelmach, 2009). Verbal and cognitive competence is required for some forms of CBT. However, residents who are more frail or impaired may benefit from pleasant events–based behavioral strategies that combine behavioral activation and pleasant event scheduling (Meeks & Depp, 2008).

CASE EXAMPLE

Ms. Betty Garrison is a 74-year-old woman who lives with her husband, Mr. James Garrison, in an apartment building for retired teachers. Both Mr. and Mrs. Garrison taught at a local community college until they retired almost 10 years ago. The couple has one daughter who lives in the area and has three-year-old twins. Mrs. Garrison has been very helpful to her daughter in caring for the active twins since her daughter is divorced and works full-time. Several years ago, Mr. Garrison started to become more forgetful.

He now has difficulty finding his way around the apartment building alone. He forgets the names of other residents, cannot remember when to take his diabetes medication, and has been unable to pay the bills for about a year. Several months ago, Mr. Garrison was diagnosed with Alzheimer's disease. Mrs. Garrison has not told anyone about the diagnosis. Throughout her life, Mrs. Garrison was a very positive and optimistic woman. However, she has begun to experience increasing periods of depression.

Mrs. Garrison, who has been trying to keep up with the needs of her husband and watch the twins two afternoons of the week, is starting to feel overwhelmed. Two weeks ago, she shut herself in the bathroom and began to cry. When she was teaching, she had been able to juggle her school-related activities, raise her daughter, and volunteer at her church. People often commented on how organized she was and sought her out to chair committees. But now she is beginning to feel that she is no longer the capable woman she once was. She remembers back to when she was teaching and raising her daughter and asks herself why she can't be as organized and competent as she once was. Last week while she was watching the twins, she fell asleep while they were playing together. When she awoke she was horrified. She couldn't believe that she had been so irresponsible and began to further doubt her abilities! She did not tell her daughter what occurred. When driving home, she was overwhelmed with feelings of helplessness. During a visit with Mr. Garrison to his doctor the following day, the doctor noticed that Mrs. Garrison appeared near tears and referred her to a social worker.

During the initial visit, the social worker, Ruth, listens to Mrs. Garrison's account of the challenges she has been facing and to her expressions of depression and helplessness, and also attends to the thoughts that she expresses. Ruth educates Mrs. Garrison about the relationship between events, thoughts, and feelings, and explains the process used in cognitive behavioral therapy. She also provides Mrs. Garrison with written materials on CBT that she can read and take home. Mrs. Garrison agrees to this approach and the two begin working together.

During the assessment of Mrs. Garrison's situation, Ruth notices several statements that may represent cognitive distortions. These include "I'm no longer the capable woman I once was" (black–white thinking); "Why can't I be as organized and competent as I once was?" (comparison); and "I can't believe I was so irresponsible as to fall asleep when baby-sitting the twins!" (labeling). As an initial step, Ruth focuses on Mrs. Garrison's comment that "I'm no longer the capable woman I once was" and asks what evidence she has to support this claim. Mrs. Garrison quickly points to falling asleep when babysitting the twins, and she also reports that she has been having problems keeping up with Mr. Garrison and her various appointments. She states that she completely forgot about her dentist appointment last week and didn't even bother trying to get herself and Mr. Garrison ready for church this past Sunday. When asked if there could be any reasons other than "no longer being capable" for the difficulties she has been experiencing, Mrs. Garrison replies, "I know I'm doing a lot but I've always been able to handle things in the past."

As a next step, Ruth asks Mrs. Garrison to list all of her activities for a typical week, including everything she does for Mr. Garrison. As Mrs. Garrison lists her activities, Ruth asks Mrs. Garrison to elaborate, so that she thoroughly describes all of the activities required for each task. Ruth lists each of these on a flip chart. Both women note the large number of items that fill the page, and Mrs. Garrison reports that she hadn't been aware that she had been doing so much. When Ruth asks Mrs. Garrison if the reason that she fell asleep while babysitting and has missed appointments could be because of the large number of tasks she is handling rather than being incompetent, Mrs. Garrison agrees that this is possible. Ruth explains the use and purpose of the Automatic Thought Record, and together they complete an ATR form, recording both Mrs. Garrison's original and new adaptive thoughts, along with her corresponding feelings. For home practice, Ruth asks Mrs. Garrison to notice automatic thoughts related to "not being competent" that may occur, to record these along with the event and related feelings, and to write down an alternate thought on the ATR.

At the next session Mrs. Garrison reports that her daughter asked her to babysit one evening because she had to work late. The twins were rambunctious and her husband repeatedly called her to ask when she was coming home. Thoughts of "I should be able to handle this" (should statement) and "maybe I just don't have what it takes to help any more" (black–white thinking) resurfaced. Mrs. Garrison reports that she felt stressed and angry with both herself and with Mr. Garrison. She was so flustered that she wasn't able to think of alternate thoughts at the time and she didn't have time the following day to write down her thoughts. Ruth suggested that they complete the Automatic Thought Record together in the office, and provided Mrs. Garrison with an ATR form. They discussed the event and Mrs. Garrison identified and recorded the thoughts "I should be able to handle this!" which upon reflection she recognizes as a should statement, and "I can't do anything anymore" (black–white statement). She rated the strength of the thoughts and the associated feelings. Together with Ruth, she developed alternate thoughts—"I can do many things well. But I can't babysit at night any more because of Mr. Garrison's illness." Then she re-rated her thoughts and feelings (see Table 3.5).

In following weeks, Mrs. Garrison continued to monitor and record her thoughts at home. Mrs. Garrison kept all of her ATRs in a binder that she took to her sessions with Ruth. Due to her continued stress, Ruth broached the possibility of Mrs. Garrison cutting back on her babysitting to one day per week. When considering this possibility, Mrs. Garrison confronted thoughts related to "failing my daughter who needs me" (black–white statement) and "letting my daughter down" (mind-reading). Ruth noted Mrs. Garrison's pattern of engaging in black and white thinking, especially related to situations that threatened her sense of competence. Ruth asked Mrs. Garrison what "being competent" (i.e., "handling things") means. Mrs. Garrison replied, "I guess, handling things means keeping everything in order, in control. Not handling things

TABLE 3.5 BETTY'S AUTOMATIC THOUGHT RECORD

Event	Automatic Thoughts (%)	Feelings (%)	Adaptive Response	Outcomes (%) Re-rate Belief in ATs; Re-rate Feelings and Probably of New Behavior
Evening babysitting for the twins; Jim calling multiple times	1) I should be able to handle this! (80%) 2) I can't do anything anymore. (45%)	1) Stressed (90%) 2) Anger at Jim (30%) 3) Anger at self (70%)	1) I can do many things well. (65%) 2) But I can't babysit at night any more because of Jim's illness. (95%)	Automatic thoughts 1) 40% 2) 20% Feelings 1) 80% 2) 25% 3) 45%

means that things could fall part" (underlying assumption). When asked what "falling apart" meant, Mrs. Garrison responded, "That I'm not safe" (core belief). Over the next couple of weeks, Ruth and Mrs. Garrison further explore thoughts related to Mrs. Garrison's underlying assumption that if things are not under control, everything will fall apart.

In order to test these assumptions, Mrs. Garrison engaged in small experiments. She ordered dinner from a take-away restaurant rather than cooking, asked a neighbor to pick up a prescription for her at the pharmacy, and finally informed her daughter that she needed to cut back her babysitting to one time per week. Ruth and Mrs. Garrison processed her expectations prior to, and her thoughts following, each experiment. As a result and with continued practice, Mrs. Garrison became more adept at addressing negative distortions related to being incompetent and letting others down when these thoughts arose. As a result, she was able to confront her assumption that she must handle everything herself or "things would fall apart."

In spite of reducing her time babysitting, Mrs. Garrison reported that she continued to feel stressed. Ruth had Mrs. Garrison complete an Activities Schedule, which revealed that Mrs. Garrison spent all her time caring for others and doing chores. Ruth asked Mrs. Garrison to use the Activity Schedule to include at least two pleasurable activities per week. Together they brainstormed how Mrs. Garrison could find the time for such activities. As a result, Mrs. Garrison contacted her local Alzheimer's Association and arranged for respite care for one morning a week so that she could leave the house and visit with friends. After confronting thoughts of failure and concerns related to unnecessary use of funds, Mrs. Garrison decided to hire a housekeeper to come once a week. As a result, one afternoon a week while Mr. Garrison naps, she now takes a couple of hours to relax and read rather using this time to clean.

At the end of their time together, Ruth reviewed the progress Mrs. Garrison made and all that she accomplished. As a result of this work, Mrs. Garrison felt less stressed, more in control, and better able to recognize and challenge distorted cognitions. To sustain the positive change, two "booster sessions" were scheduled 2 weeks apart. At their final booster session, Mrs. Garrison revealed that she still felt stressed at times and that when this occurred her negative thoughts resurfaced. But she noted that she could handle that situation. She also reported that she had joined a caregivers' support group, which provided further support, companionship, and advice.

CONCLUSION

Cognitive behavioral therapy is an evidence-based treatment that is widely used with older adults. Based on the premise that feelings and mood states are heavily influenced by an individual's thoughts and beliefs, CBT is effective for addressing long-standing, as well as later-life, problems. The strengths of CBT include its short-term nature, use of both cognitive and behavioral strategies, adaptability for use with a range of issues and in a variety of settings, and the availability of existing treatment forms and materials (Steinman et al., 2007). Those using CBT with older adults should be familiar with issues related to later life such as loss; the relationship between medical illness, functional impairment, and depression; and concerns about independence and competence. Adaptations—including slowing the pace of therapy, use of written materials as well as verbal instruction, practicing the use of forms in the office before assignment for home practice, accommodating cognitive decline through greater use of behavioral techniques, and paying special attention to the termination process—serve to improve the efficacy of CBT when used with older clients.

REFERENCES

Anderson, T., Watson, M. & Davison, R. (2008). The use of cognitive behavioral therapy techniques for anxiety and depression in hospice patients: a feasibility study. *Palliative Medicine, 22,* 814–821.

Bandura, A. (1969). Social learning theory of identificatory processes. In D. A. Goslin (Ed.), *Handbook of socialization theory and research* (pp. 213–262). Chicago: Rand McNally.

Beck, A. T., Rush, A. J., Shaw, B. F., & Emery, G. (1979). *Cognitive therapy of depression.* New York: Guilford Press.

Beck, J. S. (2011). *Cognitive therapy: basics and beyond.* New York: Guilford Press.

Butler, A. C., & Beck, A.T. (1995). Cognitive therapy for depression. *The Clinical Psychologist, 48,* 3–5.

Chand, S., & Grossberg, G. T. (2013). How to adapt cognitive-behavioral therapy for older adults. *Current Psychiatry, 12,* 10–15.

Clarke, D. M., & Currie, K. C. (2009). Depression, anxiety and their relationship with chronic diseases: a review of the epidemiology, risk and treatment evidence. *Medical Journal of Australia, 190*, S54–S60.

Coon, D. W., & Thompson, L. W. (2003). The relationship between homework compliance and treatment outcomes for older adult out-patients with mild to moderate depression. *American Journal of Geriatric Psychiatry, 11*, 53–61.

Cully, J. A., & Teten, A. L. (2008). *A therapist's guide to brief cognitive behavioral therapy*. Houston: Department of Veterans Affairs, South Central Mental Illness Research, Education, and Clinical Center.

Dobson, D., & Dobson, K. (2009). *Evidence-based practice of cognitive behavioral therapy*. New York: Guilford Press.

Freeman, S. M. (2011). Cognitive behavioral therapy within the palliative care setting. In K. H. Sorocco & S. Lauderdale (Eds.), *Cognitive behavior therapy with older adults: innovations across care settings* (pp. 367–387). New York: Springer.

Gallagher-Thompson, D., & Thompson, L. W. (2010). *Treating late-life depression: a cognitive-behavioral therapy approach. Therapists guide*. New York: Oxford University Press.

Jameson, J. P., & Cully, J. A. (2011). Cognitive behavioral therapy for older adults in the primary care setting. In K. H. Sorocco & S. Lauderdale (Eds.), *Cognitive behavior therapy with older adults: innovations across care settings* (pp. 291–316). New York: Springer.

Karlin, B. E. (2011). Cognitive behavioral therapy with older adults. In K. H. Sorocco & S. Lauderdale (Eds.), *Cognitive behavior therapy with older adults: innovations across care settings* (pp. 1–28). New York: Springer.

Konnert, C., Dobson, K., & Stelmach, L. (2009). The prevention of depression in nursing home resident: a randomized clinical trial of cognitive-behavioral therapy. *Aging & Mental Health, 13*, 288–299.

Martin, G., & Pear, J. (2007). *Behavior modification: what it is and how to do it* (8th ed.). Upper Saddle River, NJ: Pearson Prentice Hall.

Meeks, S., & Depp, C. A. (2008). Pleasant events-based behavioral intervention for depression in nursing home residents. *Clinical Gerontologist, 25*, 125–148.

Miller, G. A. (2003). The cognitive revolution: a historical perspective. *Trends in Cognitive Science, 7*, 141–144.

Mitchell, M. D., Gehrman, P., Perlis, M., & Umscheid, C. A. (2012). Comparative effectiveness of cognitive behavioral therapy for insomnia: a systematic review. *BioMedical Central, 13*, 1–11.

Pinquart, M., & Sörensen, S. (2001). How effective are psychotherapeutic another psychosocial interventions with older adults? A meta-analysis. *Journal of Mental Health & Aging, 7*, 207–243.

Satre, D, Knight, B. G., & David, S. (2006). Cognitive-behavioral interventions for older adults: integrating clinical and gerontological research. *Professional Psychology: Research and Practice, 37*, 489–498.

Serfaty, M. A., Haworth, D., Blanchard, M., Buszewicz, M., Murad, S., & King, M. (2009). Clinical effectiveness of individual cognitive behavioral therapy for depressed older people in primary care: a randomized controlled trial. *Archives of General Psychiatry, 66*, 1332–1340.

Sorocco, K. H., & Lauderdale, S. (2011). *Cognitive behavior therapy with older adults: innovations across care settings*. New York: Springer.

Steinman, L. E., Frederick, J. T., Prohaska, T., Satariano, W. A., Dronberg-Lee, S., Fisher, R., . . . Snowden, M. (2007). Recommendations for treating depression in community-based older adults. *American Journal of Preventive Medicine, 33*, 175–181.

Veehor, M. M., Oskam, M. J. Schreus, K. M., & Bohlmeijer, E. T. (2011). Acceptance-based interventions for the treatment of chronic pain: a systematic review and meta-analysis. *Pain, 152,* 553–542.

Watson, J. B. (1913). Psychology as the behaviorist views it. *Psychological Review, 20,* 158–177. doi:10.1037/h0074428.

Westbrook, D., Kennerley, H., & Kirk, J., (2011). *An introduction to cognitive behaviour therapy: skills and applications.* London: Age Publication LTD.

Zarit, S. H., & Zarit, J. M. (2007). *Mental disorders in older adults: fundamentals of assessment and treatment.* New York: Guilford Press.

4

COGNITIVE BEHAVIORAL THERAPY
EVIDENCE-BASED PRACTICE

As presented in Chapter 3, cognitive behavioral therapy (CBT) is an extensively researched therapeutic approach that possesses a solid evidence base. Studies conducted over the past 40 years document the effectiveness of CBT for the treatment of multiple disorders and problems, including depression, anxiety, symptoms of schizophrenia, trauma, insomnia, personality disorders, bulimia, anorexia, substance abuse, post-traumatic stress disorder (PTSD), obesity, and obsessive-compulsive disorder (OCD) (INSERM, 2004). While research on the effectiveness of CBT with older populations is not as encompassing, nonetheless it is substantive and more advanced than that of most other psychotherapeutic interventions used with older adults (Steinman et al., 2007).

To examine the effectiveness of CBT for use with older adults, a comprehensive literature review was conducted. PubMed, PsychINFO, Social Science Abstracts, Social Service Abstracts, and Sociological Abstracts were the databases searched. Search terms included the following: cognitive behavioral therapy or CBT and "older adult," elderly, senior, or geriatric, and meta-analysis or systematic review. Only studies meeting the following criteria were included in this review: (1) CBT or interventions derived from CBT principles were specifically included as a target of study; (2) age of participants in at least one arm of the study was 60 years and older; (3) consisted of a meta-analysis or systematic review; and (4) published between 2000 and 2015.

Fifteen studies meeting these criteria were identified. The most developed body of research on CBT effectiveness with older adults focuses on individuals with depression and anxiety. The case of Betty Garrison in Chapter 3 provides an example of the effectiveness of CBT with a depressed older client. A considerable, but more restricted, group of studies target CBT use for older adults with insomnia (CBT-I). The following review examines the results of five meta-analyses of CBT for older adults with depression and six for anxiety. Two meta-analyses and one systematic review that investigate the application of CBT-I to older individuals are also included.

DEPRESSION

Six meta-analyses indicate that CBT is an effective therapy for treating older adults with both major and minor depression (see Table 4.1). Krishna, Honagodu, Rajendra, Sundarachar, Lane, and Lepping (2013) conducted a meta-analysis of randomized controlled trials (RCTs) investigating the effectiveness of group CBT in reducing depressive symptoms among older adults with subclinical depression. Studies that met the following criteria were included: (1) randomized or cluster-randomized control trials; (2) participants were at least 50 years of age and had clinically relevant depressive symptoms, as indicated on a standardized measure; and (3) treatment occurred in a group setting with at least three participants. Studies with participants who had dementia, psychosis, a primary mental illness, or a substance abuse disorder were excluded. Four studies met the full criteria. Three studies drew participants from volunteers in the community, while the fourth study took place in a nursing home. Two trials compared group CBT with a wait-list control group. One compared group CBT with a wait list plus a computerized CBT comparison group, and the final study compared group CBT with a computerized CBT comparison group.

Results revealed that older adults with sub-threshold depression in the group CBT condition had a greater reduction in depressive symptoms than did wait-list members. No significant difference in outcomes was found between the group and the computerized CBT. The overall effect size was modest. The authors concluded that group CBT reduces depressive symptomology in older adults with sub-threshold depression and that computerized CBT is as effective as group CBT. They noted that larger effect sizes are difficult to achieve with this population due to the lower levels of depression at baseline.

The effectiveness of CBT for both minor and major depression in older adults was explored by Gould, Coulson, and Howard (2012). Twenty-three studies were included in their meta-analyses, although three of these were follow-up studies. The studies focused on adults 50 years of age and older who had diagnoses of major or minor depression or dysthymia, or who scored in the clinical range on depression measures. Participants could not have a concomitant neurodegenerative, neurological, or severe psychiatric disorder. Each study was a peer-reviewed RCT that contained a control group or compared CBT with either pharmacotherapy or psychotherapy. Ten of the studies employed non-active controls, three used active controls, three used both, and four contained comparison groups. One comparison group received pharmacotherapy. Six studies focused on group, 13 on individual, and one on combined group and individual formats. Participants' mean age was 68.4 yrs.

Study	Inclusion/Exclusion Criteria	Description of Interventions	Number and Description of Participants	Outcomes	Findings
Krishna, Honagodu, et al., 2013 Meta-analysis 4 RCTs	Participants ≥ 50 years. Clinically relevant depressive diagnosis. Treatment occurred in a group setting with at least 3 participants. Excluded studies with dementia, psychosis, primary mental illness or substance abuse disorder.	Two studies compared group CBT with WL. One compared group CBT with WL + a computerized CBT group. Final study compared group CBT with computerized CBT.	Number of participants not specified. Participants in 3 community-based studies: 55 years and older. Participants in 1 nursing home study: 60 years and older.	Group CBT: greater reduction in depressive symptoms than WL. Overall effect size was small. No significant difference between group CBT and computerized CBT.	Group CBT reduces depressive symptoms in older adults with sub-threshold depression. Group CBT does not reduce incidence of major depression. Computerized CBT is as effective as group CBT.
Gould, Coulson, & Howard, 2012 Meta-analysis 23 RCTs (3 were follow-up studies)	Participants ≥ 50 years. Major or minordepression, dysthymia, or depressive symptoms. No concomitant depression, neurodegenerative neurological, or severe psychiatric disorder.	6 group CBT, 13 individual CBT, 1 group + individual CBT. CBT compared to non-active controls, other treatments, or both.	Number of participants not specified. Mean age was 68.4 years.	CBT: significantly greater odds of clinically significant improvement than TAU or WL. No significant differences in efficacybetween CBT and other treatment (pharmacotherapyand other psychotherapies).	CBT for depression in older people is more effective than WL or TAU. Greater efficacy than other treatment has not been demonstrated.
Krishna, Jauhari, et al., 2011 Meta-analysis 18 RCTs	Participants ≥ 55 years. Diagnosis of depression. Excluded those with significant cognitive impairment (< 23 on MMSE) and psychosis.	Group based on CBT compared to WL or other types of therapies (reminiscence, etc.). M # of sessions per treatment: 12.8.	Number of participants not specified. Study participants were recruited from community, nursing home, geriatric hospital. M age range: 66–84.3 years.	Group CBT effective compared to control groups with results maintained at follow-up. No difference between group CBT and other interventions.	Group cognitive behavioral therapy is effective in older adults with depression.

(continued)

TABLE 4.1 (CONTINUED)

Study	Inclusion/ Exclusion Criteria	Description of Interventions	Number and Description of Participants	Outcomes	Findings
Peng, Huang, Chen, & Lu, 2009 Systematic review 14 RTCs	55 years of age or older. Patients with depression. Concomitant physical illness allowable. Dementia and primary psychiatric diagnoses were excluded.	CBT, reminiscence, and general psychotherapy, compared with placebo, WL, antidepressant medication, or another type of psychotherapy.	705 participants; 347 were included in the CBT, reminiscence, and GPT conditions; 360 participated in no intervention, antidepressants alone, placebo, or antidepressants + psychotherapy.	CBT, reminiscence, and general psychotherapy more effective than placebo/WL. No significant difference between CBT and reminiscence.	CBT, reminiscence, and general psychotherapy all effective for depression in older patients.
Pinquart, Duberstein, & Lyness, 2007 Meta-analysis 57 studies	Mean or median age ≥ 60 years. Subjects met criteria for major or minor depression or dysthymia according to ICD-10, DSM-III, IIIR, or IV. Comparison group contained an untreated control condition.	CBT, psycho-education, brief dynamic psychotherapy, exercise, reminiscence, and interpersonal therapy (IPT). 61.7% used a group format; 23.4% focused on inpatients. M # of sessions per treatment:15.2.	Studies included 1,956 treated participants. M age: 71.8 years (5.4); 67% were women and 43.3% were married.	All interventions, except IPT, significantly reduced depression. Effect sizes largest for CBT and reminiscence. CBT, reminiscence, and exercise had small to medium long-term effects. Smaller effect sizes found for those with major depression.	CBT is effective in reducing depressive symptoms in older adults. The effectiveness is not reduced with increasing age. No advantages were found for treatments of longer duration.
Gregory, Canning, Lee, & Wise, 2004 Meta-analysis 29 studies	Age 13 to over 60. Intervention target was depression. Bibliotherapy included some reading and applying the materials on subjects' own time.	Bibliotherapy incorporated CBT materials. M weeks of treatment: 7.4 (3.1).	Number of participants not specified. 9 studies with older individuals; 15 with adults age 25—59, and 5 with adolescents age 13—19. Older adults less depressed at pre-test.	Large effect size for bibliotherapy. No significant difference between group and self-administered bibliotherapy. Much smaller effect size for older adults.	Bibliotherapy is an effective, immediate, and inexpensive treatment for depression. If pre-test depression had been the same across age groups, no probable difference in effect sizes would exist.

WL = wait list; TAU = treatment as usual; MMSE = Mini-Mental Status Exam.

No significant differences in efficacy were found between CBT and any of the other the treatments (psychotherapies or pharmacotherapy). CBT, however, did show significantly greater odds for the remission of, or clinically significant improvement in, older adult depression than did those in the wait-list conditions at the studies' conclusion and also at 6-month follow-up. In sum, CBT was more effective than non-active control conditions for reducing depression in older people. However, greater efficacy than other treatments was not demonstrated.

In 2011, Krishna, Jauhari, Lepping, Turner, Crossley, and Krishnamoorthy completed a meta-analysis of 18 studies that examined the impact of group psychotherapy for depressed older adults. RCTs with participants aged 55 years and older who had been diagnosed with depression and who participated in group therapy, defined as having three or more members, were included. Participants were recruited from the community, nursing homes, and a geriatric hospital. All the group interventions were based on CBT practice principles. Studies having participants with comorbidities and from all treatment settings were allowable. Studies with participants who had significant cognitive impairment (< 23 on MMSE) and psychosis were excluded. No criteria were established for length of treatment or number of group sessions. The group interventions were compared to waiting conditions and/or other psychotherapeutic interventions (reminiscence, problem-solving, etc.). The mean number of sessions for all treatments was 12.8.

There was an overall significant effect of group CBT compared to control group conditions, with this effect maintained at follow-up. The reported benefits of group intervention in comparison to other active interventions, however, did not reach statistical significance. The results of this meta-analysis indicate that group CBT is an effective intervention for depressed older adults in comparison to no treatment and is equally as effective as other psychotherapeutic interventions.

A meta-analysis of 14 RCTs was conducted by Peng, Huang, Chen, and Lu (2009) to assess the effects of psychotherapy on depressed older individuals. CBT, reminiscense, and general pscyhotherapy (GPT) were compared to wait-list, antidepressants, and placebo conditions or to another type of psychotherapy. Studies that included depressed male or female patients 55 years of age and older were selected. Concomitant physical illness was allowable. Primary psychiatric diagnoses and dementia were excluded. Over 700 subjects participated in the 14 studies, with 138 participating in CBT, 109 in reminiscence therapy, and 100 in general psychotherapy. In the non-active control conditions, 260 participants received no intervention or a placebo. In the comparison groups, 51 subjects received antidepressants plus psychotherapy and 49 received antidepressants alone.

Results indicate that CBT, reminiscence, and GPT were all more effective in reducing depression than were the no treatment and placebo conditions. Additionally, there was no significant difference in efficacy between CBT and reminiscence therapy. Study results confirm the efficacy of these three forms of therapy for treating depression in older adults.

Pinquart, Duberstein, and Lyness (2007) studied the effectiveness of CBT and other psychotherapeutic and behavioral interventions on clinically depressed older adults. In their meta-analysis they included studies that contained the following criteria: (1) participants were adults 60 years and older; (2) participants met criteria for major or minor depression or dysthymia according to International Classification of Diseases (ICD-10) or the *Diagnostic and Statistical Manual of Mental Disorders* (DSM-III, IIIR, or IV); and (3) the comparison study contained an untreated control condition. Fifty-seven studies met full criteria for inclusion in the meta-analysis; CBT, psycho-education, brief dynamic psychotherapy, exercise, reminiscence, and interpersonal therapy (IPT) were represented in this study. The majority of the treatments utilized group formats (61.7%), and the average number of sessions per treatment condition was 15.2 (SD = 12.8). In all, the studies included 1,956 treated participants. Nearly one-quarter (23.4%) focused on inpatients. The mean age of the participants was 71.8 (SD = 5.4), 67% were women, and 43.3% were married.

All interventions, except IPT, significantly reduced depressive symptoms. The treatment effect sizes were the largest for CBT and reminiscence therapy. CBT had stronger effects than IPT. CBT, reminiscence, and exercise also had small to medium long-term effects. Smaller effect sizes were found for participants with major depression. Additionally, the analysis indicated that the effect sizes were smaller for patients who had physical and/or cognitive comorbidities, interventions of moderate duration (i.e., 7–19 sessions) had larger effect sizes than did those of briefer or lengthier duration, and significant differences in outcomes by age were not found. The study results suggest that CBT is effective in reducing depressive symptoms in older adults and that therapeutic effectiveness is not reduced with increasing age.

Bibliotherapy based on CBT principles for the treatment of depression was the focus of a meta-analysis conducted by Gregory, Canning, Lee, and Wise (2004). In cognitive bibliotherapy, clients use structured written or computerized materials grounded in CBT to help reduce distress. Materials often include books such as David Burns's *Feeling Good* (1980) and other CBT self-help guides. Clients use the CBT materials either on their own or in a group. To be included in the current meta-analysis, the cognitive bibliotherapies under study had to (1) incorporate some element of participants reading and applying the materials on their own time; (2) focus on depression; (3) encompass both a treatment and a wait-list control group or a single treatment group with pre- and post-test data; and (4) contain participants who were 13 years of age and older. For analysis purposes, three age groups were identified: adolescents (13–19 years), adults (20–59 years), and older adults (60 years and older). Although not required for inclusion in the meta-analysis, the authors noted that "virtually all" (p. 276) of the studies screened clients for psychotic features, suicidal tendencies, drug problems, personality disorders, and serious health problems, and used rigorous diagnostic procedures for depressive disorder. Twenty-nine studies were included in the meta-analysis. Slightly more than half (15) of the studies were conducted in a group format. Nine of the studies contained older adults, 15 focused on adults, and five targeted adolescents.

Results revealed that cognitive bibliotherapy with older adults yielded an average effect size. However, it was significantly smaller than the effect sizes for the adolescent and adult groups. The authors noted, however, that the smaller effect size among older adults was most likely due to the lower levels of depression found among the older adult group at pre-test. The impact of group versus self-administered format was also assessed, and no difference was found in effect sizes by format. The researchers concluded that cognitive bibliotherapy is an effective, inexpensive, and noninvasive route to treatment that contains no threat of stigmatization and may be used alone or to augment other treatments.

ANXIETY

Multiple different diagnoses comprise the spectrum of anxiety disorders observed among older adults, including generalized anxiety disorder (GAD), panic disorder, phobias, OCD, and PTSD. Generalized anxiety disorder and phobias represent the majority of anxiety disorders in older adults, followed by OCD, PTAS, and panic disorder (Lichenberg, 2010). As a result, meta-analytical studies examining the effectiveness of CBT for use with anxious older adults focus on GAD or on GAD and other anxiety disorders (see Table 4.2).

Goncalves and Byrne (2012) conducted a meta-analysis of controlled psychotherapeutic and pharmacological studies for GAD in older adults. Those studies that met the following criteria were included: (1) participants were 55 years of age and older, and the mean or median age was 60 years or older; (2) GAD was the primary diagnosis of study participants; (3) studies had control or comparison groups; and (4) studies were of "established" interventions (pharmacological, psychological, lifestyle) with "sufficient detail to be replicated" (p. 2). Participants were drawn from community, nursing home, and inpatient settings. Fourteen of the studies were of pharmacological and 13 were of psychotherapeutic interventions, with CBT being employed in at least one arm of the latter studies. Separate analyses were conducted for the pharmacological and psychotherapeutic interventions. The average age of the participants was 65–75 years.

Results indicated that both the psychotherapeutic (CBT) and the medication interventions were significantly more effective than the control or wait-list group. Treatment effects were better for psychotherapeutic trials that used a passive control condition (wait-list or minimal contact/care as usual) than for the pharmacological trials that used a placebo condition. No significantly greater treatment effects could be demonstrated for psychotherapeutic trials that used an active control or comparison condition. The authors concluded that both pharmacologic and psychotherapeutic interventions are effective for GAD in older adults and suggested that non-pharmacologic interventions such as CBT may be more beneficial for older, rather than younger, adults.

The application of CBT to reduce pathological worry among those with GAD was explored in 2008 by Covin, Ouimet, Seeds, and Dozois. All study participants had GAD

TABLE 4.2 META-ANALYSES AND SYSTEMATIC REVIEWS: CBT FOR ANXIETY IN OLDER ADULTS

Study	Inclusion/Exclusion Criteria	Description of Interventions	Number and Description of Participants	Outcomes	Findings
Goncalves & Byrne, 2012. Meta-analysis 27 RCTs	Age 55 or older with M or median age ≥ 60 years. GAD primary diagnosis. Established treatments with enough detail to be replicated.	14 pharmacology and 13 psycho-therapy interventions compared to WL, TAU, or active controls (e.g., discussion groups). 12 interventions included a CBT condition.	2,373 baseline participants M # participants per pharmacology condition: 132; M # psychotherapy condition: 40. M age range: 65–75 years. Participants from community, nursing home, and inpatient settings.	Significant results for intervention compared to WL or TAU. No significant difference between psychotherapy and active controls.	Psychotherapeutic/pharmacological interventions yielded significantly greater reduction in GAD symptoms compared to WL and placebo.
Covin, Ouimet, Seeds, & Dozois, 2008. Meta-analysis 10 studies	GAD diagnosis in DSM-III or DSM-IV. Studies using PSWQ as an outcome measure. CBT defined as having both cognitive and behavioral components.	Some studies used group format and some used individual format. Seven studies contained control groups: WL, no treatment, or nonspecific treatment (e.g., supportive therapy). M # of sessions (CBT): 13.5.	Number of participants not specified/ M age: 50.8 years. 72.06% female. Younger participants M age: 38.9 years; M age of older subjects: 68.1 years. M duration of GAD: 19.5 years.	Large effect size for CBT compared to control group. Pathological worry was greatly reduced for both age groups. Younger adults responded more favorably to CBT at post-treatment relative to older adults.	CBT for GAD is highly effective in reducing pathological worry for both younger and older adults. Greater use of group formats for treatment of GAD in older adults may explain superior results in younger subjects.
Gould, Coulson, & Howard, 2012. Meta-analysis 12 RCTs	Age 55 or older (mean age 68.2). Panic disorder, GAD, agoraphobia, phobia, PTSD, OCD, or anxiety disorder not otherwise specified. CBT lasting longer than 2 session as at least one of the "treatment arms" of the individual study.	9 individual and 3 group CBT formats. M # of sessions: 12.6 studies had concurrent pharmacotherapy (or combination); 6 studies had WL or minimal contact TAU conditions.	Number of participants not specified. M age: 68.2 years. M years education: 14.2 Most common diagnosis: GAD. M % comorbid psychiatric diagnosis: 41.5%.	CBT significantly and modestly more effective at reducing anxiety and depression symptoms than TAU or WL. At 6-month (but not 3- or 12-month) follow-up, CBT was significantly more effective at reducing anxiety symptoms than an active control.	CBT treatment is effective at reducing anxiety disorders in older adults. CBT aimed at alleviating anxiety can also be beneficial in reducing depression.

Study	Inclusion criteria	Focus	Participants	Results	Conclusions
Thorpe et al., 2008 Meta-analysis 19 RCTs	Psychotherapeutic intervention for anxiety disorders/symptoms; M age: 65 or older, no younger than 55 years. Include at least 5 subjects. Treatment length at least 2 sessions. Sufficient data for calculating effect sizes.	CBT alone, CBT with relaxation training, relaxation training alone. 15 studies included non-active or active control. 11 studies focused on individuals and 8 on group intervention.	Number of participants not specified. M age range of participants: 63.2–73 years. Participants in 8 studies suffered from GAD, 5 from mixed anxiety disorders, and 1 from panic disorder. Subjects in 5 studies complained of anxiety symptoms.	CBT, CBT-RT, and RT alone reduced anxiety and depression. Only CBT-RT was more effective than active control at reducing anxiety. Only CBT-RT was more effective than non-active controls in reducing depression.	CBT is effective for older adults with anxiety disorders and symptoms. CBT augmented with relaxation therapy achieved best results.
Hendriks, Oude Voshaar, Keijsers, Hoogduin, & van Balkom, 2008 Meta-analysis 9 RCTs	M age: ≥ 60 years. Diagnosis of GAD, panic disorder, social phobia, or agoraphobia according to the ICD-9, ICD-10, DSM-III, DSM-IIIR, or DSM-IV. Inclusion of treatment arm with CBT.	Use of CBT in late-life anxiety disorders. CBT compared to WL or active control (any treatment that provided contact frequency comparable with the CBT condition).	Total of 297 participants: 114 subjects in CBT / WL,73% female. M age: 68 years. 183 subjects in CBT vs. active control. 77% female. M age: 69 years.	CBT was more effective in reducing level of anxiety than either non-active or active controls. CBT was more effective in reducing depression than active controls and more effective in reducing worry than non-active controls.	CBT is highly efficacious in treating anxiety disorders in later life. CBT is also effective in treating the concurrent symptoms of worry and depression.
Pinquart & Duberstein, 2007 Comparative meta-analysis 32 studies	Mean or median age: ≥ 60 years. ICD-10 or DSM-III, III-R, or IV criteria for GAD, phobic disorders, panic disorder, OCD, PTSD, mixed anxiety and depression, other anxiety disorders.	19 pharmaco-therapy and 12 behavioral interventions (CBT, counseling, social support, exercise); 1 investigated both. M duration: 11 weeks; 27 studies involved outpatients, 5 involved inpatients.	2,484 total subjects: 69.8% female; 53% were married. Average length of illness: 19.1 years. M age: 69.4 years	Psychopharmacology and behavioral interventions did not differ in outcomes on anxiety and depression. CBT was more effective than other behavioral treatments; SSRIs more effective than behavioral approaches. Studies with older participants had higher effect size.	Pharmacotherapy and behavioral interventions are reasonably effective. Pharmacotherapy may be the first choice of treatment as long as medical conditions and patients' preferences do not preclude this form of treatment; pharmacotherapy CBT would be a satisfactory alternative.

GAD = generalized anxiety disorder; RT = relaxation therapy; PSWQ = Penn Sate Worry Questionnaire; WL = wait list; TAU = treatment as usual.

as diagnosed using DSM-III or DSM-IV criteria. Only studies using the Penn State Worry Questionnaire (Meyer, Miller, Metzger, & Borkovec, 1990) as an outcome measure and CBT interventions containing both cognitive and behavioral components were included. Ten trials were employed, seven of which contained control groups. Some studies used group formats, while others involved individual sessions. Almost two-thirds (72.1%) of the participants were female. Study members were divided into two age groups: younger (M = 38.9 years) and older (M = 68.1 years) adults.

Both groups experienced greatly reduced pathological worry following treatment, with worry falling from the clinical into the normal range at post-treatment. This gain remained at both 6- and 12-month follow-ups. Further analysis revealed that age modified participants' response to CBT, with younger adults responding more favorably. In their discussion the authors noted that CBT was very effective for reducing pathological worry among both younger and older adults, and proposed the more frequent use of group, rather than individual, formats with older adults as a possible reason for the greater improvement displayed by younger clients.

Researchers have also investigated the effectiveness of CBT to treat a wider range of anxiety disorders among older adults. Gould, Coulson, and Howard (2012), for example, conducted a meta-analysis in which participants had a diagnosis of panic disorder, GAD, agoraphobia, phobia, PTSD, OCD, or anxiety disorder not otherwise specified. They included those studies which were peer-reviewed RCTs that contained active or non-active controls, had a treatment arm that consisted of CBT lasting longer than two sessions, had at least five participants in each condition, utilized evidence-based anxiety measures, and focused on adults 55 years of age and older. Twelve studies were included in the meta-analysis. Nine utilized individual formats. Six of the studies contained an active control condition (pharmacotherapy) while six studies had a wait list or minimal contact condition. The average participant was 68.2 years old and had 14.2 years of education. The most common anxiety disorder was GAD, while 41.5% had a comorbid psychiatric disorder. Older adults participated in a mean 12 CBT sessions, most of which were delivered in an individual format.

As previously found, the CBT condition was significantly more effective in reducing anxiety than was the non-active control condition, with a moderate effect size favoring CBT. There was a small effect size that approached significance (p = .06) in favor of CBT over active controls. Small to moderate effect sizes in favor of CBT were also found at 3-, 6-, and 12-month follow-ups, although these were not always significant. The researchers also tested the impact of CBT on depression among older adults in these studies. A significant, but modest, reduction in depression post-treatment was found compared to wait-list and treatment as usual conditions. These results suggest that CBT interventions aimed at relieving anxiety in older adults may also serve to assuage depressive symptoms.

Thorpe, Ayers, Nuevo, Stoddard, Sorrell, and Wetherell (2008) also conducted meta-analyses to examine the benefits of CBT for a range of late-life anxiety disorders. The following inclusionary criteria were employed: (1) psychotherapeutic intervention for anxiety disorders/symptoms; (2) mean age 65 or older, with no participant younger than 55 years; (3) subjects reported, at least, subjective anxiety symptoms; (4) at least five subjects were included in the study; (5) treatment length at was least two sessions; (6) sufficient data existed for calculating effect sizes; and (7) established anxiety or depression measures were used. The researchers compared effect sizes from 19 studies. Fifteen of the studies included non-active or active control (e.g., supportive counseling, group discussion, psycho-education) conditions. The interventions tested in these studies included CBT alone, CBT with relaxation training (CBT-RT), and relaxation training (RT). Eight studies focused on older individuals with GAD, five on those with mixed anxiety disorders (predominantly GAD and panic disorder), five on subjects who complained of anxiety symptoms, and one on older adults with a primary diagnosis of panic disorder. The mean ages of study participants ranged from 63.2 years to 73 years of age.

Results indicated that CBT, CBT-RT, and RT had large effect sizes and were more effective in reducing anxiety symptoms than were the wait-list conditions. Only CBT-RT was statistically more beneficial than the active controls in reducing anxiety. When examining depression only the CBT-RT treatment exhibited significantly larger effect sizes than the wait-list condition. The researchers concluded that compared to active controls, CBT, CBT-RT, and RT had relatively large effect size for depression and an even larger effect size for anxiety.

The effectiveness of CBT for use with late-life anxiety disorders was also examined by Hendriks, Oude Voshaar, Keijsers, Hoogduin, and van Balkom (2008). Nine RCTs with participants 60 years of age and older who had a diagnosis of GAD, panic disorder, social phobia, or agoraphobia according to the ICD-9, ICD-10, DSM-III, DSM-IIIR, or DSM-IV were included. The inclusion of a treatment arm with CBT was required. Open trials, case series, and case reports were excluded. A total of 297 older adults engaged in the studies. The CBT versus active control condition contained 183 participants, 77% of whom were females with a mean age of 69 years. Somewhat fewer (114) participated in the CBT versus wait-list conditions. Of these, 73% were female and the mean age was 68 years. Five of the nine studies featured group therapy treatments. The number of sessions for all treatment ranged from eight to 15. The primary outcome variable was level of anxiety, while worry and depressive symptoms were secondary outcome variables.

Study results indicate that CBT was significantly more efficacious in reducing anxiety levels than were non-active and active control conditions. CBT yielded superior results in decreasing worry and depression than did the wait-list condition. In addition, CBT demonstrated significantly greater effects in depression reduction than did the active control conditions. In sum, CBT was found to be effective in reducing anxiety, worry, and depression among older adults with a DSM-IV diagnosed anxiety disorder. The authors note that due to the side effects of pharmacological interventions, especially benzodiazepines and antidepressives in older adults, psychotherapeutic treatments such as CBT may be considered the treatment of choice when working with anxious older adults.

Finally, Pinquart and Duberstein (2007) compared the use of behavioral and pharmacological interventions to treat anxiety disorders among older adults. Participants in the studies had a mean or median age of 60 years or older and either met the ICD-10 or DSM-III, III-R, or IV criteria for GAD, phobic disorders, panic disorder, OCD, PTSD, mixed anxiety and depression, or other anxiety disorders, or scored 18 or above on the Hamilton Rating Scale for Anxiety (HAMA) with symptom duration lasting more than 6 months. Uncontrolled studies were eligible for inclusion. Thirty-two studies were included in the meta-analysis, 19 of which investigated pharmacological treatment, 12 assessed behavioral interventions, and one contained both types of interventions. The majority of behavioral interventions were CBT in nature. Eighty-four percent of the studies focused on outpatients, while the remainder targeted inpatients. Participants' mean age was 69.4 years, two-thirds were women, and slightly over half were married.

Initial results indicated no significant difference between pharmacological and behavioral interventions in the reduction of anxiety or depression symptoms. The researchers then compared the impact of specific medication classes and different behavioral interventions on the reduction of anxiety symptoms. Selective serotonin reuptake inhibitors (SSRIs) were superior to CBT and the other behavioral interventions, while benzodiazepines were more effective than the other behavioral interventions but not CBT. Larger effect sizes were found in studies with older participants. The authors note that the findings suggest that pharmacological interventions are more effective than behavioral treatments in reducing late-life anxiety, and that the statistical superiority of CBT over other types of behavioral interventions was not supported.

INSOMNIA

Primary insomnia and other sleep disorders are common among older individuals, with 36%–50% reporting sleep difficulties. The gravity of this issue is highlighted by research linking difficulty sleeping to increased morbidity and mortality (Hidalgo, Bravo, Martínez, Pretel, Lapeira, & Gras, 2012; Neikrug & Ancoli-Israel, 2010). CBT for insomnia (CBT-I) came into use in the 1980s. However, it was not until two decades later, when treatment for comorbid insomnia (i.e., insomnia related to a medical illness) became more prevalent, that studies began to focus on the efficacy of CBI-I for use with older adults. Core components of CBT-I include cognitive strategies and behavioral techniques including sleep restriction (following a strict sleep schedule), stimulus control (using the bed only for sleeping or sex), sleep hygiene (creating conditions for optimal sleep environment), and relaxation training (Rybarczyk, Lund, Garroway, & Mack, 2013). Multiple randomized control trials have been conducted to examine the effectiveness of CBT for insomnia. However, only two meta-analyses and one systematic review have been conducted that include older adults (see Table 4.3).

Okajima, Komada, and Inoue (2011) completed a meta-analysis on the use of CBT-I for primary insomnia in Japan. Included studies were RCTs that focused on primary

Study	Inclusion / Exclusion Criteria	Description of Interventions	Number and Description of Participants	Outcomes	Findings
Okajima, Komada, & Inoue, 2011 Meta-analysis 14 RCTs	Interventions for the treatment of primary insomnia. CBT-I that included cognitive and multiple behavioral strategies.	Treatment conditions: used multi-component CBT-I; 9 individual and 5 group formats. Control conditions: 6 placebo, 5 WL, 1 TAU, and 2 education groups.	Number of participants not specified. Overall *M* age range: 38–71.4 years. Subjects in 8 studies had *M* age ≥ 50 years.	Effect sizes for CBT-I ranged from medium to large, except TST, which had a small effect size. Effect sizes for CBT-I compared to control groups also had medium to large effect sizes except for TST.	CBT-I is effective for treating primary insomnia at end of treatment and at follow-up.
Montgomery & Dennis, 2009 Systematic review 6 RCTs	At least 80% of subjects ≥ 60 years. Diagnosed with a sleep problem via a standardized measure. Excluded depression, sleep apnea, dementia, and secondary insomnia.	All forms of CBT (sleep hygiene, stimulus control, muscle relaxation, sleep restriction, and cognitive therapy). Control groups included no treatment, WL, sleep medication, and placebo.	282 participants, with 224 used in the review.	All gains were mild to modest at post-test. At 3-month and 1-year follow-ups, some gains were maintained.	CBT for older adults with insomnia is modestly effective. Some results erode over time.
Irwin, Cole, & Nicassio 2006 Meta-analysis 23 RCTs	Primary diagnosis of insomnia. At least one arm was CBT or recognized variant.	*M* age ≥ 55 years: 15 studies. *M* age < 55 years: 8 studies. 3 types of CBT: CMT-I, relaxation-based, and behavioral only.	Number of participants not specified. No participant information provided.	Most sleep outcomes similar for all 3 treatment groups, yielding medium effect sizes. CBT more effective than relaxation for sleep efficiency.	CBT is effective for treatment of chronic insomnia. Similar results for middle age and older adults for most sleep outcomes.

CBT-I = CBT for insomnia; TST = total sleep time; WL = wait list; TAU = treatment as ususal.

insomnia and utilized CBT-I that incorporated not only cognitive but also multiple behavior techniques. Fourteen studies met the inclusionary criteria. Nine of the CBT-I treatments were individual in format, while the remaining five were group designs. The control group consisted of both active and non-active control, six placebo, five wait-list, two educational, and one treatment as usual conditions. The mean age of participants in eight of the 14 trials was 50 years of age or older, while the mean age of those in the remaining studies ranged from 38 to 49 years. The following outcomes were examined: (1) sleep onset latency (SOL); (2) total sleep time (TST); (3) total wake time (TWT); (4) wake time after sleep onset (WASO); (5) early morning awakening (EMA); (6) time in bed (TIB); (7) sleep efficiency (SE); and (8) changes in objective sleep measures.

Initially, the authors examined just the impact of CBT-I, and then compared the effectiveness of CBT-I with the control group, on the outcomes listed in the preceding paragraph. Among the CBT-I trials, the mean effect sizes for SOL, TWT, WASO, EMA, TIB, and SE ranged from medium to large. All effect sizes, except for TIB, were maintained at follow-up. Comparison of CBT-I and the control conditions indicated that the effect sizes for CBT-I were significantly larger than those for both active and non-active control groups for SOL, TWT, WASO, EMA, TIB, and SE. These results were sustained at the 12-month follow-up for SOL. WASO and SE and point to the immediate and long-term effectiveness of CBT-I on reducing multiple indicators of chronic insomnia. While the authors did not analyze the results by age, the fact that the majority of trials included in this study focused on older adults suggests CBT-I treatment efficacy with the older population.

In 2009, Montgomery and Dennis conducted a systematic review of CBT interventions for older adults with sleep problems. Studies targeting a broad range of CBT interventions were accepted for their study, including those that consisted of sleep hygiene, stimulus control, relaxation therapy, and/or sleep restriction therapy. All of the studies contained in the review were RTCs. At least 80% of all study participants were 60 years of age or older and had been diagnosed with sleep problems as measured with a standardized scale. Studies that did not specifically screen out those with dementia and/or depression were excluded, as were studies that contained participants with sleep apnea and comorbid medical illnesses. Six studies containing 224 participants were included in the review. Only two studies incorporated cognitive strategies as part of the interventions employed. Sleep latency, WASO, TWT, sleep duration, early morning waking (EMW), and sleep efficiency were the six outcome variables examined by the authors.

The effect estimates for sleep efficacy, efficiency, WASO, and EMW were modest. However, for those studies where TWT, sleep latency, and duration were examined, effects were very mild but significant. Treatment effects were not consistently maintained across outcomes or studies. While this review is informative, the majority of the studies did not contain an intervention that employed cognitive techniques, and no comparison was made between the outcomes of the behavioral-only treatments and those employing both cognitive and behavioral strategies.

A meta-analysis conducted by Irwin, Cole, and Nicassio (2006) specifically compared the effectiveness of behavioral intervention trials for use with middle-aged and older adults. Inclusionary criteria consisted of (1) diagnosis of primary insomnia; (2) use of some form of CBT in one arm of the study (variants such as CBT-I, relaxation, sleep restriction, stimulus control, and biofeedback were accepted); and (3) contained at least one of five sleep outcomes: sleep quality, sleep latency, TST, SE, and WASO. Twenty-three trials met the required criteria, 15 of which focused on middle aged (mean age < 55 years), while eight targeted older adults (mean age ≥ 55 years). The interventions were broadly divided into three categories: CBT-I, behavioral interventions, and relaxation therapy.

Results indicate that all three treatments categories were effective in improving all outcomes, excluding TST. The only difference found among treatments was significantly enhanced sleep effectiveness for those who participated in CBT, compared to those in the relaxation therapy group. When comparing treatment outcomes by age, the findings revealed equivalent improvements in sleep quality, latency, and WASO. However, middle-aged adults experienced significantly greater increases in TST and sleep efficiency.

CONCLUSION

This review confirms the efficacy of CBT for use with older adults. Many individual studies suggest the usefulness of CBT across a wide range of late-life disorders. Nonetheless, a solid body of evidence, as established by meta-analyses, demonstrates that CBT effectively reduces symptoms of depression, anxiety, and insomnia in older individuals.

For decreasing depression, all studies found that CBT was an efficacious treatment and resulted in decreased symptomatology when compared to non-active control conditions. All studies also found that CBT was as beneficial as other types of treatments, whether they be psychotherapeutic or pharmacological in nature. It should be noted, however, that just one meta-analysis compared medication trials with CBT interventions. CBT in multiple formats—individual, group, computerized, and bibliotherapy—and in both community and nursing home settings was found to be efficacious in reducing depression among older adults. Only one study reported that CBT was superior to other psychotherapeutic interventions, specifically interpersonal therapy. Results from these studies cannot be generalized to all older adults. All studies, save one, explicitly excluded trials that contained older adults with dementia, psychosis, substance abuse, severe mental illness, and/or a primary medical illness. Therefore, based on the findings of these meta-analyses, one can state with reasonable certitude that CBT is an effective intervention for alleviating non-comorbid depression among older adults. However, its superiority over other psychotherapeutic interventions has not been effectively demonstrated.

Studies further reveal that CBT is as effective as, but not always superior to, other psychotherapeutic interventions for the treatment of depression and insomnia in older adults. The research findings cited in the preceding, however, do indicate that CBT performs better than other psychotherapeutic interventions in decreasing the negative impacts of anxiety in older populations. Findings from this review also support claims concerning the flexibility of CBT. CBT interventions with demonstrated effectiveness include those that are offered in individual and group formats, are conducted in a variety of treatment settings, and employ both face-to-face and computerized designs.

Similarly, results of meta-analyses indicate that CBT is an effective treatment for reducing anxiety in older adults. Results from all studies suggest that CBT is more beneficial than non-active wait-list conditions in alleviating symptoms of GAD and other anxiety disorders. In addition, results from these meta-analyses suggest that CBT for anxiety is also effective in reducing related chronic worry and depression in older adults. Several studies also found that CBT performed better than active control conditions in decreasing the negative impacts of anxiety on older populations. Only two studies compared CBT with pharmacological interventions. While one found no significant difference between the two, the other compared the impact of specific medications with CBT and revealed that SSRIs had superior results, while CBT performed more effectively than did benzodiazepines. The choice of CBT or a pharmacological agent in the treatment of late-life anxiety may hinge on the older individual's personal preference and ability to tolerate medication side effects.

Unlike the research on depression and anxiety, there are limited reviews related to insomnia. Only two meta-analyses, thus far, have examined the benefits of CBT for use with older adults with this disorder. Interestingly, while the majority of older individuals experience insomnia related to some comorbid medical illness, all three studies focused on the benefits of CBT to treat primary insomnia in this population. All three studies examined the impact of CBT on multiple sleep outcomes. Results indicate that CBT is effective in improving sleep latency, TWT, WASO, EMA, TIB, and SE, and that mild to large effect sizes were found when CBT was applied to these conditions. CBT was found to have greater efficacy than non-active control conditions and greater efficacy than relaxation therapy, in at least one meta-analysis. Comparisons of the benefits of CBT for older and middle-aged adults revealed similar outcomes for sleep quality, latency, and WASO, and more beneficial outcomes in TST and efficacy for the middle-aged. It must be noted that not all of the studies specifically focused on CBT-I. Rather, they often included a wide variation of CBT interventions. Additional research on the effectiveness of CBT-I for use with older adults is warranted.

While these data consistently affirm the benefits of CBT for the treatment of older adult depression, anxiety, and insomnia, limitations exist on the conclusions that may be drawn from this research. The majority of studies have been conducted in outpatient settings, or in mixed settings, without disaggregating results by environment type. Therefore, it is not possible to determine if CBT performs equally well in community-based, inpatient, and nursing homes settings. The majority of studies exclude those with cognitive impairment and comorbid psychological and medical disorders. None of the studies examined outcomes by race, gender, or socioeconomic status (SES), and none contained information concerning the racial or SES composition of participants. Thus, while considerable research has been conducted concerning the effectiveness of CBT for use with older adults, these limitations seriously constrain the generalizability of the findings. Additionally, only one study investigated outcomes by age. This study found no difference in intervention outcomes with advancing age. However, most of the studies defined older adults as those 50 years of age and older, and the mean age of participants tended to be in the lower range of the older adult population.

As the number of adults who join the ranks of the oldest-old continues to grow, additional studies that explore the benefits of CBT with the over 80 age group are needed. Also necessary are additional RCTs that examine the efficacy of CBT for older adults with a wider range of disorders, such as alcohol and medication misuse, OCD, and pain. To reliably establish the promise of CBT for the growing population of older adults, further research addressing these questions is essential.

REFERENCES

Burns, D. D. (1980). *Feeling good.* New York: Avon.

Covin, R., Ouimet, A. J., Seeds, P. M., & Dozois, D. J. A. (2008). A meta-analysis of CBT for pathological worry among clients with GAD. *Journal of Anxiety Disorder, 22,* 108–116.

Goncalves, D. C., & Byrne, G. J. (2012). Interventions for generalized anxiety disorders in older adults: systematic review and meta-analysis. *Journal of Anxiety Disorder, 26,* 1–11.

Gould, R. L., M. C. Coulson, Howard, R. J. (2012). Efficacy of cognitive behavioral therapy for anxiety disorders in older people: a meta-analysis and meta-regression of randomized controlled trials. *Journal of the American Geriatrics Society, 60,* 218–229.

Gregory, R. J., Canning, S. S., Lee, T. W., & Wise, J. C. (2004). Cognitive bibliotherapy for depression: a meta-analysis. *Professional Psychology: Research and Practice, 35,* 275–280.

Hendriks, G J., Oude Voshaar R. C., Keijsers, G. P. J., Hoogduin, C. A. L., & van Balkom, A. J. L. M. (2008). Cognitive-behavioural therapy for late-life disorders: a systematic review and meta-analysis. *Acta Psychiatrica Scandinavica, 117,* 403–411.

López-Torres Hidalgo, J., Bravo, B. N., Martínez, I. P., Pretel, F. A., Lapeira, J. T., & Gras, C. B. (2012). Understanding insomnia in older adults. *International Journal of Geriatric Psychiatry, 27,* 1086–1093.

INSERM Collective Expertise Centre. (2004). INSERM Collective Expert Reports [Internet]. *Psychotherapy: three approaches evaluated.* Paris: Institut national de la santé et de la recherche médicale. Retrieved August 21, 2015 from http://www.ncbi.nlm.nih.gov/books/NBK7123/.

Irwin, M. R., Cole, J. C., & Nicassio, P. M. (2006). Comparative meta-analysis of behavioral interventions for insomnia and their effectiveness in middle-aged and older adults 55+ years of age. *Health Psychology, 25,* 3–14.

Krishna, M., Honagodu, A., Rajendra, R., Sundarachar, R., Lane, S., & Lepping, P. (2013). A systematic review and met-analysis of group psychotherapy for sub-clinical depression in older adults. *International Journal of Geriatric Psychiatry, 28,* 881–888.

Krishna, M., Jauhari, A., Lepping, P., Turner, J., Crossley, D., & Krishnamoorthy, A. (2011). Is group psychotherapy effective in older adults with depression: a systematic review. *International Journal of Geriatric Psychiatry, 26*, 331–340.

Lichtenberg, P. A. (2010). *Handbook of assessment in clinical gerontology* (2nd ed.). Boston: Academic Press.

Meyer, T. J., Miller, M. L., Metzger, R. L., & Borkovec, T. D. (1990). Development and validation of the Penn State Worry Questionnaire. *Behaviour Research and Therapy, 28*, 487–495.

Montgomery, P., & Dennis, J. A. (2009). Cognitive behavioral interventions for sleep problems in adults 60+ (Review). *The Cochran Collaboration.* Hoboken, NJ: John Wiley & Sons.

Neikrug, A. B., & Ancoli-Israel, S. (2010). Sleep disorders in the older adult: a mini-review. *Gerontology, 56*, 181–189.

Okajima, I., Komada, Y., & Inoue, Y. (2011). A meta-analysis on the treatment effectiveness of cognitive behavioral therapy for primary insomnia. *Sleep and Biological Rhythms, 9*, 24–34

Peng, X. D., Haung, C. Q., Chen, L. J., & Lu, Z. C. (2009). Cognitive behavioral therapy ad reminiscence techniques for the treatment of depression in the elderly: a systematic review. *The Journal of International Medical Research, 37*, 975–982.

Pinquart, M., Duberstein, P. R., & Lyness, J. M. (2007). Effects of psychotherapy and other behavioral interventions on clinically depressed older adults: a meta-analysis. *Aging & Mental Health, 11*(6), 645–657.

Rybarczyk, B., Lund, H. G., Garroway, A. M., & Mack, L. (2013). Cognitive behavioral therapy for insomnia in older adults: background, evidence, and overview of treatment protocol. *Clinical Gerontologist, 36*, 70–96.

Steinman, L. E., Frederick, J. T., Prohaska, T., Satariano, W. A., Dronberg-Lee, S., Fisher, R., . . . Snowden, M. (2007). Recommendations for treating depression in community-based older adults. *American Journal of Preventive Medicine, 33*, 175–181.

Thorpe, S. R., Ayers, C. R., Nuevo, R., Stoddard, J. A., Sorrell, J. T., & Wetherell, J. L. (2008). Meta-analysis comparing different behavioral treatments for late-life anxiety. *American Journal of Geriatric Psychiatry, 17*, 105–115.

5

PROBLEM-SOLVING THERAPY
THEORY AND PRACTICE

Problem-solving therapy (PST) is a psychological intervention that teaches people to cope with the stress of "here-and-now" problems to reduce negative health and mental health outcomes. Within this perspective, a person's problem-solving ability is understood as a moderator of the relationship between challenges and emotional stress responses. Therefore, effective problem-solving skills are thought to mitigate the probability of experiencing negative health and mental health outcomes when confronted with difficult and challenging events (Gellis et al., 2008).

In PST, clients are trained to overcome major obstacles that inhibit effective coping and heighten stress by means of effective problem identification, generation of solutions, solution implementation, and post-implementation evaluation. The goal of PST is not to solve all of the client's problems, but rather to teach the client to effectively engage in problem resolution (Hegel & Areán, 2012). Effective problem-solving involves the ability to develop adaptively and to match solutions to life problems while taking into account the specific internal and external factors that are present (Nezu et al., 2013).

One area in which older clients benefit from PST is modifying behaviors that are creating poor health outcomes. For instance, Mrs. Thompson's physician warned her about her need to lose weight, as she suffers from debilitating back pain from a severe automobile accident that took place a few years ago. Mrs. Thompson, a 68-year-old woman, has been unsuccessful at losing the 40 pounds that the doctor recommends. She reports that she is stressed and depressed by her inability to control her weight.

In working with a therapist who used a problem-solving approach, several factors were revealed about her current situation. Her husband did not survive the accident, and being a widow altered her life in many ways. She does not like to cook for herself, so she frequently eats at fast food restaurants. Further exploration revealed that she was unsure of what her nutrition consumption goals should be and had a very limited knowledge about nutrition. Because she was in constant pain, she no longer exercised, which added to the weight problem.

Together, she and the therapist devised a plan to deal with these two major issues of her weight gain. She made specific decisions about her dietary habits, including eating out less and choosing different restaurants that offered healthier selections. In addition, she joined a low-impact exercise class at her local YMCA. While this helped her activity level, the class also provided a place for her to meet others and gain support in her weight-loss goals.

HISTORY AND BACKGROUND

Problem-solving was originally conceptualized as a means of improving social competence and psychological adjustment (D'Zurilla, 1984). PST falls under the cognitive-behavioral umbrella of therapeutic treatments. This intervention approach is a general problem-solving model for stress reduction, in which clients are taught skills to enhance coping abilities (D'Zurilla & Nezu, 1999; Nezu, Nezu, & D'Zurilla, 2013).

PST is rooted in the early work of Thomas D'Zurilla and Marvin Goldfried (1971), who were the first researchers to publish an article dealing with problem-solving in a therapeutic context. Titled "Problem Solving and Behavior Modification," their seminal article was a "comprehensive review of the relevant theory and research related to real-life problem solving" (Nezu et al., 2013, p. 6). While the concepts of problem-solving and behaviorist approaches existed prior to this early article, these researchers were the first to thoughtfully consider combining problem-solving and behavior modification into an actual therapeutic intervention.

A number of factors were influential in the emergence of PST as an important therapeutic modality. First, PST is generally considered a type of cognitive behavioral therapy (CBT), in that both approaches look at maladaptive and ineffective coping behaviors and their corresponding negative social and psychological consequences (D'Zurilla & Goldfried, 1971; D'Zurilla & Nezu, 2010). Against this backdrop, the development and swift expansion of CBT aided PST in gaining a foothold as a unique therapy. A second influential factor was the emergence of interest in nurturing creativity and promoting problem-solving ability, which gave rise to the social competence approach to therapy. As opposed to the extant medical model of mental health, emerging therapies rooted in the social competence approach focused less on pathologizing those receiving therapy, and more on developing their coping and problem-solving skills (D'Zurilla & Nezu, 1999). While still incorporating theoretical aspects of social problem-solving and stress, the social competence approach centered on problem-solving, self-control, decision-making, and overall social competence in practical, real-world settings.

THEORETICAL FOUNDATION

PST developed as a form of therapy that viewed clients in a positive, strengths-based light. The *process* of solving a given problem was seen as having greater import than the problem itself. This idea was influenced by Lazarus's transactional/relational model of stress, which viewed stress in terms of one's coping abilities (cf., Lazarus & Folkman, 1984). The influence of the transactional/relational model of stress is apparent in PST, as the greatest consideration in therapy is how a person solves problems and responds to stress (D'Zurilla & Nezu, 1999). While PST is now used to address multiple problematic issues, utility in treating depression continues to be one of its best-known and supported applications (Nezu et al., 2013).

D'Zurilla and Goldfried described the foundational concepts of PST as defining the problem, problem-solving, and implementing a solution. A *problem* is defined as any life situation that requires an adaptive coping response for which no solution is readily identifiable due to the presence of barriers (D'Zurilla & Nezu, 1999; Hegel & Areán, 2012). As defined, a problem may occur in an individual's social environment, external environment, or in both. Problems may also stem from internal issues (e.g., fear of confronting tension in a relationship with a daughter because of the need to rely on her for assistance). Problems commonly occur in the following situations: (1) a new or novel situation (e.g., moving from home to an assisted living facility); (2) an ambiguous circumstance (e.g., not knowing whether a child will be able to help with caregiving responsibilities); (3) lack of control (e.g., loss of a driver's license); (4) conflicting goals (e.g., wanting to be independent and wanting to be safe); (5) personal skill deficits (e.g., not knowing how to manage money following the death of a spouse); and (6) insufficient resources (e.g., not having enough funds to pay for in-home care for a spouse with dementia).

Problem-solving is the cognitive-behavioral process used by an individual to identify, develop, and implement effective solutions in response to problems in everyday life (D'Zurilla & Nezu, 1999; Hegel & Areán, 2012). In PST, problem-solving is often referred to as "social problem-solving." The term "social" does not refer to solving difficulties in interpersonal relations, but rather to solving problems that occur within the individual's social environment. Social problem-solving can be understood as both a skill-based application and a learning process. In PST, a client learns the cognitive and behavioral skills, and the specific techniques needed, to solve a particular problem. Moreover, each time a client successfully solves a problem, her problem-solving abilities and self-confidence increase. As a result, she is more likely to apply the problem-solving skills to new situations and experience continued growth in skill development. For example, Mrs. Goldberg had always relied on her husband to initiate social situations for the couple. Following her husband's death, she was anxious and hesitant about reaching out to others on her own. She decided to attend a luncheon at her temple, but was fearful about walking in by herself. She managed anticipatory anxiety by engaging in deep breathing exercises. In addition, she offered to drive a friend to the luncheon so she would not have to walk in on her own. After successfully participating in this outing, she is more likely to use these skills and techniques to engage in future social gatherings.

In PST, an effective *solution* is one that achieves the individual's goal in relationship to the identified problem. This process involves the implementation of effective coping responses (cognitive and/or behavioral) while maximizing benefits and minimizing negative consequences to oneself and others. As exemplified in the vignette of Mrs. Goldberg, a solution may consist of behavioral skills, cognitive skills, or a combination of the two. While minor problems may involve the application of one strategy, more complex problems require the implementation of multiple skills and tactics (Nezu et al., 2013).

PRACTICE APPROACHES AND APPLICATION

Multiple methodologies are used within PST. Clients are taught problem-solving skills through verbal instruction, written materials, participating in exercises, and completing assigned homework. The Socratic method is also employed to elicit ideas and suggestions for problem solutions from the clients. To be clear, PST therapists *do not* provide solutions. Instead, they engage in discussions and formulate questions that encourage clients to come to their own conclusions (D'Zurilla & Nezu, 1999).

Two overarching treatment goals exist for those involved in PST. First is the acquisition of a positive orientation toward problems that arise in one's life. Second is development of the ability to effectively employ specific problem-solving behaviors (Nezu et al., 2013).

PROBLEM ORIENTATION

The nature of one's problem orientation strongly influences the degree to which one is able to effectively tackle life problems. Problem orientation is defined as the "set of relatively stable cognitive-affective schemas that represent a person's generalized beliefs, attitudes, and emotional reactions about problems in living and one's ability to successfully cope with such problems" (Nezu et al., 2013, p. 11). While earlier iterations of PST acknowledged the importance of problem orientations, there was a greater focus on training clients in practical problem-solving skills. More recent approaches, however, give equal consideration to both problem orientation and problem-solving style.

Problem orientations are categorized as either positive or maladaptive approaches. A positive or adaptive orientation yields a greater probability for reaching a successful resolution to problems. Those with a positive orientation are more likely to demonstrate competence as they confront problematic situations in their lives, develop realistic solutions, persist in solution implementation in spite of difficulties, and as a result, successfully resolve stressful life issues. Characteristics of a positive orientation are (1) the willingness to recognize a problem, rather than responding with denial or avoidance;

(2) the aptitude to see a problem as a challenge, rather than a threat; (3) the ability to correctly identify the causes of a problem, rather than attributing problems to either a personal defect or features outside of oneself; (4) the capacity to view negative emotional reactions to problems as natural responses that can be managed; (5) an attitude of realistic optimism concerning the existence of a solution; (6) the belief in one's own ability to deal with problems (i.e., self-efficacy); (7) an understanding that some problems are not easily solved and that persistence is required for success; and (8) a commitment to engage in the process of dealing with one's problems.

Individuals possessing maladaptive orientations are more easily confounded and ultimately are overcome by life's challenges. Three types of maladaptive orientations have been identified—negative, impulsive, and avoidant (Nezu et al., 2013). Those with a *negative orientation* see problems as a direct threat to their well-being, doubt their ability to effectively deal with problems, and tend to become emotionally overwhelmed and distraught when confronting problems. Individuals with an *impulsive orientation* react quickly without thinking through consequences. They exhibit difficulty seeing the broader context (i.e., they settle on a limited view of the problem), and are careless and incomplete in their problem-solving attempts. Finally, individuals with an *avoidant orientation* often deny the existence of a problem, procrastinate in dealing with the problem, hope the problem will go away on its own, and rely on others to fix the problem. Maladaptive orientations undermine individuals' capacity to engage in the problem-solving process.

STAGES OF PROBLEM-SOLVING THERAPY

Problem-solving therapy involves six stages, with each having significant goals and outcomes for the work between client and therapist. The first stage of PST is to explore and address clients' *problem orientation*. If clients have avoidant orientations, for example, then helping to recognize and acknowledge the particular problem is the initial step. When exploring problem orientations, therapists and clients address the problem perception, attribution, appraisal, and specific beliefs about personal control (Areán, Raue, & Julian, 2011). In problem attribution, therapists and clients work together to discern a realistic understanding of the cause of the clients' problems in living. Some clients may overly focus on internal issues and see the root of problems encountered as stemming from personal deficits. Other clients may attribute the development of problems to factors outside of themselves (e.g., lack of public transportation to get to work).

While internal and external factors may both be involved in the development of a particular problem, overemphasis on either set may represent underlying negative assumptions and schema that distort the client's perception of the actual factors contributing to the problem. For example, a new resident in an assisted living facility contents that other residents' ignorance and small-mindedness are the cause of her difficulty in developing friendships. This perspective focuses on her social environment and does not prompt her to examine any factors related to her behaviors (e.g., wearing a scowl, avoiding eye contact with others).

Problem appraisal involves the individual's perception of the problem as either a challenge or a threat. The view that a problem is a threat to future well-being may increase client anxiety and inhibit the ability to effectively employ problem-solving skills. For example, a husband's belief that "I can't survive if my wife dies" may promote avoidance behavior in response to her cancer diagnosis, as well as heighten his depressive symptoms. The notion of personal control involves clients' understanding that while there are situations that they can control, there exist some factors, such as the behavior of others, that they cannot change (Nezu et al., 2013). For example, a client's acknowledgment that she cannot change her mother's overbearing personality allows her to focus on strategies that she can implement to shape her mother's involvement with her teenage children. When a maladaptive orientation does exist, the therapist's exploration of negative features during the introductory PST session may be sufficient to promote a more positive mindset. However, negative orientations stemming from distorted underlying assumptions, or schema, may require multiple sessions before the client is able to move on and effectively engage in the actual problem-solving process.

The second stage of PST, *problem definition*, is critical to the success of clients' problem-solving endeavors. If a client is unable to clearly and concretely identify a problem, then the probability of an effective solution generation is greatly reduced. The problem definition step begins with the therapist asking the client to select one problem that is important. At times, a client may be confronting multiple problems with varied and complex elements. It is important to examine problems, or aspects of problems, one at a time. In order to promote the likelihood of success in initial problem-solving, the first issue selected should be one that is not emotionally charged.

The exploration and clarification of the problem are necessary elements of problem definition and constitute the information-gathering phase of this intervention. Clients should gather all the information they can about the problem and draw from as many perspectives as possible. Pertinent data include tasks that one must accomplish to effectively function in the day-to-day world. In addition, social-behavioral information related to the client's goals, needs, expectations, and desires is identified. When collecting this type of information, the client should consider the following questions:

- What makes this situation a problem?
- When does the problem occur?
- Where does the problem occur?
- Who is involved with the problem?
- How often does the problem occur?
- What solutions have been tried and how did they work?
- Is this a problem over which you have control?

When answering the preceding questions, the client needs to be able to distinguish between assumption and fact. When a client's statements are vague, the therapist should encourage the client to look for "evidence." This step is similar to helping a client investigate a cognition to determine if it is accurate or distorted. For example, Mrs. Hathaway is distressed by the conflict arising in the church choir, a group that she has belonged to for 18 years and that represents her major social network. Among other changes, a new choir director has reassigned some members, including Mrs. Hathaway, to new vocal groups. Mrs. Hathaway sees this change as an attempt by the new director to drive her and others out of the choir. Her assumption may be incorrect and may prevent her from effectively coping with the changes that a new choir director presents. The therapist helps the client explore the accuracy of her contention by asking her what other reasons there could be for the choir director's actions. Using this approach, PST therapists work with clients to identify and correct distorted cognitions that arise in response to specific triggers and, thus, contribute to problem development.

Because factors contributing to the problem may be both internal and external, problem-solving often requires multifaceted coping responses. Often, problems are composed of distinct but interrelated parts. Complex problems should be broken down into smaller and more manageable parts. Instead of attempting to find a solution for the entire problem, the client is taught to examine and develop solutions for one part of the problem at a time.

Consider the case vignette of Mrs. Thompson, presented at the beginning of the chapter, about her inability to lose weight as her physician recommended. After breaking the larger problem into these discrete parts, Mrs. Thompson decided that the most useful problem to initially target was finding social support for weight loss endeavors, and she joined a low-impact exercise class at her local YMCA. Expressing the problem in a clear and concrete manner is essential for the later development of effective solution generation. Mrs. Thompson initially stated that "I just need other folks' help somehow to lose weight." While this statement indicates a desire for support with the process, specificity and clarity were missing. As a response, the therapist assisting Mrs. Thompson in further exploration regarding types of "help" that would be most valuable to her, and as a result she decided to join an exercise class with others who were trying to loss weight.

Solution generation is the third stage of PST. During this stage of treatment, the therapist works with the client to develop realistic, feasible, and concrete goals (D'Zurrila & Nezu, 2010; Hegel & Areán, 2012). In the previous stage, the problem was concretely stated; this stage involves the clarification of goals. For example, a goal of "getting my blood sugar under control" is too vague and may require multiple behaviors. In addition, this goal may not be entirely within the client's power to accomplish individually. However, working more closely with a doctor about diabetes management and practicing more consistent blood sugar testing are concrete goals that are within reach.

While some clients may be able to readily identify a solution once they have clearly defined the problem, others may have great difficulty with this process. In such cases, the therapist uses *brainstorming* to help the client generate as many potential solutions as possible. During brainstorming, the therapist encourages the client to come up with ideas and does not offer solutions. If a client asks the therapist to share ideas, the therapist turns this task back by explaining that the client is the one who best understands the identified problem.

To facilitate brainstorming, therapists cover several important points before the session begins. First, the therapist explains that the goal is not to produce one right solution, but to come up with as many different ideas for solutions as possible. The best solution may not be the first that comes to mind, or the one that is the most easily accomplished. By brainstorming, helpful ideas emerge that the client might not have considered otherwise. Second, the therapist explains that the client should be as creative and open as possible, and avoid internally screening out ideas because they seem silly or lack feasibility. Third, the therapist instructs the client to avoid making judgments since this curtails the process and results in the generation of fewer ideas.

Once sufficient solutions have been identified, the therapist works with the client on stage four of PST, which is *decision-making*. During this stage, the client assesses the potential success of each generated solution and makes a final decision about which to implement. To effectively weigh the pros and cons of each solution, the client thoughtfully considers the benefits and the costs of each. During this process, the client is encouraged to first review potential benefits. Focusing initially on the benefits promotes optimism, while conversely, starting by considering objections can lead to negativity and premature rejection of ideas. During this analysis, the client is asked to consider four areas: (1) the contribution of the solution to the client's short-term goals; (2) the contribution of the solution to the client's long-term goals; (3) the impact of the solution on the client; and (4) the impact of the solution on others. When weighing options, the client should consider aspects such as the feasibility of the solution, barriers to successful resolution that may exist, and the likely impact of the solution. Multiple areas of cost should also be considered. For example, will there be a financial cost involved? If so, is it affordable? What is the cost in terms of time and energy for the client and others?

Once the client has evaluated each solution, it is time to weigh these against one another and to pick a final solution. This phase is one of the most critical of the problem-solving process, and helps promote growth in critical thinking. Since one goal of PST is to train the client in skills needed to solve future problems, it is vital that this stage be given adequate time and attention. To be clear, the best solution is the one that most effectively meets the client's goals while engendering the least cost to the client and others.

In the following example, a client devises and then weighs the benefits and costs of several possible solutions. Mr. Roberts is a 68-year-old man who has failing eyesight and is no longer able to drive. He is having trouble getting to the grocery store and to doctors' appointments. While he lives close enough to walk to church, he is unable to do so during bad weather conditions. As a result, he feels angry, depressed, and helpless. When working with the therapist to develop solutions, the first idea that comes to Mr. Roberts' mind is to ask his daughter to serve as his driver. This would be easy and convenient for him, and would allow him to spend more time with his daughter, which he would enjoy. However, his daughter has three young children. Mr. Roberts believes that driving him multiple times a week would create too much stress for her. Alternately, public transportation is a possibility, as the bus runs right outside his house. This solution is low cost, but his poor eyesight and lack of familiarity with the bus system created an uncomfortable situation for Mr. Roberts. If he could be trained on the public transportation system, this may be a possible solution, but it would be time-consuming and would be unhelpful in the short term. Taxis are not a viable option due to cost. All of these options seemed costly or labor intensive.

A feasible option seemed to be a friend or neighbor who could drive Mr. Roberts. He identified a friend from church who drives and who is retired. Mr. Roberts voiced that he is hesitant to ask his friend until he realized that he could address this barrier with an offer to pay his friend for driving. While this would be a new expense, he believes that it would be within his means and would give his friend an opportunity to make some money. His daughter might be able to act as a backup driver, since it would only be on occasion.

The fifth stage of PST is to *implement a solution*. Once the particular solution has been chosen, it is time to carefully plan out the steps required to carry it out. While it is the client's job to come up with these details, it is the therapist's task to make sure that the client does plan out the required steps and decides how each of these will be accomplished. If the client has difficulty with this step, the therapist should ask questions such as "What will you need in order to _____? When will you do this? Where will you do this? Will you need anyone's help and, if so, whose? How much will this cost?" Once again, each step and related task should be stated in clear measurable language. In Mr. Roberts's case, the task of "contacting my friend" would be insufficient. Along with the therapist's support, Mr. Roberts identified his tasks as the following:

1. Check my calendar to see how many appointments I have in a typical week and how many I have each week for the next month. I will do this tonight.
2. Check my finances to see how much I could pay per month. I have a doctor's appointment tomorrow (Wednesday), so I will do this on Thursday.
3. Speak to my friend, Roger, at church on Sunday at the 10 a.m. service.
4. Talk to my daughter—I'll do this after I talk to Roger and find out what he says.

The therapist and Mr. Roberts agree that Mr. Roberts will carry out steps 1–3 before they meet again the following week.

Prior to ending a session, the PST therapist asks the client to identify any obstacles that could occur during the implementation phase. If any are identified, it is critical that methods of dealing with these obstacles are discussed and developed. If the client does not feel confident in his or her ability to carry out each step of the plan, this may be an indication that the identified tasks are not truly suitable. In such a case, the therapist and client should return to their consideration of what is feasible. Sometimes helping the client write out a script, or engaging in a role-play, is sufficient to bolster the client's confidence.

Evaluating the outcomes is the sixth and final stage of PST. During this stage, the therapist and client work together to evaluate two components of solution outcomes. First, they examine the progress the client has made in accomplishing the identified solution by examining each task separately. When a client has successfully completed a task, the therapist provides positive feedback and asks if the client faced any challenges. If so, the therapist further explores with the client how he or she overcame these challenges. This type of discussion helps the client build self-efficacy by focusing on accomplishments. If the client has been unable to accomplish a task, the therapist helps the client examine the barriers. Once the barriers are identified, brainstorming takes place concerning methods of overcoming the barriers. If a barrier cannot be surmounted, then a new task is developed.

From the preceding example, Mr. Roberts was able to determine the number of appointments he had in a typical week and the precise number he had in the coming month. He was able to speak with his friend at church, who was very willing to drive Mr. Roberts to his appointments. However, Mr. Roberts was not able to go through his finances to calculate how much he could afford to pay someone. He found that due to his poor eyesight he could not clearly read the monthly statements he received from the bank. After discussing this obstacle, Mr. Roberts decided to call his daughter to see if she could come by for a few hours the coming weekend to help him go through his papers and determine how much he could offer to pay his friend. Mr. Roberts stated that he would call his daughter that evening after she came home from work. At the next session Mr. Roberts reported that, together with his daughter, he was able to determine how much he could pay to have someone act as his driver. Additionally, after discussing the finances with his friend, they had reached an agreement. In subsequent sessions following the enactment of this solution, the therapist and Mr. Roberts examined the degree to which the solution actually met Mr. Roberts's goal. In this case, Mr. Roberts reported that the solution fully met his goal. At this point the therapist worked with Mr. Roberts to review all the steps he had taken to effectively identify and meet his goal.

As stated previously, the aim of PST is not to solve all of the client's problems, but rather to train the client to effectively engage in the problem-solving process. In the concluding sessions of PST, the therapist works with the client to articulate the steps taken, review the challenges met, and acknowledge the success achieved. The client is then encouraged to apply the problem-solving skills learned in therapy to future challenges.

PROBLEM-SOLVING THERAPY WITH OLDER CLIENTS

PST can be a very useful therapy for clients who are older and for those who have mild cognitive impairment because the steps involved in PST are structured, concrete, and clearly laid out. In addition, older adults who are uncomfortable with the concept of psychotherapy often are more open to the skills-training approach employed in PST. When using PST with older adults, some adaptations of this intervention are recommended (Arean et al., 2011; Demiris et al., 2012).

Initially, it is critical to take the time needed to socialize the client into therapy. Because older clients may doubt the usefulness of "talk therapy," it is helpful to inform the client that through PST they will learn skills that will help them to more effectively solve their own problems. Furthermore, the therapist's job will be to act as a teacher and supporter during this process.

In addition, the therapist needs to employ a variety of educational techniques. Older adults are more likely to grasp and retain information when it is presented in multiple formats. Therefore, the therapist should explain information verbally, present written materials that highlight key concepts, and practice PST skills in session with the client. Many figures, forms, and worksheets that could prove useful when conducting PST with older clients may be found in the supplemental section of *Problem-Solving Therapy: A Treatment Manual* (Nezu et al., 2013).

PST includes homework, and the older client needs to understand the importance of completing assigned activities. The therapist should explain the homework process and rationale. In addition, a good strategy is to have the therapist demonstrate how to correctly complete the first homework assignment. This in-session demonstration and practice will help promote older clients' ability to successfully complete later homework assignments on their own.

A direct and uncomplicated approach is best with older clients. For example, if an older client is unable to come up with clear problem definitions, goals, or solutions, the therapist may need to offer suggestions. Some older clients may not have the cognitive ability, or the independence, to address complicated problems. However, tackling smaller and more manageable problems can lead the way to early success.

As appropriate, the therapist should involve family members. Family caregivers can play crucial roles as sources of information and active participants in some aspects of PST, with client approval. Family members can also help remind the older client of assigned homework and provide support with homework completion.

CONTEXT AND IMPLEMENTATION

Similar to CBT, PST is a flexible approach that can be implemented in numerous settings with older adults. Often used as a treatment approach in geriatric depression, PST has been successfully implemented in long-term care settings, as well as with community-based samples in individuals' home environment and community agencies (e.g., outpatient clinics). To date, studies about the effectiveness of this approach in acute care settings has not been reported.

PST also demonstrates flexibility as a practice approach. Outcomes studies have reported that PST is effective when delivered in face-to-face formats, as well as over the telephone. In addition, this approach can be offered as an individual treatment or within a group setting.

Due to the complex nature of caregiving, PST has also been employed with care providers as well as with older adults themselves. The approach assists caregivers with resolving problems associated with care demands, as well as the emotional aspects involved in the role. In particular, PST can assist caregivers involved in dementia care, who often face multiple and ongoing decision-making.

CASE EXAMPLE

Mr. Chernitsky is a 63-year-old widower who lives in his own home with his 14-year-old grandson. He and his wife had been caring for the grandson since he was an infant because of his mother's problems with drugs. Mr. Chernitsky's wife died from cancer 2 years ago. In addition, Mr. Chernitsky lost his job as a middle manager at an industrial facility when it went through downsizing 11 months ago. Mr. Chernitsky had developed a painful rash on his arms, legs, and head. Due to the pain, Mr. Chernitsky consulted with his doctor, who prescribed a medication for the rash, which he believed was stress induced. During his appointment Mr. Chernitsky admitted to high levels of stress and growing depression. As a result, the doctor referred Mr. Chernitsky to the behavioral health specialist at the clinic.

During the pre-treatment assessment phase, the PST therapist gathered information concerning Mr. Chernitsky's current life problems and stresses, steps he had already taken to deal with the problems, consequences that had occurred as a result of the problems, and his emotional reactions. The therapist also assessed Mr. Chernitsky's problem orientation, which included some avoidant tendencies, especially ignoring problems. For example, Mr. Chernitsky reported that he had known that the downsizing was coming but hadn't wanted to believe that it would really impact him, and so he wasn't prepared when he was finally laid off. He also noted that he had taken the same approach when his rash occurred. He put off seeing a doctor until the rash had become so painful that he couldn't deal with it any more. Upon further exploration of this tendency with the therapist, Mr. Chernitsky acknowledged that his denial had not served him well in either situation, and that he now needed to face up to his problems. During the initial session, the therapist explained to Mr. Chernitsky the rationale and course of PST and gave him printed material about PST that he could review at home. For homework, the therapist asked Mr. Chernitsky to develop and prioritize a list of the problems he was experiencing.

During the second session, the therapist and Mr. Chernitsky reviewed the problem list he had generated. These problems included the following: (1) no one wants to hire a 63-year-old man; (2) I can barely pay all my bills each month; (3) I can't contribute to my grandson's college fund; (4) I'm bored; I sit at home all day on my couch. The therapist and Mr. Chernitsky discussed each problem to examine which were short- versus long-term, which were based on assumptions and which on fact, and the consequences of each. During this process the therapist examined with Mr. Chernitsky's assumption that "no one will hire a 63-year-old." After discussing this assumption and the emotional consequences stemming from this thought (feeling hopeless and depressed), Mr. Chernitsky was able to reframe this negative assumption as a clear problem that could now be addressed, "I can't find a job." After further discussion, Mr. Chernitsky re-prioritized his problem list to (1) I can't find a job; (2) I'm bored; I sit on the couch all day (the latter was re-categorized by Mr. Chernitsky as number two since, through discussion, he recognized that boredom was a major contributor to his feeling of depression); (3) his problem with respect to paying bills each month was moved down on this list because he was actually able to pay all of his bills (he just had very little left over for anything extra); (4) although still a major concern, his grandson's college fund was identified as a longer-term problem that did not need to be solved immediately.

In this new context, Mr. Chernitsky identified not being able to find a job as his major problem, and one that he could creatively address. However, after further discussion with the therapist, the two agreed that Mr. Chernitsky should first work on his problem of boredom. Mr. Chernitsky readily acknowledged that his lack of activity substantively contributed to his depression. Since he had always been an active man, he further realized that with support he could make progress in this area quickly. Through targeted questioning, the therapist helped Mr. Chernitsky identify an activity he could preform in the coming week (i.e., walking the dog in the morning after breakfast for at least 15 minutes).

During the next session the therapist and Mr. Chernitsky reviewed his week. Mr. Chernitsky reported that he had walked the dog each day and that during the last 2 days he had walked for almost a half-hour. He felt pleased, not only about accomplishing this goal, but also for slightly exceeding it. He agreed to continue walking every morning during the coming week. During this session Mr. Chernitsky agreed that it was time to begin addressing his problem of finding a job. For homework the therapist asked Mr. Chernitsky to write down everything he had attempted in his search for a job and all the factors that he could think of that contributed to the inability to secure one. During the next session, Mr. Chernitsky reported that he had continued to walk each morning. He and the therapist then turned to his homework. Mr. Chernitsky reported that he had taken the following steps in trying to find a job: (1) wrote a resume; he noted that this was very a difficult exercise but with help from a friend he was able to do so; and (2) reviewed the employment section of the paper every day for managerial positions in industrial plants for which he felt well qualified and was able to apply.

Despite this improvement in problem-solving, he received no responses to his applications since there were very few positions available. In the next step, he broadened his search beyond employment at manufacturing plants and applied for any managerial position that he could find. Once again, there were few jobs available. When looking at factors that presented barriers to his finding a job, Mr. Chernitsky identified his age and layoffs at other factories creating a large supply of middle managers on the job market. During this session the therapist continued to ask probing questions to help Mr. Chernitsky delve more deeply into the factors contributing to his problem. Mr. Chernitsky finally came to the conclusion that the major factors inhibiting his ability to be rehired in the manufacturing industry were external factors beyond his control. At this point, the therapist and Mr. Chernitsky worked together to redefine the problem he was facing.

Mr. Chernitsky redefined his problem definition, observing that "because there are very few jobs left in the manufacturing business and because of my age, I cannot find a managerial job in this industry." Although Mr. Chernitsky reported that he felt sad acknowledging this reality, he also felt more positive because "now I can stop beating my head against the wall and getting nowhere." For homework, the therapist asked Mr. Chernitsky to come up with a list of alternate solutions to his problems.

During the next session Mr. Chernitsky presented the following solutions: (1) take early retirement; (2) take a lesser job in the plant; and (3) find a job outside of the industry. After looking at the pros and cons of each solution, Mr. Chernitsky decided he would rather look for a job outside of the manufacturing industry. As homework for the following week, Mr. Chernitsky looked to determine the types of positions that were available in his town. Mr. Chernitsky used the problem-solving skills he had learned and during the week identified the types of available jobs, weighed the pros and cons of each, and made a decision about the type of job he wanted. In addition, he realized that he did not want to try for managerial positions in other industries because of his lack of background, and that he did not want to retrain for a job in a field such as IT due to his age. He did report, however, that he was now willing to take a lesser job in the service field. In Mr. Chernitsky's decision-making phase, the best solution was not easily reached. But in light of realities beyond his control, there was still a best solution that most effectively met his needs while engendering the least cost to himself and others.

Together, Mr. Chernitsky and his therapist identified his job needs: (1) salary—Mr. Chernitsky realized that he could take a sizable pay cut and still pay his bills with funds to contribute something to his grandson's college fund and still have a little left over; (2) physical demands—he could not stand on his feet all day; and (3) environmental demands—he did not want to be in a high stress environment. With this information, Mr. Chernitsky and the therapist could plan the steps required to implement this solution. The following tasks were identified: (1) redo his resume to emphasize more generalizable skills; (2) submit at least two job applications in the coming week; and (3) reach out to two friends he identified who might know of service jobs in the area. Mr. Chernitsky carried out all these tasks in the following week.

During the next couple of weeks, he continued to send out resumes and meet with the therapist to discuss the results of his efforts. Although he had received three phone calls, he had not been invited for any interviews. The therapist then asked Mr. Chernitsky to describe everything that had occurred during the job-related phone calls. When discussing the calls, Mr. Chernitsky realized that he may have spoken too much about his previous work experience and supervisory role, revealing too little about his willingness to engage in new tasks that required less skill and experience. The therapist and Mr. Chernitsky then engaged in role-plays to enhance his ability to effectively communicate with poten-tial employers. A week later, one of Mr. Chernitsky's friends called to let him know of an opening at the hardware store where his friend worked. Mr. Chernitsky applied and was hired. He reported to his therapist that he would never have thought of looking for a job in a hardware store and probably would not have been open to the idea in the past. Although the job required less skill and paid less than his previous job, he was happy to be earning some income and to have the opportunity to interact with people every day. When asked, he stated that he felt that this solution had met his goal. During their last session, the therapist asked Mr. Chernitsky to recount all of the steps he had taken to effectively identify and meet his goal. With prompts from the therapist, Mr. Chernitsky was able to recount each step. They also discussed how Mr. Chernitsky overcame the obstacles he had encountered. Mr. Chernitsky reported that he was proud of what he had been able to accomplish. The therapist encouraged Mr. Chernitsky to continue using the skills he had learned in PST to tackle new problems as they arose in the future.

Mr. Chernitsky had learned skills to solve one problem in a manner that enhanced his overall problem-solving abilities and increased his self-confidence. With this experience of success, concomitant with the therapist's explicit encouragement, he had an increased likelihood of applying these problem-solving skills to new situations, generalizing their application to varied circumstances, and continuing to develop his array of problem-solving skills on a path toward greater competence.

CONCLUSION

In conclusion, problem-solving therapy is an approach that has important uses with older clients. Due to the focus on skill development, the treatment has utility for working with those individuals who are experiencing life transitions, are depressed, or have insufficient coping abilities. Because of this orientation, PST may be appealing to older clients who might resist a more therapeutic approach to problem resolution.

REFERENCES

Areán, P. A., Raue, P., & Julian, L. (2011). *Social problem solving therapy for depression and executive dys-function*. Old Age Project. Retrieved June 1, 2015 from http://pstnetwork.ucsf.edu/sites/pstnetwork.ucsf.edu/files/documents/Social%20Problem%20Solving%20Therapy%20ED.Final_.pdf.

Demiris, G., Oliver, D. P., Wittenberg-Lyles, E., Washington, K., Doorenbos, A., Rue, T., & Berry, D. (2012). A noninferiority trial of a problem-solving intervention for hospice caregivers: in person ver-sus videophone. *Journal of Palliative Medicine, 15*, 653–660.

D'Zurilla, T. J. (1984). This week's citation classic. *Citation Classics/Life Sciences, 50*, 24.

D'Zurilla, T. J., & Goldfried, M. R. (1971). Problem solving and behavior modification. *Journal of Abnormal Psychology, 78*, 107–126.

D'Zurilla, T. J., Nezu, A. M. (1999). *Problem-solving therapy: a social competence approach to clinical inter-vention* (2nd ed.). New York: Springer.

D'Zurilla, T. J., & Nezu, A. M. (2010). Problem-solving therapy. In Dobson, K. S. (Ed.), *Handbook of cognitive-behavioral therapies* (3rd ed.) (pp. 197–225). New York: The Guilford Press.

Gellis, Z. D., McGinty, J., Tierney, L., Jordan, C., & Misener, E. (2008). Randomized controlled trial of problem-solving therapy for minor depression in home care. *Research on Social Work Practice, 18,* 596–606.

Hegel, M. T., & Areán, P. A. (2012). *Problem-solving treatment for primary care (PST-PC): a treatment manual for depression.* University of Washington Psychiatry and Behavioral Sciences. Retrieved June 4, 2015 from http://impact-uw.org/tools/pst_manual.html.

Lazarus, R. S., & Folkman, S. (1984). *Stress, appraisal and coping.* New York: Springer.

Nezu, A. M., Nezu, C. M., & D'Zurilla, T. J. (2013). *Problem-solving therapy: a treatment manual.* New York: Springer.

6

PROBLEM-SOLVING THERAPY
EVIDENCE-BASED PRACTICE

Over the decades, a body of research has emerged that documents the effectiveness of problem-solving therapy (PST) for use with those experiencing a variety of issues. These include *mental health* disorders, such as schizophrenia, social phobias, and substance abuse, as well as *health* problems, such as cancer and arthritis (D'Zurilla & Nezu, 1999). The use of PST for combating depression among these populations continues to be one of its best-known and supported applications (Nezu, Nezu, & D'Zurilla, 2013). More recent meta-analyses comparing PST to other psychotherapies and psychotropic medications for the treatment of depression have also displayed largely favorable results (Bell & D'Zurilla, 2009; Cuijpers, van Straten, & Waarmerdam, 2007). As with other psychotherapeutic interventions, however, fewer research studies have been conducted that examine the use of PST with older populations.

The following literature review was conducted to examine the extant research base of studies focused specifically on the effectiveness of PST for use with older clients. The search terms employed in this review include problem-solving, problem-solving therapy, older adults, elderly, and geriatric. Search engines used in the search included Google Scholar, Academic Search Premier, Science Direct, and PsychINFO. Additionally, *The Journal of the American Medical Association* (JAMA) and the *Journal of the American Geriatrics Society* databases were searched directly. Only those studies meeting the following criteria were included in the review: (1) intervention of focus involved the key components of the problem-solving model; (2) age of participants in at least one arm of the study was 60 years and older; (3) consisted of a meta-analysis or systematic review; and (4) was published between 2000 and 2015. The initial search yielded a preliminary total of 28 research articles. However, 12 of these were excluded for the following reasons: (1) did not focus specifically on problem-solving therapy (e.g., the focus was problem-solving but not problem-solving *therapy*); (2) contained no actual therapeutic intervention; (3) did not employ true randomization; (4) not yet published in peer-reviewed journal; (5) intervention employed several forms of therapy and PST could not be considered distinctly; and (6) mean age of study participants was too low.

Following the exclusion of these studies, 16 articles remained that met the inclusion criteria, one meta-analysis and 15 randomized controlled studies. The sole meta-analysis examined the effectiveness of PST for the treatment of major depression. The remaining studies are all RCTs and are categorized by client population. One category of studies is community-based, with outcomes of decreased depression, enhanced quality of life, and coping with health-related conditions. Mr. Chernitsky, the client in the case example presented in Chapter 5, would fall into this category, as he was depressed after being widowed and losing his job. The second category of studies is those conducted within home settings of older adults. In this set, the older participants were all medically frail and were experiencing depression. In the final category of studies, PST was evaluated with care providers of older adults. The outcomes evaluated in caregiver studies included decreased depression and anxiety, enhanced quality of life, and increased problem-solving skills.

META-ANALYSIS

Kirkham, Seitz, and Choi (2015) conducted a meta-analysis to examine the effectiveness of PST for the treatment of major depressive disorder (MDD) in older adults (see Table 6.1). In all, nine studies were included, with a total of 569 participants ($n = 290$ PST, $n = 279$ control). Studies meeting the following criteria were included: (1) randomized controlled trials (RCTs) comparing PST to a control condition (wait list, usual care, psychoeducation controls, and psychotherapy modalities); and (2) average age of participants was 60 years and older. A majority of the trial participants were diagnosed with MDD. Studies that only evaluated other depressive disorders were excluded. The median sample size for each study was 44. There was a preponderance of women in each study that reported gender, and the mean age range for each study was 65.2–80.5 years. A majority of participants were recruited from community outpatient programs. Four of the nine studies included patients with some degree of executive cognitive impairment. All studies, but one, excluded patients with dementia. PST was provided individually in all studies, with the exception of one that implemented PST in a group setting. One study employed PST via telephone, while the others studies used in-person PST. A majority of the studies delivered PST weekly, varying from 5 to 12 sessions.

The researchers found a significant reduction in depression scores from PST as compared to alternate treatments as measured by a variety of scales frequently used with older adults. Two of the nine studies examined the effects that PST had on disability. A significant reduction in disability was found for participants treated with PST as compared to those in control groups. In conclusion, this review found PST to be an effective treatment for MDD in older adults. However, there is a relatively small number of studies available

TABLE 6.1 PST META-ANALYSIS

Study	Inclusion/Exclusion Criteria	Description of Interventions	Number and Description of Participants	Outcomes	Findings
Kirkham, Seitz, & Choi, 2015 Meta-analysis	RCTs only. Comparing PST to control or other treatment conditions. All participants 60 or older. Majority of participants diagnosed with major depressive disorder (MDD).	PST: delivered in person by trained mental health professionals. Treatment lasted between 5–12 sessions. Control group: Wait list or usual care, psychoeducation, or other psychotherapy modalities.	9 studies Median group size: 44 participants. Most participants recruited from community: $n = 569$. PST condition: $n = 290$. Control conditions: $n = 279$. M age = 65.2–80.5 years.	Significant reduction in depression with large effect size for PST when compared to control groups using a variety of depression measures. In three studies examining disability, significant decrease in disability for subjects treated with PST compared to controls.	PST is an effective treatment for older people with MDD. Support found for reduction in disability due to PST. PST can be delivered by a variety of health-care practitioners in different formats and to a range of patient populations with MDD.

in this area. The changes in depression severity were consistent with clinically significant improvements in depression as determined by various measures. PST appears to be effective in reducing disability and treating depression in older adult populations both with and without underlying executive impairments. This review supports the use of PST as treatment for MDD in older adults.

COMMUNITY-BASED STUDIES

Six RCTs included community-based samples of older adults (see Table 6.2). Areán et al. (2010) conducted a study comparing the effectiveness of PST with supportive therapy to reduce depression among older patients with executive dysfunction. Individuals with executive dysfunction display lack of insight and behavioral difficulties, including trouble with goal-setting, planning, and sequencing behavior. The researchers hypothesized that the structured format of PST would enhance problem-solving ability and reduce stress and depression. To be included in this study, all participants were required to meet the DSM-IV criteria for major depression, score higher than 20 on the Hamilton Depression Rating Scale (HAM-D), higher than 24 on the Mini-Mental State Examination (MMSE), and less than 33 on the initiation/preservation subscale of the Mattis Dementia Rating Scale. Exclusionary criteria included current treatment for depression with psychotherapy or antidepressants, high risk for suicide, any axis I disorder other than unipolar major depression and generalized anxiety disorder, an acute medical condition, and inability to perform one or more activities of daily living. All participants in this study ($n = 221$) were aged 60 years and older with major depression and executive dysfunction. One hundred and ten patients ($M = 72.8$ years; $M = 15$ years education) participated in the PST condition, while the remaining 111 patients received supportive therapy ($M = 73.2$ years; $M = 15.5$ years education). Participants were randomly assigned to 12 weekly sessions of PST or supportive therapy, and were assessed at weeks 3, 6, 9, and 12. Individuals receiving PST were taught a five-step problem-solving process, including development of a relapse prevention plan. Those in the supportive therapy condition received weekly individual sessions during which the therapist provided active listening and support, but did not engage in any therapeutic strategies.

At the conclusion of the first 6 weeks of treatment, reduction of depressive symptom severity was comparable for participants in both treatment conditions. At weeks 9 and 12, however, those in the PST group had greater reduction in symptom severity, a superior response rate, and a better remission rate than those in supportive therapy. This study provides support indicating that PST is effective in reducing depressive symptoms and producing robust treatment response and remission rates among older patients with major depression and executive dysfunction.

In a Hong Kong study, the effectiveness of screening followed by brief problem-solving treatment in primary care (PST-PC) to improve health-related quality of life was explored (Lam et al., 2010). Participants for this RCT were recruited from two

TABLE 6.2 COMMUNITY-BASED PST STUDIES

Study	Inclusion/Exclusion Criteria	Description of Interventions	Number and Description of Participants	Outcomes	Findings
Areán et al., 2010 RCT PST vs. supportive therapy to treat depression in those with executive dysfunction	Inclusion = Age: 60 years and over; evidenced depression and executive dysfunction on screening measures. Exclusion = Current psychotherapy or antidepressants; psychotic depression; high suicide risk; axis I disorder other than unipolar major depression and GAD.	Participants randomly assigned to 12 weekly sessions of PST or supportive therapy and assessed at weeks 3, 6, 9, and 12. PST group participants taught a five-step problem-solving model including relapse prevention. Supportive therapy group: Active listening and support provided.	n = 221. PST group: n = 110; M age = 72.8; 15.0 years education; 7.4% had GAD. Supportive therapy group: n = 111; M age = 73.2; M = 15.5 years education; 6.3% had Generalized Anxiety Disorder.	Reduction of depressive symptom severity comparable for both treatment groups during the first 6 weeks of treatment, but at weeks 9 and 12 PST group had greater reduction in symptom severity, superior response rate, and better remission rate than supportive therapy group.	PST effective in reducing depressive symptoms and leading to improved treatment response and remission rate in older patients with major depression and executive dysfunction. PST may be a treatment alternative in an older patient population likely to be resistant to pharmacotherapy.
Lam et al., 2010 Hong Kong RCT PCT-PC vs. comparison group to improve health-related quality of life (HRQOL) and reduce consultation rates among community-dwelling older adults.	Inclusion = age 60 or above; consulting the two general outpatient clinics of one district in Hong Kong; screened positive on a depression and anxiety scale. Exclusion = diagnosed psychological disorder; history of psychotropic meds; suicidal plans or strong suicidal thoughts; psychotic symptoms; cognitive impairment.	PST-PC: 3 PST-PC sessions to identify problem, promote change in mood, thoughts, and behavior, and reinforce coping. Comparison group: Watched health education videos on healthy diet, exercise, and physical and psychological health in clinic. All subjects continued to receive their usual medical care.	n = 299. PST-PC: n = 149; M age = 71.6 years; 55% female; 44.3% no education; 65.8% married, living with spouse. Comparison group: n = 150; M age = 72 years; 58.7% female; 48.7% no education; 61.3% married, living with spouse.	PST-PC resulted in short-term (6- and 12-week) improvements to scores measuring HRQOL; benefits not found in the comparison group. HRQOL benefit became insignificant by week 26 and 52.	PST-PC health benefits were modest and transient. Only 3 sessions of PST-PC may have been insufficient. Influence of culture may have been a factor. PST-PC may be best used with depressed or anxious patients who do not respond to other treatment.

(continued)

TABLE 6.1 CONTINUED

Study	Inclusion/Exclusion Criteria	Description of Interventions	Number and Description of Participants	Outcomes	Findings
Robinson et al., 2008 RCT Compared impact of PST, escitalopram (medication), and placebo (comparison) on number of depression cases in post-acute stroke patients.	Inclusion: Ages: 51–89 years; within 3 months of an index stroke (either ischemic or hemorrhagic). Exclusion: major or minor depression; severe comprehension deficits; impaired decision-making; occurrence of stroke secondary to complications from intracranial aneurysm, arterial-venous malformation, intracranial tumor, etc.	12-month intervention period. PST group: Manualized PST with 6 treatment sessions over first 12 weeks and 6 reinforcement sessions in next 8 months. Medication group: 10 mg/day for those < age 65; 5 mg/day for patients age ≥ 65. Comparison group: Pills and administration identical to medication group.	n = 176. PST group: n = 58; M age = 67.3; 50.8% male; 45.8% married; 14.2 M years education. Medication group: n = 59; M age = 61.3; 64.4% male; 57.6% married; 13.5 M years education.	Comparison patients significantly more likely to develop depression than those in medication and PST groups. All patients evidenced improvement in ADLs over time.	Study authors concluded that both medication and PST were effective in decreasing depression and disability among post-stroke patients.
Downe-Wamboldt et al., 2007 – Canada Prospective RCT Assess comparative effect and expense of telephone PST vs. usual care to prevent depression among cancer patients.	Inclusion = Age ≥ 50; surgery within past 3 months; access to a telephone; aware of their diagnosis. Women with breast cancer; men with prostate cancer and those with non-small cell lung cancer.	3-month intervention period. Telephone PST + usual care: offered at participant's convenience during 3-month interval; identified health-related concerns, developed solutions, and monitored consequences. Usual care control group: Diagnostic and follow-up care at 3-month intervals, conducted through physician/ oncologists' offices.	n = 149; 60% female; 91% White; 51% breast cancer; 16% lung cancer; 33% prostate cancer. Telephone PST: n = 76; 52.6% breast cancer; 15.8% lung cancer; 31.6% prostate cancer. Control group: n = 73; 49.3% breast cancer; 16.4% lung cancer; 34.3% prostate cancer.	PST telephone counseling improved use of positive coping behaviors, prevented development of clinically important (but not statistically significant) depression and poor psychosocial adjustment. PST results associated with greater total per person per annum expenditure for use of health and social services compared with the control group.	PST telephone is effective in preventing depression in cancer patients; but, due to the expense of treatment, recommend targeted PST for those with significant psychological distress or at heightened risk of developing such distress.

Study / Design / Purpose	Inclusion / Exclusion	Intervention	Sample	Results	Conclusions
Alexopoulos, Raue, & Areán, 2003 RCT PST vs. supportive therapy (ST) to treat depression in those with executive dysfunction.	Inclusion = Age: ≥ 65 years; evidenced depression and executive dysfunction on screening measures. Exclusion = Current psychotherapy or antidepressants; psychotic depression; high suicide risk; Axis I disorder other than unipolar major depression and GAD.	Interventions administered by therapists trained in PST and ST. PST group: 12 weekly sessions; duration not specified. ST group: 12 weekly sessions; duration not specified.	n = 25; M age = 74.1 years; 52% female; 76% White; 52% education: M = 13.7 years. PST group: n = 12. ST Group n = 13.	PST group had significant improvement in depression and disability scores compared to ST group; effects most evident on subjects with most pronounced executive dysfunction.	PST was more effective than ST in inducing remission and reducing depressive symptoms and disability in older adults with major depression and executive dysfunction.
Williams et al., 2000 RCT Compared effectiveness of PST, paroxetine (medication), and comparison group in reducing depression and improving functioning among primary care patients.	Inclusion = Age 60 and over; dysthymia or minor depression evidenced by DSM-III-R criteria or depression screen. Exclusion = Major depression, psychosis, schizophrenia, bipolar substance abuse, antisocial or borderline personality disorders; serious suicidal risk; moderate to severe cognitive impairment.	PST-PC Group: Manualized PST; problem identification and definition, and solution generation; 6 visits over 11 weeks; antidepressants prohibited. Medication group: Paroxetine plus six 15-minute visits for support and monitoring of adverse side effects; psychological treatment prohibited. Comparison group: Inactive medication plus six 15-minute visits for support and monitoring of adverse side effects; psychological treatment prohibited.	n = 415; M age = 71 yrs.; 41.5% women; 21.8% minorities; medical conditions: M = 3.4; minor depression:49.2%; dysthymia: 50.8%; clinical and SES characteristics similar for all three conditions.	Medication group showed greater symptom resolution than comparison group; PST-PC group did not show more improvement than comparison group, but their symptoms improved more rapidly (weeks 2–11) than those of comparison group during later treatment weeks. Mental health functioning in patients with dysthymia was not significantly improved by PST-PC; mental health functioning in patients with minor depression improved by medication and PST-PC in those with lowest baseline functioning.	Benefits for PST-PC participants were smaller and more subject to site differences (4 different sites used in this study) than for those in the medication group. Weak, inconsistent positive results from this study prevent recommendation of PST-PC.

government-funded general outpatient clinics. All patients aged 60 or older were initially invited to participate. Patients were excluded if they had a diagnosed psychological illness, past year history of taking psychotropic medicine, suicidal plans or ideation, psychotic symptoms, or cognitive impairment. All participants were screened with the Hospital Anxiety and Depression Scale, with those screening positive being accepted into the study. In all, 299 older adults participated in the study. The group receiving PST-PC (n = 149) were primarily female and had a mean age of 71.6 years. Likewise, those in the comparison group (n = 150) had a higher percentage of females and a mean age of 72 years. The SF-36, a measure of quality of life, and consultation rates were used to assess trial outcomes. Each member of the PST-PC group received three sessions conducted by a family medicine trainee who had attended PST-PC workshops. The PST-PC sessions focused on the development of a problem definition, promoting change in mood, thoughts, and behavior, and reinforcement of coping behaviors and positive thinking. The comparison group participants were invited to attend the clinic in groups of three to watch health education videos focused on healthy diet, exercise, and physical and psychological health. All subjects continued to receive their usual medical care.

PST-PC resulted in short-term (6- and 12-week) improvements in health-related quality of life, while no benefits were found in the comparison group during this time frame. PST-PC participants' health benefits were only modest and transient, however. By weeks 26 and 52, the quality of life benefit had become insignificant. Thus, in the end, this study found no difference in outcomes between the treatment and control groups. Treatment failure may have been due to insufficient dosage, influence of culture (i.e., PST-PC was originally developed in the United Kingdom and was used in Western cultures), and/or use of a screen for identifying participant depression and anxiety, rather than a diagnosis of a depression or anxiety disorder. The researchers conclude that PST-PC may be best used with depressed or anxious patients who do not respond to other treatment, rather than administering this intervention to all patients who screen positive.

In 2008, Robinson et al. completed a study to determine whether PST or a medication (escitalopram) would decrease the number of depression cases among post-acute stroke patients at 12 months. Patients were enrolled through university departments of neurology and recruited via newspaper advertisements. Those included in the study were between the ages of 50 and 90, within 3 months of an index stroke, and had had either an ischemic or hemorrhagic stroke. Exclusionary criteria included a diagnosis of major and minor depressive disorders, severe comprehension deficits or impaired decision-making capacity, stroke-related considerations, life-threatening heart or respiratory failure, cancer, and neurodegenerative disorders. Study participants (n = 176) were randomly assigned to one of three conditions. The PST group consisted of 58 participants (M = 67.3 years) while the escitalopram group had 59 participants (M = 61.3 years). Fifty-eight participants were assigned to the comparison group (M = 63.9 years). There were no significant differences in group membership by age, sex, socioeconomic status (SES), marital status or education. Those in the PST group participated in a manualized version of PST for treating medical patients with depression. Therapists trained in PST administered the treatment, which consisted of six sessions over the first 12 weeks and six reinforcement sessions during the following 8 months. The medication group received escitalopram, and the comparison group received identical-looking pills throughout the 12-month period.

At the 1-year interval, participants in the medication and PST groups were significantly less likely to have developed depression than the comparison group. All patients experienced improvement in ADLs over time, particularly during the first 3 months. As a result of the findings, the study authors concluded that both medication and PST were effective in decreasing depression in post-stroke patients.

Downe-Wamboldt et al. (2007) conducted a research study in Canada to assess the comparative effectiveness and expense of telephone PST counseling and usual cancer care. Cancer patients were recruited through private oncologists and urologists' offices and from an Academic Center Cancer clinic. Those included in this study were 50 years or older, had had surgery within the past 3 months, were receiving care from an Academic Center Cancer clinic, and were aware of their diagnosis. Participants were women with stage I or II breast cancer, men with prostate cancer, and those with non-small cell lung cancer. Subjects receiving chemotherapy were excluded from this study. Patients were randomly assigned to individualized telephone PST (n = 76) or a usual cancer care control group (n = 73). The telephone PST group received counseling sessions offered at their convenience and administered by trained registered nurses over a 3-month period. Nurses worked with the participants to identify health-related concerns, develop alternate solutions to address concerns, and evaluate the consequences of these solutions. Slightly less than one-half of the participants received 1 to 4 sessions (42.3%), while the others received 5 or more sessions (57.7%). The control group received diagnostic and follow-up care at 3-month intervals.

As compared to usual care, findings revealed that PST telephone counseling significantly improved the use of positive coping behaviors, and prevented the development of depression. For PST group participants, however, these favorable results were also associated with a greater total per person expenditure for use of all other health and social services compared with the control group. Due to this increased expense, the researchers' recommendations included targeting PST treatment at those experiencing significant psychological distress or at heightened risk of developing such distress.

The comparative effectiveness of PST and supportive therapy (ST) depression reduction among older adults with executive dysfunction was evaluated (Alexopoulos, Raue, & Areán, 2003). To be included in this study, participants had to be 65 years or older, meet the DSM-IV criteria for unipolar major depression, and score one standard deviation below the mean on tests of executive function. Exclusionary criteria included having a history of other psychiatric disorders, suicidal ideation, severe or acute medical illness within 3 months of the study, a neurological disorder, and a score below 24 on the MMSE. Twenty-five participants were enrolled in the study (M = 74.1 years of age). The highest percentage of participants was white and female. These older patients were randomly assigned to the PST ($n = 12$) and supportive therapy ($n = 13$) conditions. The interventions were administered by therapists trained in both PST and supportive therapy. Treatment fidelity was monitored. All patients were assessed at baseline and at the end of the 12-week study.

Results indicate that the PST group evidenced significantly greater reductions in depression scores and disability than did the ST group. In addition, the effects of PST were most evident in participants who had the most pronounced executive dysfunction. Although the number of subjects in this study was small, the findings do offer preliminary evidence of the efficacy of PST in reducing major depression and impairment in older adults with executive dysfunction.

Williams et al. (2000) sought to examine the relative effectiveness of PST, an antidepressant medication, and a comparison condition in reducing depressive symptoms and improving functional status among older primary care patients suffering from minor depression and dysthymia. Participants were recruited from four primary clinics chosen for their geographic and patient population diversity. Patients included in the study were 60 years of age or older, met the DSM-III-R criteria for dysthymia or minor depression, and scored 10 or higher on the Hamilton Depression Rating Scale (HAM-D). Patients with major depression, psychosis, schizophrenia, bipolar disorder, substance abuse, antisocial or borderline personality disorder, serious risk of suicide, and moderate or severe cognitive impairment were excluded from this study. Of the 415 older patients ($M = 71$ years of age), the majority were female and almost half had minor depression. Mental health and physical function was markedly impaired for all participants. Regardless of the treatment, all patients were scheduled to participate in six visits over 11 weeks. Of the total participants, 338 (81.4%) attended at least four treatment sessions, and 311 (74.9%) completed all the scheduled treatment sessions. Those in the PST-PC group ($n = 138$) received manualized PST administered by trained mental health professionals. The PST counseling involved helping patients link their symptoms to everyday problems, identifying and defining problems, and developing problem solutions. Sessions lasted about 1 hour for the first visit and 30 minutes for each subsequent visit. Individuals in the medication ($n = 137$) and the comparison ($n = 140$) groups participated in approximately 15-minute visits designed to provide general support and monitoring for adverse side effects. Specific psychological treatment was prohibited for both groups.

Overall, antidepressant medication made the biggest impact in depression. The medication group showed greater symptom reduction than did the comparison group. While those in the PST-PC group did not show more improvement than the comparison group, their symptoms did improve more rapidly than those in the comparison group. Mental health functioning in patients with dysthymia improved for patients in the medication, but not in the PST group. Antidepressant medication enhanced the mental health functioning of patients with minor depression; however, only those with lowest baseline functioning in the PST-PC group received similar benefit. Due to the weak, inconsistent results from this study, the researchers were unable to recommend PST-PC.

IN-HOME STUDIES

Five RCT studies examined the impact of PST implemented in in-home settings with older adults (see Table 6.3). Choi et al. (2014) conducted a study to evaluate the acceptance and preliminary efficacy of in-home tele-health delivery of PST (tele-PST) among depressed low-income homebound older adults. The inclusion criteria for this study were (1) non-Hispanic White, Black, or Hispanic; (2) English-speaking; (3) adults over the age of 50; and (4) score of 15+ on the Hamilton Rating Scale for Depression (HAMD). Of the 124 older adults who met the criteria, 121 agreed to participate in the study. The highest percentages of participants were White, with the majority being female. The tele-PST intervention was compared to in-person PST and telephone support calls. All intervention arms consisted of six sessions. The 43 participants receiving tele-PST had a 60-minute first session, followed by five 30-minute sessions, while those in the in-person PST condition (n = 42) received six 60-minute PST-PC sessions. Finally, the 36 participants receiving telephone support calls had six 30-minute sessions. The baseline and follow-up assessments were conducted in person, and 6-month booster sessions were conducted by telephone. The HAMD was given at 12 and 24 weeks to assess for change.

No significant difference was found between tele-PST and in-person PST in their treatment effects on depression severity. However, participants who received tele-PST and in-person PST had symptom severities significantly lower than those participants who received telephone support calls at the 12-week follow-up. This study found that all participants had extremely positive attitudes toward tele-PST at the 12-week follow-up. The researchers concluded that tele-PST is an efficacious treatment modality for depressed homebound older adults.

Gellis and colleagues conducted three studies to examine the effectiveness of PST on the mental health functioning of home-care clients. Gellis and Bruce (2010) conducted an RCT to determine whether elderly home health patients with heart disease receiving problem-solving therapy in home care (PST-HC) would experience greater short-term improvements in depression and anxiety scores, improved health functioning, and greater satisfaction with treatment than those in a usual care plus education (UC+E) treatment. To be included in this study, patients had to be 65 years of age or older, homebound, have cardiovascular disease, be cognitively intact, and meet the DSM-IV criteria for sub-threshold depressive symptoms. Adults who had coexisting chronic conditions such as cancer, coronary artery disease requiring surgery or angioplasty, renal disease on dialysis, dementia, or psychotic disorders were excluded, as were those with major depression. In all, 36 individuals were included in this study. Eighteen participants (M = 75.6 years) received PST-HC. The other 18 participants (M = 76.2 years) received UC+E. The majority of participants in both treatment conditions were female,

TABLE 6.3 IN-HOME PST STUDIES

Study	Inclusion/Exclusion Criteria	Description of Interventions	Number and Description of Participants	Outcomes	Findings
Choi et al., 2014 RCT Comparison of Tele-PST to In-Person PST and telephone support for depressed low-income homebound older adults	Inclusion = Over age 50; non-Hispanic White, Black, or Hispanic; English speaking; score of 15+ on depression screen. Exclusion = high suicide risk, dementia, bipolar disorder, psychotic symptoms or disorder; substance abuse; current involvement in psychotherapy.	All treatment conditions consisted of 6 sessions. Tele-PST: First session was 60-min PST-PC, followed by five 30-minute sessions. In-Person PST: Six 60-minutes PST-PC sessions. Telephone support calls: Six 30-minute sessions.	$n = 121$. 77.7% female; 41.3% White, 33.9% Black, 24.8% Hispanic. Two-thirds met criteria for major depressive disorder. Tele-PST: $n = 43$. In-Person PST: $n = 42$. Telephone support: $n = 36$.	No significant difference between Tele-PST and In-Person PST participants in their treatment effects on depression severity. Symptom severities significantly lower among participants in either Tele-PST or In-Person PST than those in telephone support at 12-week follow-up.	Tele-PST is as effective as In-Person PST in reducing depressive symptoms in home-bound older adults. Tele-PST participants had extremely positive attitudes toward the treatment. Tele-PST is an effective and acceptable intervention for the homebound population.
Gellis & Bruce, 2010 RCT PST-HC vs. usual care (UC) to treat depression and anxiety in home health care patients with heart disease.	Inclusion = Age: ≥ 65 years and older; homebound; cardiovascular disease; cognitively intact; DSM-IV criteria for subthreshold depression symptoms. Exclusion = cancer, coronary artery disease, renal disease on dialysis, dementia, psychotic disorder, major depression.	12-month study period. PST-HC: 6 weekly 1-hour sessions in patients' homes focused on problem identification and orientation, thought stopping, and problem-solving techniques. UC+E: 6 routine nurse case manager home visits with 2 educational sessions on heart disease and depression; called twice over 6-week period for brief check-in; no counseling offered.	$n = 36$. PST-HC 9: $n = 18$; M age = 75.6 years; 94.4% female; 94.4% White; 88.9% living alone; # medical conditions: $M = 5.1$. UC+E: $n = 18$; M age = 76.2 years; 88.8% female; 94.4% White; 88.9% living alone; # medical conditions: $M = 5.4$.	PST-HC group reported significantly larger decrease in depressive symptoms, significant increases in mental health and emotional role functioning, and greater overall satisfaction with time with staff and treatment delivery.	PST-HC intervention had significant positive effects on older home health care patients with cardiovascular disease. PST-HC offers potentially sustainable service delivery approach by home care agencies.

Study	Inclusion/Exclusion	Intervention	Sample	Results	Conclusion
Gellis et al., 2008 RCT Compared PST-HC and treatment as usual (TAU) for reducing depression among medically ill home health patients.	Inclusion = Age: ≥ 65 years or older; acute home care patients; minor depression. Exclusion = major depression, schizophrenia, bipolar disorder, substance abuse, psychosis, personality disorder, serious suicidal risk, cognitive impairment; current receipt of either psychotherapy or drug treatment for depression.	PST-HC 6 weekly1-hour sessions of home-based PST focused on problem-definition and selection, solution generation, and evaluation, plus standard acute home health care for medical treatment. TAU: Standard acute home health care and referral for medication assessment to PCP, augmented with educational literature.	n = 62. M age = 77.4 years. PST-HC: n = 30 M age = 77.3; 88% female; 85% White; 80% living alone; 3 or more medical conditions: 55%. TAU: n = 32 M age = 78; 87% female; 85% White; 80% living alone; 3 or more medical conditions: 55%.	PST-HC subjects had significantly lower levels of depressive symptoms, significantly higher problem-solving ability scores; but not significantly higher quality of life scores compared to TAU; PST-HC results maintained at 3 and 6 months after treatment ended.	PST-HC appears to be an effective brief psychosocial intervention to treat depressive symptoms in older home care patients with minor depression.
Gellis et al., 2007 Pilot RCT PST-HC compared to usual care (UC) for medically ill, depressed older home care patients.	Inclusion = Age: ≥ 65 years or older; acute home care patients; screened positive for depression and ≥ 24 on MMSE. Exclusion = Acute suicidal behavior, psychosis, bipolar disorder, or substance abuse within past month; current receipt of either psychotherapy or drug treatment for depression.	PST-HC: Manualized treatment of 6 weekly 1-hour sessions focused on problem-solving skills; completed two pleasurable activities per day; psycho-education about depression; UC: Standard acute home health care and referral for antidepressant medications from PCP; educational literature about depression. No direct counseling provided.	n = 48 initial. PST-HC: n = 20; M age = 79.7 years; 85% female; 80% White; 60% living alone; medical conditions: M = 2.8. UC: n = 20; M age = 80.1 years; 80% female; 85% White; 60% living alone; medical conditions: M = 2.7.	PST-HC patients reported significantly lower levels of depressive symptoms, higher quality of life, and higher problem-solving ability compared to UC group. Positive effects maintained at 3 and 6 months after treatment.	Brief home-based problem-solving intervention is feasible and associated with significantly lower depressive symptoms, increased quality of life, and increased problem-solving abilities relative to UC.

(continued)

TABLE 6.3 (CONTINUED)

Study	Inclusion/Exclusion Criteria	Description of Interventions	Number and Description of Participants	Outcomes	Findings

Ciechanowski et al., 2004
 	
RCT
 	
Home-based PEARLS (Program to Encourage Active, Rewarding Lives for Seniors) vs. usual care (UC) to treat minor depression or dysthymia among older adults.
	Inclusion = Age: ≥ 60 years or older; receiving services from senior service agencies or living in senior public housing; DSM-IV minor depression or dysthymia diagnostic criteria.
	
	Exclusion = no depression; major depression, bipolar disorder, psychosis, substance abuse, cognitive impairment.
		PEARLS intervention:
		
		Eight 50-minute in-home problem-solving treatments, social and physical activation, and recommendations to physicians regarding antidepressants, as needed.
		
		UC:
		
		No additional services, but letters sent to patients' physicians and social workers reporting depression diagnoses with recommendations to continue usual care.
			n = 138.
			
			PEARLS intervention:
			n = 72;
			M age = 72.6 years;
			82% female;
			racial/ethnic minority: 42%;
			dysthymia:61%;
			minor depression: 38%.
			
			UC:
			n = 66;
			M age = 73.5 years;
			76% female;
			racial/ethnic minority: 43%;
			dysthymia: 35%;
			minor depression: 65%.
				PEARLS intervention resulted in significantly lower severity and greater remission of depression, greater health-related quality of life, and improved functional well-being and emotional well-being compared to usual care at 6 and 12 months.	PEARLS significantly reduced depressive symptoms and improved health status in chronically medically ill older adults with minor depression and dysthymia.

white, and widowed. Those participating in PST-HC received six weekly 1-hour sessions conducted over a 6-week period. During these sessions, patients were taught problem-solving coping skills, including problem identification and orientation, thought stopping, and problem-solving techniques. Participants were also instructed to complete two pleasurable activities per day. Those in the UC+E condition received six weekly routine nurse case manager home visits (including two educational sessions on cardiovascular disease and receipt of a depression brochure). These participants were also called twice over the 6-week period for a brief check-in. No counseling was offered to these patients. All services were provided in the patients' homes.

Study outcomes revealed that the PST-HC group experienced a significantly larger decrease in depressive symptoms than did those in the UC+E group. PST-HC participants also experienced statistically significant increases in mental health and emotional role functioning, while UC+E participants did not. Finally, the PST-HC group reported greater satisfaction with time spent with staff, accessibility, communication, interpersonal manner, and an overall satisfaction with treatment delivery. No significant impact on anxiety was found for either treatment condition. Overall, this study found that PST-HC had significant positive effects on older home health care patients with cardiovascular disease, and that PST-HC offered a potentially sustainable treatment approach for home care agencies working with older medically ill patient.

In 2008, Gellis et. al. examined the effectiveness of PST versus treatment as usual (TAU) for reducing depression among medically ill home health patients. The inclusion criteria for this study were (1) adults 65 years or older; (2) acute home care patients; and (3) having minor depression, as indicated by a score of 11 or higher on the Hamilton Rating Scale for Depression. Individuals were excluded from the study if they were too ill to participate; had major depression, psychosis, schizophrenia, schizoaffective disorder, bipolar disorder, alcohol or other substance abuse in the last 6 months; were at serious suicidal risk; had moderate to severe cognitive impairment; or were current recipients of either psychotherapy or drug treatment for depression. Sixty-two individuals, ranging in age from 65 to 99 years, participated in this study. Of the 62, 30 participated in the PST-HC. The remaining 32 participants received TAU. The highest percentages of both groups were female and white. The PST-HC intervention consisted of six weekly sessions of home-based PST, with each session lasting an hour. The PST skills of problem-definition, solution generation, weighing pros and cons, problem selection, and solution evaluation were reviewed during each weekly session. Participants also received home health care for their medical treatment, referral for medication assessment to their primary care physician, and educational materials describing depression. Individuals participating in TAU received standard acute home health care for their medical treatment, referral for medication assessment to their primary care physician, and educational literature on depression. They were also contacted weekly to assess need for crisis management or mental health referral, but no direct counseling was provided. All participants received follow-up interviews post-treatment at 3 and 6 months.

Study findings revealed that older adults in the PST-HC condition had significantly lower levels of depressive symptoms and significantly higher problem-solving ability scores than did those in TAU. Those in the TAU condition did not experience any significant changes on any measure from baseline to post treatment. PST-HC results were maintained at 3 and 6 months after treatment ended. This study provides support for the effectiveness of PST in reducing depressive symptoms in older home care patients with minor depression.

Gellis, McGinty, Horowitz, Bruce, and Misener (2007) implemented a pilot program to compare the effects of PST with usual care (UC) for medically ill, depressed older adults. Participants were recruited through a home-care agency, and met the following criteria: (1) 65 years or older; (2) scored a 22 or higher on the CES-D; (3) scored a 24 or lower on the MMSE; and (4) spoke English. Those with acute suicidal behavior, diagnosis of psychosis, bipolar disorder, or substance abuse within the past month were excluded, as well as those currently receiving psychotherapy or drug treatment for depression. All 40 participants included were receiving at-home care for medical problems and had depressive symptoms. Twenty participants (M = 79.7 years) received PST-HC. The remaining 20 participants (M = 80.71years) received usual care. The majority of both groups were female and white. Those in the PST-HC group received training in problem-solving skills and psycho-education about depression, were asked to complete two pleasurable activities per day, and were given homework related to each step in the PST process. The vast majority of participants in the PST-HC group (93%) completed their weekly homework. UC participants received the usual home health care for their condition, literature concerning depression, and referral to their physician for medication assessment.

Study results indicated that PST-HC patients achieved significantly lower levels of depression, higher quality of life, and higher problem-solving ability, as indicated by standardized measures, compared to the UC group. UC patients did not experience any significant changes on any measure from baseline to post-treatment. Positive effects for PST participants were maintained at 3 and 6 months after treatment. Study findings provide support for the claim that PST is both feasible and effective in lowering depressive symptoms and increasing quality of life and problem-solving abilities among depressed older home-care patients.

Ciechanowski et al. (2004) examined the impact of a home-based PST program for detecting and managing depression among older adults. The study compared the Program to Encourage Active, Rewarding Lives for Seniors (PEARLS) to usual care (UC). To be included in this study, participants had to be 60 years of age or older and receiving services from senior service agencies or living in senior public housing. Subjects also met the DSM-IV criteria for minor depression or dysthymia. Adults with no depression, major depression, bipolar disorder, psychosis, substance abuse, or cognitive impairment demonstrated by the Mini-Mental State Examination were excluded. In all, 138 older adults were included in the study. Participants (M = 73.0 years) were 79% female and had an average of 4.6 (SD = 2.1) chronic medical conditions.

Seventy-two participants received the PEARLS intervention, while 66 received usual care. The PEARLS intervention consisted of problem-solving treatment, social and physical activation, and potential recommendations to patients' physicians regarding antidepressant medications. The intervention contained eight 50-minute in-home problem-solving sessions over 19 weeks. PST sessions were modified to provide greater emphasis on social and physical activation. The goal of physical activity was duration of 30 minutes for at least 5 days per week. Group activities encouraging peer support were given highest priority. Usual care participants received no additional services. However, letters were sent to the patients' regular physicians and social workers, reporting their depression diagnosis with recommendations to continue usual care. Depression and quality of life were assessed at baseline and at 12 months.

The PEARLS intervention resulted in significantly lower severity, and greater remission, of depression compared with usual care at 6 and 12 months. At 12 months, PEARLS patients were more likely to have at least a 50% reduction in depressive symptoms, achieved complete remission from depression, and have greater health-related quality of life improvements in functional well-being and emotional well-being than those in the UC condition. Relatively few patients initiated antidepressants, and no net increase in antidepressants was found in either group. The PEARLS intervention significantly reduced depressive symptoms and improved health status in chronically medically ill older adults with minor depression and dysthymia. As a result, the authors assert that by partnering with community agencies, it is possible to target and treat depressed, frail elderly adults with non-pharmacological treatments such as PST.

CAREGIVING

Four studies examined PST in relation to caregiving (see Table 6.4). Garand et al. (2014) examined the effectiveness of PST for reducing the likelihood of depression among caregivers of individuals with mild cognitive impairment (MCI) or early dementia. Employing a sample of 73 predominantly White, female caregivers with a mean age of 65 years, the authors compared a two-phase PST group to a nutrition comparison group. Of these 73 caregivers, 43 were caring for individuals with MCI (23 in the PST group and 20 in the nutrition group) and 30 for those with early dementia (13 in the PST group and 17 in the nutrition group). The first phase of the PST intervention consisted of six sessions of PST that lasted about 1.5 hours each, took place in the caregiver's home, and were set about 2 weeks apart. The second phase included three 45-minute telephone contacts set 2 weeks apart. The nutrition group was matched to the PST group in terms of the number and duration of sessions. Nutrition group participants received guidelines and information about nutrition.

In assessing depression, anxiety, and problem-solving orientation at months 1, 3, 6, and 12 following treatment, the authors found that enhancing problem-solving skills for caregivers resulted in positive mental health outcomes. Skill attainment was most

TABLE 6.4 PST CAREGIVER STUDIES

Study	Inclusion/Exclusion Criteria	Description of Interventions	Number and Description of Participants	Outcomes	Findings
Garand et al., 2014 RCT PST vs. nutritional group to reduce likelihood of depression among caregivers of individuals with mild cognitive impairment or early dementia.	Inclusion = Live with person with new diagnosis of MCI or early dementia; live in community setting; live within 300-mile radius; understand English.	PST Two phases of treatment 6 sessions of about 1.5 hours each, in caregiver's home, about 2 weeks apart; then, 3 telephone contacts of about 45 minutes each, about 2 weeks apart. Nutrition education: Same as PST in terms of number and duration of sessions; given DHHS guidelines about nutrition.	Caregivers: n = 73; M age = 65 years; 78.1% female; 98.6% White; years in relationship with care recipient: 34.8 M; live alone with care recipient: 32.8%; Care recipients: M age = 75.5 years; 35.6% female; MCI: 43; early dementia: 30.	PST led to significantly reduced depression symptoms, particularly among early dementia caregivers, lowered caregivers' anxiety levels, and led to lessening of negative problem orientation compared to nutrition group.	Enhanced problem-solving skills resulted in positive mental health outcomes when learned early diagnosis, especially in those caring for those with dementia. PST was feasible and acceptable to family caregivers of older adults with new cognitive diagnoses.
Pfeiffer et al., 2014 Germany RCT PST vs. control group to treat depression and improve competence and problem-solving skills among stroke caregivers.	Inclusion = Stroke survivors: Age: ≥ 60 years or older at time of most recent stroke; in need of care or supervision; no terminal disease; did not plan to move into a nursing home within the next 6 months. Caregivers: Reside in the metropolitan area; at least 18 years old; understand and speak German.	PST Group: 2 home visits (initial and at month 4), 18 60–150 minute telephone calls delivered over 3 month intervention period and 9-month maintenance period. Control group: Received monthly information letters in addition to usual care.	n = 122. PST group n = 60. Caregivers: M age = 66.7 years; M months caregiving = 30; 76.7% female; 85% German. Care recipients: M age = 73.4 years; 31.7% female; Control group: n = 62. Caregivers: M age = 65.6 years; M months caregiving = 26; 79% female; 79% German.	Caregivers of PST group showed significantly lower levels of depressive symptoms after 3 and 12 months, but no better sense of competence compared to the control group. No effects found on caregivers' social problem-solving abilities.	Although beneficial effects were observed among caregivers in the PST group, the lack of effects on problem-solving abilities implies that other characteristics of the intervention might account for these benefits.

Study	Inclusion/Exclusion	Intervention	Sample	Results	Conclusions
Demiris et al., 2012 Randomized trial Effectiveness of PST delivered face-to-face vs. videophone PST for hospice primary caregivers.	Inclusion = Enrolled as family/informal caregiver of hospice patient; 18 years or older; no or only mild cognitive impairment without functional hearing loss or with hearing aid that allows participant to conduct phone conversations; access to a standard telephone line at home. Exclusion = Score of less than 7 on Short Portable Mental Status Questionnaire.	Both interventions began within 20 days of hospice admission, and employed manualized PST. PST face-to-face: 3 visits lasting about 45 minutes each. PST via videophone: 3 calls lasting about 45 minutes each.	n = 126. M age = 59.6 years. PST face-to-face: n = 77; M age = 59.5 years; 71.4% female; 13% HS education; 40.3% college degree; 89.6% White. PST via videophone: n = 49; M age = 59.7 years; 79.6% female; 83.7% White.	PST delivered via video was not inferior to face-to-face delivery. The observed changes in quality of life, problem-solving, and anxiety scores were similar for each group. Caregiver quality of life improved and state anxiety decreased under both conditions.	Intervention delivered in both modalities was associated with improvement in caregiver quality of life and problem-solving ability, and reduction of Anxiety. Audiovisual PST is effective and provides a solution to geographic barriers that inhibit treatment.
Grant et al., 2002 RCT In-person plus telephone social problem-solving partnerships (SPTP) vs. comparison and control groups for caregivers of stroke survivors.	Inclusion = Primary caregiver for stroke survivor; provide at least 6 hours of care per day; were related by blood or marriage; 18 years of age or older; were reachable by telephone.	SPTP treatment: Initial 3-hour face-to-face session with trained nurse in home, followed by weekly telephone contacts at weeks 2, 3, and 4 after discharge and biweekly telephone contacts at weeks 6, 8, 10, and 12 after discharge. Comparison group received same number of weekly and biweekly telephone contacts as SPTP group; asked to identify professional and skilled health services received by stroke survivor since last contact. Control group: Usual discharge planning services only.	Participants: n = 74. Caregivers: M age = 58 years; 74% White; 41% spouses; 36% daughters. Stroke survivors: M age = 73 years; 74% White.	SPTP group had significantly better social problem-solving skills, significantly less negative orientation and impulsivity/carelessness, but more rational problem-solving skills, significantly greater caregiver preparedness, and less depression than comparison or control group. No significant differences among the groups regarding caregiver burden.	Problem-solving training by telephone was beneficial and acceptable for family caregivers of stroke survivors after discharge from rehabilitative facilities.

prominent soon after diagnosis, especially for dementia caregivers. PST treatment lowered the caregivers' levels of anxiety and resulted in a significant lessening of negative problem orientation. In addition, PST reduced depressive symptoms significantly, especially for dementia caregivers. Conversely, participants in the nutrition group displayed anxiety levels that were higher than those of the PST group, as well as levels of depression that remained elevated when compared to those of the PST group. Overall, the authors found PST to be a feasible and acceptable intervention for caregivers of older adults following a cognitive diagnoses.

Pfeiffer at al. (2014) studied the effects of a problem-solving intervention (PSI) for caregivers of stroke survivors residing in Germany. The authors employed a sample of 122 caregivers over a 3-month intervention period, followed by a 9-month maintenance period. For inclusion in the study, caregivers were required to have provided at least 10.5 hours of care per week for 6 months to 5 years after the care recipient's last stroke. Caregivers were also required to have reported distress associated with caregiving, as well other logistical criteria, such as being able to speak German. Stroke survivors were 70% male, had a mean age of 72.9 years, received care at home, required a minimum of 1.5 hours of care or supervision per day on average, and were not suffering from a terminal disease. The 60 caregivers in the PST group ($M = 66.7$ years, $M = 30$ months of caregiving) received two home visits during the initial and fourth months of the study, 18 telephone calls over the 3-month intervention and 9-month maintenance period, and monthly information letters in addition to usual care. Each telephone call lasted from 60–150 minutes, and four additional calls could be provided during the maintenance period in case of crisis. The 62 caregivers in the control group ($M = 65.6$ years; $M = 26$ months of caregiving) received only monthly information letters in addition to usual care.

Findings indicated that caregivers in the PSI group showed significantly lower levels of depressive symptoms after 3 and 12 months compared to the information-only control group. However, the PSI group displayed no greater sense of competence when compared to the control group, nor were any effects found on the caregivers' social problem-solving abilities. The authors posit that this lack of effect on problem-solving abilities may be attributable to other characteristics of the intervention. Ultimately, the authors concluded that the "relative intensity and therapeutic contact during the first 3 months of the intervention" (Pfeiffer at al., 2014, p. 628) may be of particular help in reducing depressive symptoms among the caregivers of stroke victims.

Demiris et al. (2012) examined the effectiveness of PST delivered face to face as compared to PST administered via videophone for hospice primary caregivers. A total of 126 hospice caregivers ($M = 59.6$ years) were included in the study, with each caregiver providing care for one patient only. Both the face-to-face PST group of 77 participants and the videophone PST group of 49 patients were similar in demographics ($M = 59.5$ years, 71.4% female, and 89.6% White; and $M = 59.7$ years, 79.6% female, and 83.7% White, respectively).

The face-to-face PST intervention consisted of three visits lasting about 45 minutes each, and PST via videophone consisted of three video calls of 45 minutes each. Both interventions took place within 20 days of the care recipients' admission into hospice care. Participants in each condition also received an exit interview after the third and final call or visit. The authors assessed quality of life, problem-solving, and anxiety, and found that the observed changes in scores were similar for both groups: quality of life for caregivers improved, and state anxiety decreased under both conditions, prompting Demiris and colleagues to conclude that PST delivered via video was not inferior to PST delivered face to face.

Grant, Elliott, Weaver, Bartolucci, and Giger (2002) conducted an RCT to explore the efficacy of telephone PST delivered to family caregivers of stroke survivors after discharge from rehabilitation facilities. The initial sample size included 74 caregivers, with 63 completing the intervention (85%). The caregivers had a mean age of 58 years and were 74% White; 41% were spouses of the stroke survivors, and 36% were daughters. The stroke survivors had a mean age of 73 years and were also 74% White. Referring to the PST intervention as "social problem-solving telephone partnerships" (SPTP), the authors compared the SPTP group to a control group and a comparison group over an 18-month intervention period. All three groups received usual discharge planning services provided by the hospitals included in the study. Data were collected 1–2 days before discharge, at 5 and 9 weeks during the intervention, and at 13 weeks following the intervention. For the SPTP group, there was an initial 3-hour face-to-face session with a trained nurse in the caregiver's home, followed by weekly telephone contacts at weeks 2, 3, and 4 after discharge. These were followed by biweekly telephone contacts at weeks 6, 8, 10, and 12 after discharge. The comparison intervention group received the same number of weekly and biweekly telephone contacts as the SPTP group. Caregivers in this group were asked to identify professional and skilled health services that the stroke survivor received since the last contact was made. The control group received only the usual discharge planning services.

At the end of the 18-month study period, researchers reported the SPTP group had significantly better social problem-solving skills than did the comparison or control group. In addition, the SPTP group had more rational problem-solving skills and demonstrated significantly fewer negative and impulsivity/carelessness orientation characteristics. The SPTP group had lowered depression and significantly greater caregiver preparedness than did the comparison intervention or control groups. While there were no significant differences among the groups regarding caregiver burden, caregivers' satisfaction with healthcare services decreased over time for the control group and remained comparable for both the SPTP and comparison groups. On the whole, the authors conclude that problem-solving training by telephone may be useful for family caregivers caring for stroke survivors after discharge from rehabilitative facilities.

CONCLUSION

Compared to the overall research focused on PST, far fewer studies have been conducted on the efficacy of this approach with older adults. However, the majority of these studies do support its utility in treating depression in older adult populations both with and without underlying executive impairments. The majority of studies indicate that PST is at least as effective as psychotropic medications and other psychotherapies in improving problem-solving, coping, and mental well-being among community-dwelling and homebound older adults.

In addition to decreasing depression, PST is also effective in enhancing medical care. This process assists older patients in dealing with health issues such as managing cancer care. Research indicates that PST is effective in decreasing symptom severity, which enhances patients' and care providers' quality of life. With the increasing probability of health-related issues in the older population, the use of PST in acute and long-term care setting seems appropriate. Additional research on the use of this approach in different contexts and with different medical diagnoses is warranted.

In addition, PST provides another avenue for supporting those in caregiving roles. Notably, consistent support was found for the efficacy of telephone and videophone PST, indicating that these alternate means of administration may help overcome geographic barriers that prevent in-person access to therapy. Caregivers who participated in PST and related therapies had decreased depression and anxiety. Additionally, their abilities to perform in caregiving roles through better problem-solving and caregiving competence was enhanced.

While these results are promising, notable limitations exist among the studies reviewed. First, sample sizes in most studies were small. The median number of participants in the studies included in the meta-analysis was 44, while 40% of the RCTs reviewed had less than 100, and 80% had less than 200 subjects. In addition, in all studies that reported race and gender, the vast majority of the participants were White females. Studies with larger numbers of older participants who possess greater diversity are critical. Little to no information is currently available concerning the potential impact of varying cultural backgrounds on the effectiveness of PST.

In spite of these limitations, the current research does suggest that PST can be a highly beneficial treatment option. This is especially relevant due to the demonstrated flexibility of PST. Even among the limited number of studies performed with older adults, the flexibility of PST is clearly demonstrated. Studies conducted in the community, in in-home settings, and with older clients suffering from a variety of serious illnesses and their caregivers exhibit the utility of PST in reducing depression and increasing mental well-being among aging populations.

REFERENCES

Alexopoulos, G. S., Raue, P., & Areán, P. (2003). Problem-solving therapy versus supportive therapy in geriatric major depression with executive dysfunction. *The American Journal of Geriatric Psychiatry*, *11*, 46–52.

Areán, P. A., Raue, P. R., Mackin, R. S., Kanellopoulos, D., McCullough, C., & Alexopoulos, G. S. (2010). Problem-solving therapy and supportive therapy in older adults with major depression and executive dysfunction. *The American Journal of Geriatric Psychiatry, 167,* 1391–1398.

Bell, A. C., & D'Zurilla, T. J. (2009). Problem-solving therapy for depression: a meta-analysis. *Clinical Psychology Review, 29*(4), 348–353.

Choi, N. G., Hegel, M. T., Marti, N., Marinucci, M. L., Sirriani, L., & Bruce, M. L. (2014). Telehealth problem-solving therapy for depressed low-income homebound older adults: acceptance and preliminary efficacy. *The American Journal of Geriatric Psychiatry, 22,* 263–271.

Ciechanowski, P., Wagner, E., Schmaling, K., Schwartz, S., Williams, B., Dieher, P., . . . LoGerfo, J. (2004). Community-integrated home-based depression treatment in older adults: a randomized controlled trial. *Journal of the American Medical Association, 291,* 1569–1577.

Cuijpers, P., van Straten, A., & Waarmerdam, L. (2007). Problem solving therapies for depression: a meta-analysis. *European Psychiatry, 22,* 9–15.

Demiris, G., Oliver, D. P., Wittenberg-Lyles, E., Washington, K., Doorenbos, A., Rue, T., & Berry, D. (2012). A noninferiority trial of a problem-solving intervention for hospice caregivers: in person versus videophone. *Journal of Pallative Medicine, 15,* 653–660.

Downe-Wamboldt, B. L., Butler, L. J., Melanson, P. M., Coulter, L. A., Singleton, J. F., Keefe, J. M., & Bell, D. G. (2007). The effects and expense of augmenting usual cancer clinic care with telephone problem-solving counseling. *Cancer Nursing, 30,* 441–453.

D'Zurilla, T. J., Nezu, A. M. (1999). *Problem-solving therapy: a social competence approach to clinical intervention* (2nd ed.). New York: Springer.

Garand, L., Rinaldo, D. E., Alberth, M. M., Delany, J., Beasock, S. L., Lopez, O. L., & Dew, M. A. (2014). Effects of problem solving therapy on mental health outcomes in family caregivers of persons with a new diagnosis of mild cognitive impairment of early dementia: a randomized controlled trial. *The American Journal of Geriatric Psychiatry, 22,* 771–781.

Gellis, Z. D., & Bruce, M. L. (2010). Problem solving therapy for subthreshold depression in home healthcare patients with cardiovascular disease. *The American Journal of Geriatric Psychiatry, 18,* 464–474.

Gellis, Z. D., McGinty, J, Horowitz, A., Bruce, M. L., & Misener, E. (2007). Problem-solving therapy for late-life depression in home care: a randomized field trial. *The American Journal of Geriatric Psychiatry, 15,* 968–978.

Gellis, Z. D., McGinty, J., Tierney, L., Jordan, C., & Misener, E. (2008). Randomized controlled trial of problem-solving therapy for minor depression in home care. *Research on Social Work Practice, 18,* 596–606.

Grant, J. S., Elliott, T. R., Weaver, M., Bartolucci, A. A., & Giger, J. N. (2002). Telephone intervention with family caregivers of stroke survivors after rehabilitation. *Stroke, 33,* 2060–2065.

Kirkham, J., Seitz, D., & Choi, N. G. (2015). Meta-analysis of problem solving therapy for the treatment of depression in older adults. *The American Journal of Geriatric Psychiatry, 23,* S129–S130.

Lam, C. L. K., Fong, D. Y. T., Chin, W.-Y., Lee, P. W. H., Lam, E. T. P., & Lo, Y. Y. C. (2010). Brief problem-solving treatment in primary care (PST-PC) was not more effective than comparison for elderly patients screened positive of psychological problems. *The American Journal of Geriatric Psychiatry, 25,* 968–980.

Nezu, A. M., Nezu, C. M., & D'Zurilla, T. J. (2013). *Problem-solving therapy: a treatment manual.* New York: Springer.

Pfeiffer, K., Beische, D., Berry, J., van Schayck, R., Hautzinger, M., Wengert, J., . . . Elliott, T. R. (2014). Telephone-based problem-solving intervention for family caregivers of stroke survivors: a randomized controlled trial. *Journal of Consulting and Clinical Psychology, 82*, 628–643.

Robinson, R. G., Jorge, R. E., Moser, D. J., Acion, L., Solodking, A., Small, S. L., . . . Ardnt, S., (2008). Escitalopram and problem-solving therapy for prevention of poststroke depression: a randomized controlled trial. *The Journal of the American Medical Association, 299*, 2391–2400.

Williams, J. W., Jr., Barrett, J., Oxman, T., Frank, E., Katon, W., Sullivan, M., . . . Sengupta, A. (2000). Treatment of dysthymia and minor depression in primary care: a randomized controlled trial in older adults. *Journal of the American Medical Association, 284*, 1519–1526.

7

MOTIVATIONAL INTERVIEWING
THEORY AND PRACTICE

Motivational interviewing (MI) is an approach to counseling that focuses on helping clients resolve ambivalence in an effort to work toward and effect behavioral change. MI has often been termed a counseling approach, a conversational style, and a way of being with clients, rather than an explicit type of therapy (Serdarevic & Lemke, 2013). MI practitioners work with clients to elicit and enhance their intrinsic motivation to achieve the behavioral change they desire and value.

MI possesses a clear focus that is explicitly rooted in the principles of autonomy and collaboration and includes a core set of communication techniques. It does not espouse prescribed steps to achieve predetermined outcomes, however. The Center for Substance Abuse Treatment (1999) notes that MI is "any clinical strategy designed to enhance client motivation for change" (p. xviii) and further specifies that successful MI contains the following elements (p. xix–xx):

- Expressing empathy through reflective listening
- Communicating respect for and acceptance of clients and their feelings
- Establishing a nonjudgmental, collaborative relationship
- Complimenting rather than denigrating
- Listening rather than telling
- Understanding that change is up to the client
- Developing discrepancy between clients' goals/values and their current behavior and helping clients recognize the discrepancies between where they are and where they would like to be
- Avoiding arguments and direct confrontation
- Adjusting to, rather than opposing, client resistance
- Focusing on clients' strengths and supporting self-efficacy.

Motivational interviewing is a brief treatment that typically has a duration of one to four sessions, although follow-up sessions are often included. MI has been used widely in the area of addiction and other health-related areas where behavioral change in needed. However, there are other areas where this approach can help older clients become motivated to change behaviors. One example is a need for a residential relocation when informal caregiving is no longer adequate to meet the care requirement of an older adult. Consider the following situation of an older husband who is caring for his wife with Alzheimer's disease.

Mr.and Mrs. Clark have been married for 53 years and live together in their home in a medium-size metropolitan area. About 5 years ago, Mrs. Clark was diagnosed with Alzheimer's disease, and Mr. Clark has been her primary caregiver. Although he continues in this role, his own health is suffering and his wife's condition is deteriorating. Their two adult children have been a source of support, but they both have their own families and careers. One of their daughters contacted a therapist to help the family with decision-making since their father is unwilling to consider moving from their home.

In working with Mr. Clark, the practitioner understood that he was less unwilling to move than he had expressed to his daughters. However, he was quite ambivalent about the possibility. He had been thinking about the precariousness of their living arrangement and his ability to provide care for his wife for some time. Yet, he also felt great sadness about leaving the house where they raised their children and moving to unfamiliar surroundings. He was also very concerned about Mrs. Clark and how she would adjust to a new place. The practitioner empathized with Mr. Clark's feeling of loss and reflected his deep commitment to and concern for his wife. This evolved into a conversation about the adjustments Mr. Clark had been able to make, thus far, to best care for his wife and the strengths and resources he possessed that had enabled him to do so. The practitioner was able to help Mr. Clark tap into his strong motivation to provide the best environment for his wife at this time and to help him explore what this type of environment may entail.

In working with him, the practitioner was able to help Mr. Clark consider possible options without becoming overwhelmed. Unlike his two daughters, who were forceful in their discussions that their parents "had to move," the practitioner accepted Mr. Clark's ambivalence and fear about a possible relocation. She helped him discern his deepest motivation (to care for his wife) and explore alternatives that were acceptable to him for achieving his goal. At the end of four sessions with the therapist, Mr. Clark had decided that an assisted living facility (ALF) would most likely provide the best care for his wife and would also allow the couple to remain together. He agreed to talk with the ALF administrators with his daughters, and have his daughters help him consider how to place his home on the market. In the meantime, he also decided that he would have a home health agency provide in-home assistance with Mrs. Clark to help with caregiving. Through the nonjudgmental motivational interviewing approach, the practitioner was able to help Mr. Clark confront his ambivalence, get in touch with his primary desire, and embark on his journey of securing the best living situation for his wife and himself.

HISTORY AND BACKGROUND

MI was originally developed by William Miller for use with clients experiencing sub-stance abuse disorders. In the early 1980s, two events converged that led to the devel-opment of MI. The first was Miller's reflection on and articulation of his own personal counseling style in response to questions posed during a training session he presented on behavioral interventions for substance abusers. The second was emerging research indi-cating that therapist empathy and use of a client-centered interpersonal style were greater predictors of problematic drinking reduction than were specific types of substance abuse treatments.

In his own research, Miller found that interventionists' empathy had a greater impact on client drinking than did the particular interventions being investigated in the research studies (Miller & Baca, 1983). Reflecting on his own personal style, Miller noted that he also used an empathic and client-centered approach. Further, he favored language that evoked and strengthened clients' expressions of their own motivation to change. He went on to distinguish between specific styles of communication that produced *change behav-ior* talk, rather than *sustain behavior* responses, from clients. From this reflection, he devel-oped a central principle of MI: arguments for change must arise from and be expressed by the client rather than the therapist (Miller & Rose, 2009).

Miller met Stephen Rollnick, who was familiar with the use of MI for addiction treat-ment in the United Kingdom, in 1989 (Miller & Rose, 2009). The two began teach-ing motivational techniques, but soon realized that techniques alone did not capture MI. As a result, they articulated the "spirit" of MI to convey the fundamental perspec-tive that underlies the MI approach. They published the first book on MI, *Motivational Interviewing: Preparing People to Change Addictive Behavior*, in 1991. Since that time, the use of MI to treat substance abuse has grown exponentially. Motivational enhance-ment therapy (MET)—client assessment and feedback combined with motivational interviewing—emerged in the 1990s. MET is a manualized brief four-session inter-vention to treat individuals with alcohol abuse and dependence (Miller, Zweben, DiClemente, & Rychtarik, 1999). Since the 1990s the use of MI and MET have moved beyond the field of addictions. With its focus on helping clients resolve ambivalence, MI and MET are now used in the fields of health care, corrections, education, and beyond to assist clients in effecting behavioral changes to enhance their lives (Cummings, Cooper, & Cassie, 2009; Moyers & Rollnick, 2002).

THEORETICAL FOUNDATION

Theoretically, MI builds on Carl Roger's client-centered therapy (Hohman, 2012). To Miller, Roger's focus on empathy, genuineness, and unconditional acceptance described an environment that was safe and supportive enough for clients' honest exploration of their behavior and ambivalence concerning change. The MI approach is also linked to

Festinger's theory of cognitive dissonance (1957), which purports that individuals experience stress in the face of cognitive dissonance (i.e., holding two or more contradictory beliefs at the same time), and that this stress motivates the individual to engage in action to reduce conflict. When dissonance or ambivalence is due to a behavior, the individual can select among several types of actions—for example, deny, justify, or change behavior. In Miller's experience, clients who hear themselves articulate arguments for change are more likely to resolve their dissonance (ambivalence) in the favor of change than are those who hear the argument from a therapist (Miller & Rose, 2009).

MI also aligns with the transtheoretical model of change (TTM) (Prochaska & DiClemente, 1984), which is a six-stage model. Each stage has implications for understanding a client's motivation for behavioral change. Because change is a cyclical process, clients move back and forth between stages in a nonlinear fashion.

The first stage is *pre-contemplation* (lacking readiness to change). Those at this stage see no problem with their behavior and have no plans to change. Individuals may remain at this stage for months or years, or may never move beyond this stage. Those at this stage may be completely unaware that their behavior is problematic and may have not even considered the possibility of change. Others may have heard the admonitions of others concerning their behavior but see no personal need for change. There are still others who realize their behavior is problematic but are discouraged due to past failed change efforts and are not currently considering behavior alteration. Most, although not all, of those at the pre-contemplation stage have not yet experienced harsh consequences of their behavior because their behaviors have not yet escalated to a harmful level.

Stage two is *contemplation* (thinking of changing). People at this stage realize that their behavior is concerning and are considering behavior change. They are more aware of the pros and cons of their behavior and are actively weighing the costs and benefits of change. This deliberation may produce great ambivalence and, as a result, individuals may remain at this stage for prolonged periods of time (Miller et al., 1999).

In the remaining stages, individuals are beginning to focus on the change process. *Preparation* (ready to change) is the third stage. At this point, individuals have come to believe that the pros of behavioral change outweigh the cons, and that change will lead to a healthier life. They are ready, and they intend to take action. *Action* (making change) is stage four, in which individuals have taken steps to change their behaviors and have modified their environment, experiences, and behaviors in order to achieve their desired goals. Stage five is *maintenance*. At this stage, individuals intend to maintain the behavioral change and actively engage in ongoing work to sustain new behaviors and prevent relapse. Additionally, they are increasingly confident that they can maintain their behavior.

The sixth and last stage is conceptualized in two different ways. As conceived by Prochaska and DiClemente (1984, 1997), the final stage is *termination*. At this point, individuals no longer experience temptation and possess self-efficacy. An alternate way of thinking about this stage has been proposed as a time of *reoccurrence* (SAMHSA, 1999). This view is proffered due to the recognition that most people do not make steady progress through the stages of change to complete adherence to new behaviors. Rather, re-engagement in original behaviors is not unusual. However, individuals can gain important information from these experiences that lead them to more effective strategies for maintaining behavioral change in the future. Miller and Rollnick (2013) note that MI techniques align particularly well with the earlier stages of the TTM, particularly pre-contemplation, contemplation, and preparation, in which clients are less ready for change.

A foundational belief of MI, adopted from Rogerian therapy, is that all people have the desire to be happy and to develop themselves to their fullest potential, despite the barriers that might block their way (Hohman, 2012). Individuals have innate internal motivation and will engage in changes they believe are relevant to their own concerns, interests, and values. Most people, for example, do want to live healthy lives and avoid disease and disability. Taking steps to achieve this desired goal, however, is often undermined by opposing internal desires and reluctance to engage in new behaviors that are perceived as being difficult or unpleasant. Individuals contemplating change, for example, may be comfortable with their current routines, and reluctant to make changes that take effort (e.g., exercising), are uncomfortable (e.g., doing a finger prick to test blood sugar levels), and/or necessitate altering a behavior that one enjoys (e.g., eating sweets, smoking). Therefore, a major aspect of MI is working with the ambivalence that clients experience considering and adopting strategies for change within their lives.

UNDERSTANDING CLIENT AMBIVALENCE

A main goal of MI is helping clients move toward and engage in change by working through ambivalence. Ambivalence can be understood as an internal conflict between the perceived pros and cons of change (Cooper, 2012). In the past, clients who were able to perceive the benefits of modifying a behavior, yet did not take action to do so, were often labeled as "resistant." However, in motivational interviewing, ambivalence is seen as a natural part of the human experience and a normal part of the change process. Research indicates that a very large proportion of clients entering therapy are at the "pre-contemplation stage" of change. That is, they are experiencing levels of ambivalence high enough to preclude active adoption of change (Dozios, Westra, Collins, et al., 2004). A common sign of ambivalence is "yes-but" statements (see Table 7.1).

TABLE 7.1 EXAMPLES OF "YES-BUT" STATEMENTS

I really do want to lose weight—but I just love chocolate.

I know I should cut down on drinking a bit—but having a scotch when I get home from work really helps me to unwind.

I would exercise more, and I used to—but as I've gotten older my knee has started to hurt and I don't want to push it.

My husband and I should get into marriage counseling. We need it—but I'm afraid if I bring it up he'll get mad.

In order to make a decision to engage in behavioral change, individuals must resolve their ambivalence. Although frustrating for therapists, client ambivalence does indicate that clients recognize the need for change on some level. If a client did not perceive some benefits to change, no ambivalence would exist. According to motivational interviewing, the therapist's job is to draw out the motivation for change.

Approaching client ambivalence with openness, understanding, and respect is critical to the MI process. The very nature of ambivalence suggests that a person both does and does not want to change and, as a result, is experiencing an internal conflict. If the therapist argues or tries to persuade or convince the client of the "rightness" of one side of the argument (for change), this evokes a tendency for the client to argue the other side (not to change). Since people tend to believe their own arguments more than those provided by others, clients who vocalize arguments against change can talk themselves into maintaining the status quo. When therapists present the client with something that he or she is doing wrong (e.g., drinking too much, not exercising enough) and *should* change, clients often react by defending themselves and their current behavior (e.g., "I don't drink any more than most of my friends"; "I hardly drink at all during the week—only on the weekends"; "I don't have time to exercise"; "the gym is too far away"). MI recognizes that people have a natural tendency to resist being pushed in one direction, especially if it is not a direction in which they currently wish to go.

PROCESS OF CHANGE IN MOTIVATIONAL INTERVIEWING

The process of change in MI also involves various stages that are undertaken within the therapeutic relationships. MI consists of the interrelated processes of engaging, focusing, evoking, and planning (Miller & Rollnick, 2013). *Engaging* is the process in which the worker and client establish a connection and sufficient trust for the client to explore behavioral change. *Focusing* involves establishing a direction for the conversation concerning change. This direction may not be the one that the worker originally envisioned; rather, it must be based on the client's values and goals. The process of *evoking* involves eliciting the client's own motivations for change and facilitating the client's vocalization of this motivation. MI moves to the *planning* phase once the client has expressed a commitment to change. The therapist elicits change strategies from the client, and works with the client to establish a concrete and viable plan for change.

The spirit of motivational interviewing entails core beliefs concerning the therapist's "way of being" with a client that result in the development of a positive relationship conducive to calling forth clients' motivation to change. Four elements are central to the spirit of MI—partnership, acceptance, compassion and evocation (Miller & Rollnick, 2013). In previous work, Miller and Rollnick (1991) defined these elements as autonomy, collaboration, evocation, and support. The present conceptualization places even greater emphasis on the therapist's recognition of and communication to the client of her or his belief in the client's innate worth and value as a human being.

Partnership between therapists and clients is key to MI. Others therapies, such as CBT, also use partnership, or collaboration, as the basis for the worker–client relationship (Beck, 2011). In MI, however, partnership is viewed as essential for the development of a relationship that is capable of evoking clients' motivation to change.

While therapists have certain expertise related to MI processes and techniques, clients are recognized as the expert of their own lives. No one understands the clients' history, current situation, values, or desires as do the clients themselves. The therapists express *acceptance* of the clients for who they are and for where they are at the particular point in life. Acceptance in these terms reflects back to the Rogerian principle of unconditional positive regard (Roger, 1951).

Through nonjudgmental acceptance, therapists communicate to clients that their perspective is understandable and valid as viewed through their own framework. A therapist provides the support and space for clients to open up and acknowledge their true selves and situation, instead of holding on to who they may think they need to be, as perceived by others. Once individuals can acknowledge that they are struggling, or that their behaviors/situations are not all that they want them to be or believe they should be, then they can begin to explore the discrepancy between what they want and their current situation and behavior (Rosengren, 2009). For this reason, therapists do not try to dictate, cajole, or persuade the client to engage in certain behaviors. Rather, workers and clients participate in active collaborative conversation and joint decision-making. "MI is not a way of tricking people into change; it is a way of activating their own motivation and resources for change" (Miller & Rollnick, 2013, p. 15). The role of the worker, therefore, is one that consists more of guiding than directing. The old adage "you cannot make another person change" is a fundamental principle of MI. As a result, partnership is essential to the therapeutic relationship. The metaphor of "dancing rather than wrestling" has often been used to describe the worker–client relationship in MI (Miller & Rollnick, 2013). The therapist actively listens to and expresses genuine respect for the client's values and desires. This respect for and acceptance of the client is rooted in *compassion*, that is, the therapist's authentic commitment to fostering the well-being of the client (Miller & Rollnick, 2013). In the end, accepting and promoting clients' welfare are critical to the MI spirit and to the successful process of change.

The spirit of MI also focuses on recognizing and honoring client *autonomy*, which involves allocating responsibility for change to the client. Therapists often harbor the idea that if they are "good enough therapists" they will be able to make clients understand the need for change, or that they will have the skill needed to guide the client to the place where clients take necessary steps to modify behavior in the necessary direction. On the other hand, MI asserts that the worker must be detached from the client outcome, because the client is the one who must make the decision to change and carry out that change. According to MI, therapists must let go of the belief that it is their job to fix a client or that they are supposed to know, and be able to provide, all the right answers (Miller & Rollnick, 2013). Those engaging in MI practice do not coerce clients into taking a course of action that they believe is in the best interest of the clients. This type of engagement is avoided in favor of active exploration of the client's thoughts and concerns about her situation and the possibility of change.

In the end, MI practitioners support what the clients choose, even if the practitioners do not believe that the choice is in the best interest of the client (Rosengren, 2009). For example, a client may be well aware of the health risks of smoking given a COPD (chronic obstructive pulmonary disease) diagnosis, but after discussing the pros and cons of this behavior, chooses to continue smoking anyway. While the MI practitioner would not affirm this decision, the therapist would accept and respect the decision and leave the door open for further discussion. The alternative therapist behavior (i.e., trying to convince or pressure the client into smoking cessation) would likely result in the client coming to the same decision but with little openness to future discussion with the therapist.

Evocation, another key element of the MI spirit, involves drawing out clients' own desires, values, and goals and their thoughts on how they would like to accomplish their goals (Hohman, 2012). MI recognizes the strengths that clients possess. Rather than coming from a deficit viewpoint (e.g., fixing what is wrong with the client or providing what the client lacks), MI is rooted in the strengths perspective. A belief is that clients already have the needed drive and resources to engage in change. If clients are ambivalent, this provides evidence that they do have some ideas of the need for change, even if vaguely formed. From prior experience, clients also have knowledge of the skills and resources they have successfully utilized to accomplish desired goals. An essential job of the therapist is to help clients call forth their own reasons for change, their goal for behavioral change, and the methods for accomplishing this modification that best fit with their own abilities and within the context of their own lives (Rosengren, 2009). Therefore, MI involves evoking what is already present within the client, rather than installing what is lacking.

PRACTICE APPROACHES AND APPLICATION

In the practice of MI, the practitioner uses various skills and techniques to enhance the client's ability to work through ambivalence and develop a sustainable plan for action. In order to facilitate this process, the practitioner must understand the client's situation through his or her unique perspective, and must develop a relationship with sufficient trust to enable the exploration of change. Through various examples of practitioner–client dialogue, this section presents MI skills and techniques essential to this process.

PRINCIPLES OF MOTIVATIONAL INTERVIEWING

There are four principles fundamental to the practice of MI. Flowing directly from the MI spirit, these principles are expressing empathy, developing discrepancy, rolling with resistance, and supporting self-efficacy (Miller & Rollnick 2002). *Empathy* refers to the therapist's ability to understand the client's meaning and worldview. Through reflective listening, the therapist expresses this understanding and communicates respect for the client's feelings. Empathy enables the development of trust, which is necessary for the client to feel safe enough to open up and explore issues. As a result, MI therapists avoid non-empathic responses such as directing, warning, giving advice, lecturing, moralizing, judging, interpreting, or disagreeing. Non–empathic responses to be avoided also include agreeing, approving, and consoling (CSAT, 1999). Through listening and nonjudgmentally reflecting back the words and emotions expressed, trust is built, allowing the client to be more open and the therapist to better understand the client's struggles (Hohman, 2012). In the following example, a therapist (T) uses reflective listening when speaking with an older woman (C) referred for overuse of opioid medication.

C: I've been using pain medication just to function ever since I had my hip replacement.

T: The pain medication helps you to carry on with your daily activities.

C: Yes, without it, I'd be in pain all the time.

T: You don't want to be in pain.

C: Right! I never thought I'd be on it this long. But, I don't go out as much since my hip surgery and I'll be sitting at home, especially in the afternoon, and the pain just gets worse and worse!

T: The consequences of the hip surgery sound very different from what you expected. You're still in a lot of pain and you can't get out as much as did in the past.

C: I know. I have nothing to distract me from the pain. I just sit and watch TV.

The second principle of MI is the *development of discrepancy*. As discussed previously, many clients are aware, at some level, of their own ambivalence. They maintain the status quo, even though they may be unhappy or uncomfortable with some aspects of their lives. The perceived cost of initiating and engaging in change outweighs their discomfort with their behavior. The therapists' goal is to explore and amplify the ambivalence that clients feel. When the clients perceive the gap between current behavior and desired life goals or values, motivation for change increases (Cummings et al., 2009). Until clients recognize that the benefits outweigh the cost, they are unlikely to engage in change behavior. It must be noted that a therapist's approach can help promote or suppress ambivalence. Telling, lecturing, or persuading clients that their behavior is problematic often results in clients defending their behavior and engaging in "sustain" talk (i.e., expressing the pros of the status quo or the cons of change). Through the use of empathy and accurate reflective listening, the MI therapist seeks to raise the client's awareness of the negative consequences of the behavior and the discrepancy that exists between these consequences and the client's desires for the future (Miller & Rollnick, 2013). The goal is to guide the client in the transition from "sustain" talk to "change" talk and to have the client state the need for change. In the following, a therapist uses reflective listening and clarifying questions to develop discrepancy.

C: I know the doctor thinks I should lose weight, but I've always been heavy ever since I had my children and I'm fine.

T: You've been overweight for several decades and it hasn't caused any health problems so far.

C: Well, not really. The doctor says I'm pre-diabetic but that means I'm not diabetic. I gained weight after having each of my children and then I never really lost any of it. And then as you get older your body changes and you just seem to gain weight. I don't even eat that much.

T: So, you don't eat that much and you've still gained weight, and now the doctor says you're pre-diabetic.

C: I know. It just doesn't seem fair (laughing ruefully). My sister keeps telling me I need to lose weight but she's naturally thin, so she really doesn't know how hard it is.

T: Losing weight is a big challenge for you. What have you tried so far?

C: After the doctor told me I was pre-diabetic the first time, I tried walking but I really didn't like it. It's just boring. I stopped when it got hot outside and then, I don't know, I just can't get myself to do it again.

T: It sounds like when you first found out about the pre-diabetes, you were concerned enough that you tried walking even though you didn't like it.

C: Well, I was. But, fortunately, it hasn't gotten worse.

T: So, you were concerned about the pre-diabetes and you hope it won't get worse.

C: No, of course, I don't want it to get worse. The thought of it does scare me. My grandmother had diabetes and it really affected her eyesight.

T: Even though losing weight is a challenge for you, you really are concerned about diabetes and the possible consequences to your health in the future.

Rolling with resistance is the third principle of MI, which is the process of engaging in opposition to change. Resistance in the therapeutic relationship it is not viewed as the behavior of a problematic client, even though opposition may be a small or great amount (Rosengren, 2009). Rather, it is seen as an indication that the therapist's current approach is unhelpful to the client and that a different tactic is required. When the therapist and client are discussing change talk, the therapist is on the right path. If the therapist is arguing for change and the client is defending the status quo, however, this is an indication that the therapist has gotten off track.

Rather than confronting a client's resistance, the therapist seeks to explore the reasons that a client may not want to change and acknowledges the client's concerns and ambivalence. As a result, rolling with resistance decreases defensiveness and helps the client to further open up and engage in discussion (Serdarevic & Lemke, 2013). The analogy of canoeing can be used to conceptualize rolling with resistance. A person in a canoe being carried along by a strong current would probably not turn the canoe around and try to peddle upstream since this effort would most likely be both ineffective and exhausting. Likewise, the MI practitioner does not argue with the client, but strategically uses this energy to redirect and open up the conversation. MI therapists often use reflective and strategic responses to roll with resistance (Moyers & Rollnick, 2002). A reflective response is similar to reflective listening but includes an intentional element to move the client beyond opposition and toward change. In an amplified response, the therapist intentionally overstates what the client has said. Clients may then correct the therapist and, as a result, open up an avenue for positive discussion.

C: Listen—I know that my cholesterol is a little high, but I really don't think it's that bad. I mean, I'm not at risk of having a heart attack right now.

T: You know your cholesterol is somewhat high but you can't think of any reasons to lose weight right now.

C: Well, I mean, there are some reasons but nothing life-threatening.

T: So even though you're not in a life-threatening situation, you do see some reasons to lose weight. What would you say is the most important reason to you right now?

Using a strategic response, the therapist makes comments to actively shift the momentum of the conversation. For instance, a client who is arguing against change may be reminded that the decision to change is up to her and under her control.

C: I resent the fact that the doctor keeps telling me that I need to lose weight and now here I am seeing you. I like eating sweets and you're not going to make me give them up.

T: You're right. You're the only one who can make a decision about changes in your diet. What changes would *you* like to make?

Self-efficacy, the fourth principle of MI, involves the client's belief in his ability to change. A client must believe that he has the ability to make a change, before he will take steps toward change. Even if a client believes that the problem is an important one, thinks that change is necessary and wishes to change, if he doesn't believe he is capable of making the change, the odds of his moving forward are minimal (Serdarevic & Lemke, 2013). The therapist's job is to support self-efficacy by demonstrating confidence in clients' abilities to engage in the behavior change being addressed. Through "mining for affirmations," the therapist seeks to find and acknowledge the client's strengths and abilities, and to help the client mobilize these to engage in change (Motivational Interviewing Network of Trainers, 2008). For example, when working with a client who has made several unsuccessful attempts to stop smoking, the MI practitioner might state, "You've struggled with quitting smoking for several years now and here you are talking with me about it again. You have a lot of determination! How could you use this determination to take your next step?"

OARS

The techniques used in these processes combine both person-centered and directive approaches. *OARS* is an acronym used to describe the techniques—*o*pen-ended questions, *a*ffirmations, *r*eflective listening, and *s*ummary (Hohman, 2012). Non-directive

OARS techniques are initially used to establish rapport, understand the client's perspective, and get a sense of the client's goals. Once the client has expressed openness to behavioral change, more directive OARS skills are used to strengthen and confirm commitment to change, as well as establish a plan of action.

Open-ended Questions

Open-ended questions are key to helping the client build motivation, develop commitment, and establish an action plan for change. Open-ended questions that evoke change focus on four areas—desire, ability, reasonsm and need, or "DARN." *Desire questions* help the client to explore what she wishes, wants, or would like to do. For example, "How would you like your life to be different?", "What aspects of your health concern you?", "What would you like to change?" As noted earlier, however, a client is unlikely to engage in change behavior if she doesn't believe she has the ability to do so. *Ability questions* ask the client what she is able to do, has done in the past, or possibly could do in the future, such as "What do you think may be a good first step?" "What have you done when you've confronted this type of roadblock in the past?" and "How confident are you that you can get yourself to the morning walking group?" At times, clients may not possess sufficient confidence in their abilities. In such cases, the therapist can ask questions about other people's perceptions of their abilities, such as "Who in your life would know you could do this? Why do they think that?" *Reason questions* draw out from the clients their own motivations for change: "What may be the benefits of taking your medications more consistently?" "What do you see as the consequences of continuing to smoke?" "How might things change for you if you do lose weight?" Finally, *need questions* focus on what is not working as the client would like in her life. These questions may not be directed at the behaviors that clients believe they must change, but, rather, at the aspects of their lives they would like to see change. For example, a diabetic client may not recognize a need to change his diet but, upon questioning, may voice a need to "get my blood sugars under control." Questions such as "What do you think has to change?" "How important is it to you that your children don't worry about you?" "How serious do you feel this is?" address the client's need for change.

Open-ended scaling questions can also be very helpful in eliciting "DARN" responses. For instance, "On a scale of 1 to 10, with 1 being not important at all and 10 being extremely important, how important is it for you to make this change (Need)," or "On a scale of 1 to 10, with 1 be not confident at all and 10 being extremely confident, how confident are you that you'll be able to engage in one activity outside your home in the coming week (Ability)?" Clients' responses to scaling questions not only give the therapist an idea about the strength of the client's conviction, but also serve as probes for further exploration, such as "Wow, on a scale of 1 to 10 you're at a 5 for your desire to lose weight. That's pretty high. Where is that desire coming from?"

Affirmations

Many individuals who seek the help of a professional concerning a health behavior have already tried unsuccessfully to change (Rosengren, 2009). These attempts may have been modest and fleeting, or more serious. Because of unsuccessful previous efforts, clients often are discouraged and dubious about their ability to change. Affirmations are positive assertions concerning the clients' strength that support their belief in their ability to change. Affirming, however, is not the same as praising (Miller & Rollnick, 2013). Praising, which usually starts with an "I" statement (e.g., "I think you're a strong woman!"), places the therapist in the elevated position of someone who judges what is good and what is not. Affirmation, on the other hand, focuses on the client and consists of "you statements" such as "You're really a strong woman!" or "You got up and went to water aerobics even though you really wanted to stay in bed. Good for you!" Even a discussion of the client's previous failures can be reframed to an affirmation: "Even though you haven't been able to quit smoking yet, you've kept on trying. That shows a lot of persistence. You don't give up!" Following up affirmations with questions can help the client tap into her desire, ability, reasons, and/or need. A question such as, "How did you get yourself to keep trying?" could elicit responses related to any or all aspects of DARN.

Reflective Listening

As stated previously, reflective listening is a method of actively trying to understand another person's perspective and feelings, and of communicating this understanding in a nonjudgmental manner. As a result, reflective listening promotes the client's feeling of being understood and accepted.

There are several different types of reflective listening statements that MI practitioners often use. The simple reflection is content focused. In a simple reflection, the therapist makes a statement to indicate that he or she is attending to the client and hears what the client has said, for example, "You're not really sure why the doctor asked you to come see me today." A complex reflection goes beyond what the client says and reflects the therapist's understanding of the client's underlying feelings, thoughts, or values, such as, "You're confused about why the doctor asked you to see me today and this is causing you a lot of stress." A double-sided reflection reflects back the client's current statement in conjunction with a contradictory previous statement made by the client, for example, "You don't believe that your cholesterol is high enough to cause any real problems and yet you are concerned enough that you did try to diet for a little while."

Summaries

Summaries gather key pieces of information that the client has communicated during a session and offer these back for consideration. Because summaries indicate that the therapist is paying attention and cares about what the client is saying, they can also serve as affirmations. There are several different types of summaries that are helpful in MI. These include collecting summaries, which combine and integrate thoughts offered by the client related to a specific topic, such as, "So, when dealing with difficult situations in the past you've relied on several coping strategies—praying because that helps you feel centered, speaking to your wife who is typically very supportive, and going to the gym. Working out at the gym helps you to get out your pent up energy and frustrations. On the other hand, when dealing with stress you also tend to cope by smoking, which is something you really don't want to do again. Given all of this, which strategy, or strategies, do you think you want to use to help you cope right now?"

Linking summaries connect a client's comment or series of comments to things that the client has said in the past, for example, "You've been feeling down this past week and so haven't exercised at all. I remember you telling that me this has happened to you before. What did you do then to get yourself going again?" Transitional summaries bring a part of the session or the entire session to a conclusion by wrapping up the most important elements of what the client has said, such as, "You've tried to quit smoking several times in the past but haven't been successful. At times you're feeling discouraged like you just want to give up. And a part of you also feels angry because you already did give up drinking and that was a real battle for you. Now you're being asked to give up something else and, at times, that just doesn't seem fair. But you really do love your wife and she hates your smoking. You want to make her happy and have a better relationship with her. Because support from AA was so critical to your being able to stop drinking, you think that any program to help you to quit smoking that's going to be successful will need to incorporate some strong elements of support." Although summaries are commonly used in other types of psychotherapy, summaries in MI pull out key elements to help the client build motivation, commit to change, and develop an action plan.

DRUMMING FOR CHANGE

All of the OARS techniques described in the preceding can also be used to "drum for change." When "drumming for change," the therapist consciously uses a directive strategy to facilitate the client's expression of arguments for change. Preparatory change talk refers to client speech that references desire, ability, reasons, and need (DARN). The therapist fosters *preparatory change* talk by selectively using reflections and asking questions that evoke and highlight openness to change. Once motivation for change is evident, the therapist then moves toward *implementing change* talk (i.e., helping the client consolidate his or her commitment to change; Miller et al., 1999). Implementing change talk focuses on dialogue concerning commitment, activation, and taking steps (CAT). The therapist seeks to elicit from the client both DARN and CAT statements (see Table 7.2).

An important principle is to allow the client to move toward change talk without feeling rushed, or she or he may begin to back away from change. Rather, the MI practitioner recognizes when the balance of the client's statements have tipped in favor of change. If a client's statements suggest hesitancy or a lack of readiness to change, however, the practitioner further explores the client's reservations and ambivalence. Once the client's speech has tipped in favor of commitment to change, the therapist shifts from focusing on reasons for change to negotiating a plan for change. Planning for change focuses on both building commitment to change and developing steps to carry out change. Once again, the therapist relies on, open-ended questions (O), affirmations (A), reflective listening (R), and summarizing (S).

TABLE 7.2 EXAMPLES OF CHANGE TALK (DARN AND CAT)

Desire—Expression of a preference for change (I want to, I would like to, I wish)

" I want to be around for my grandkids."
"I wish I could walk up stairs without having to stop to huff and puff."

Ability—Statements about capacity for change (I can, I'm able to, I could)

"I could probably take a walk after breakfast."
"I might be able to cut down a bit."

Reasons—Reports of motives to change

"Now that our kids are grown, my wife said she'll leave me if I don't get my drinking under control."
"It's important for me to be a good example for my grandchildren."

Need—Communication about necessity of change (I have to, I need to, I should, I must)

"I need to do something to get my energy back."
"My doctor said I have to get my cholesterol down or I'm at risk for having a heart attack."

Commitment—Declaration of intention to change (I will, I'm going to)

"I'll go to that Alzheimer's Support Group on Wednesday night."
"I'm going to make an appointment with the dietician."

Activation—What the client is ready to do (I'm ready to, I'm prepared to)
"I'm ready to stop feeling so sleepy and drugged."

"I'm prepared to get my health back in gear."

Taking Steps—Statements about actions taken to change (I have, I did)

"I tested my blood sugar two times every day last week."
"I started walking in the mornings."

C: I've been smoking for 50 years. I love smoking but I guess I really have to quit.

T: In spite of the fact that you really like to smoke, you know it's time to quit. (R)

C: I do. My wife's been nagging me and now the doctor says its really affecting my health.

T: What are you prepared to do in order to stop? (O)

C: I'm going to try the patch. That seems the best way for me to start.

T: When do you think you might start with the patch? (O)

C: I'll buy it on the way home and put it on when I get home.

T: You sound really committed! You're a strong person to make this kind of change. (A)

C: Yeah, well, once I make up my mind to do something I usually can stay on track and get it done.

T: You're really persistent. Good for you! Is there anything else that will help you stay on track with quitting? (A/O)

C: Well, I guess I'll have to throw out my cigarettes. I hate to do it. But I'll do it when I get home.

T: OK. So, let's see where we are. You've really enjoyed smoking but your wife has been nagging you and now the doctor has told you that you need to stop. You've made the decision to quit. So, you're going to buy the patch on the way home and once you're home you're going to throw out your cigarettes and put on the patch. Does that sound about right?

C: Yep, that's it.

MOTIVATIONAL INTERVIEWING WITH OLDER CLIENTS

Older adults often experience threats to their health and decreases in physical well-being that necessitate behavioral adaptation to prevent disease progression and maintain maximum functioning. Long-standing patterns of alcohol consumption, for example, which previously caused no negative effects earlier in life, may require modification due to physical alterations in the body's ability to process alcohol as one ages (Center for Substance Abuse Treatment, 1999). Multiple chronic conditions such as diabetes, chronic heart failure (CHF), and pain may co-occur and require consistent observance of medication, diet, and exercise regimes over time. Likewise, acute events such as strokes and falls may unexpectedly necessitate adherence to demanding programs of physical, occupational, and/or speech therapy.

Additionally, older adults often present in settings that necessitate brief interventions, such as hospitals, medical clinics, and rehabilitation centers. For all of these reasons, a treatment such as MI, which is both brief and focuses on enhancing motivation to effect behavioral change, can prove especially useful when working with the older population (Cummings et al., 2009). Studies do demonstrate that MI is acceptable to and effective in promoting behavioral change among older adults (see Chapter 8) and that substantial modifications are not required for use of MI with this population (Serdarevic & Lemke, 2013).

Although significant adjustments to MI are not needed, there are some considerations that should be kept in mind when conducting motivational interviewing with older adults. Due to the brevity of MI, practitioners must be adept at quickly establishing trust and rapport with their clients. However, when working with older clients, it is often necessary to slow down this process. Older adults who are unfamiliar or uncomfortable with psychotherapy may require additional time to become comfortable with the therapist and to be socialized into therapy. As discussed in earlier chapters, later life cognitive changes, such as decreased cognitive speed and spontaneous recall of newly learned information (Chand & Grossberg, 2013), may also necessitate a slower pace of therapy. The traditional four sessions of the MET format, for example, may be insufficient for work with some older clients. The use of printed materials, in addition to verbal information, to reinforce learning is also recommended (Hanson & Gutheil, 2004). Using a standard drinks chart (see Figure 7.1), for example, when working with older at-risk drinkers, helps to demonstrate and concretize information concerning appropriate drinking levels. Creating scaling question flashcards (see Figure 7.2) that contain one scaling question per card in a large font and asking older clients to circle the number that indicates their response to DARN questions provides visual and tactile stimuli to amplify learning.

Older patients may be unaware of the link between problematic symptoms they are experiencing and their health behaviors. Education can be especially helpful when working with older adults who are unaware of the negative impact of their current behavior. It

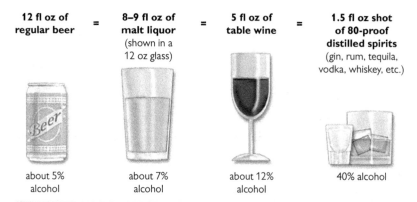

The percent of "pure" alcohol, expressed here as alcohol by volume (alc/vol), varies by beverage.

FIGURE 7.1. Standard drink chart. *Source:* National Institutes on Alcohol Abuse and Alcoholism (February 2003). Alcohol and intimate relationships: a guide for marriage and family therapists. NIH Publication Number 03-5284.

should be noted that the MI practitioner always first asks the client for permission before providing education. A question such as, "Do you mind if I give you a little information about . . . ?" opens up the door for further education but allows the client the make the final decision about receiving this information and, in doing so, taking a positive step toward change. Once a client has agreed, education concerning the specific illness or condition that brought the client into a health clinic can then be followed by a discussion that promotes the older adult's consideration of the impact of behaviors on the illness/condition. For example, an older man visits his primary care physician complaining of memory problems, dizziness, and a recent fall. A brief screen reveals an overreliance on opioids, which he refers to as "my hip medicine." After discussing the client's use and

Please Circle

On a scale of 1 to 10, **how important** is it for you to _____?

1   2   3   4   5   6   7   8   9   10

Not   Extremely
at all   Important
Important

FIGURE 7.2. Scaling question chart.

impact of opioids, the behavioral health consultant invites the older client to comment on possible connections he sees, if any, between his use of the medication and his physical and cognitive complaints.

Although factors that motivate individuals toward change are multiple and varied, certain themes are especially meaningful to many older individuals and should be kept in mind by the MI practitioner. These include the desire for independence, the importance of family, and the significance of faith (Bugelli & Crowther, 2008). Individuals are typically cognizant of changes in their physical performance as they age and wish to avoid an increase in conditions that will substantially limit their functional abilities. When working with older clients who express little or no motivation to change specific health behaviors, engaging in discussion concerning their desire for continued independence and linking this goal to the importance of treatment adherence may be especially useful. Inviting older clients to consider how the consequences of current behaviors may impact their ability to engage with their family members can also be fruitful. Goals such as "to be there as my grandchildren grow up" and to "not be a burden to my kids" can be weighed against the potential impact of their current health behaviors.

C: I really love being able to visit my daughter and grandson, but I haven't been able to see them as much as I would like lately.

T: Spending time with your daughter and grandson is really important to you and gives you a lot of pleasure, but the neuropathy in your feet is getting in your way and causing you a lot of problems in trying to see them.

C: I hate the numbness and prickly feeling in my feet. It makes me afraid that I'm going to fall, so I don't go out as much as I used to.

T: So, the pain in your feet is preventing you from seeing your daughter and grandson.

C: Yeah.

T: What has the doctor told you about the reasons for neuropathy?

C: Well, I know he said it has something to do with my sugars but I'm not sure.

T: How about we take a few minutes to look at the connection between blood sugars and that numbness and prickly feeling in your feet? Perhaps we can find something that will help with your feet so that you can get back to seeing your family more often.

C: Well, I'd like that.

CONTEXT AND IMPLEMENTATION

MI is a flexible intervention that can be successfully used in a variety of settings such as a doctor's office, mental health clinic, hospital, and at home. Research also indicates that MI can be effectively applied through face-to-face interventions, as well as via the telephone (Lilienthal, Pignol, Holm, & Vogeltanz-Holm, 2014). Regardless of where or how MI is implemented, the issue that most frequently prompts the use of MI with older adults is the promotion of positive health behaviors. MI therapists employed as behavioral health specialists in such settings, therefore, must be cognizant of common medical conditions and illnesses that occur in later life, their symptoms and consequences, and the interrelatedness of medical and mental health conditions. Knowledge of medical terminology is also necessary so that the therapist can understand medical records and communicate effectively with other members of the health-care team.

Although the main focus of an MI practitioner's work with older clients may be health related, the practitioner must be conscious of environmental, social, physical, and other factors that impact older adult functioning. Goals and strategies developed with the client should always take such factors into consideration. An assessment that focuses only on medical concerns and consequences is insufficient. Without an understanding of the environment in which the client lives, and her financial status, level of social support, and functional ability, the therapist will not be able to effectively draw on the client's strength or address her limitations. Depending upon living situation, mobility status, and pain levels, additional supports may be needed for an older adult to accomplish his or her goals. An important goal for a client may be to enhance socialization; however, mobility and transportation issues may inhibit the client's ability to achieve this goal if necessary strategies and supports are not addressed in advance (Bugelli & Crowther, 2008).

MI is often used as a "stand-alone" approach; however, it is also frequently employed as a pre-treatment (i.e., a method of engaging patients for other therapies). Research findings suggest that MI amplifies effectiveness when used in combination with other therapies. In particular, the application of MI techniques enhances outcomes of other treatments when client ambivalence and motivation present barriers to change (Miller & Rose, 2009). In such cases, MI strategies help move ambivalent clients forward and increase the probability that they will engage in CBT and other treatments (Bugelli & Crowther, 2008). For example, Cooper (2012) described the Healthy Living Program (2012) that utilized both MI and CBT to treat substance misuse and mental health problems experienced by low-income elders residing in public housing. A biopsychosocial assessment of older adults was conducted in their homes. Those screening positive for substance misuse or mental health problems received up to four sessions of MI. For many clients, these sessions were sufficient to produce the desired change. Further sessions employing CBT were used with those clients requiring additional assistance and support to resolve their issues. Case management was also employed to help older residents overcome barriers and access needed resources to achieve behavioral change.

In sum, MI can be effectively applied in a variety of settings and formats, either alone or in conjunction with other therapies and approaches. Above all, MI practitioners must be sensitive to the goals and needs of those with whom they are working and, by artfully engaging in the "dance" of MI, adjust this approach to fit the special needs of specific populations and clients.

CASE EXAMPLE

Lorna Vitali is a 67-year-old woman who has been widowed for 7 months and retired for 2 years from a job in a law office, where she worked for 25 years after her children were grown. During a pre-screen the doctor found a higher than recommended level of alcohol consumption and following the exam referred Mrs. Vitali for a follow-up appointment with the social worker.

Mrs. Vitali: I've always been a drinker. Not heavy, but I'm from a large Italian family, my husband was too, and we always had wine in the evenings with dinner.

T: Having a couple of glasses of wine in the evenings has been your routine for a long time.

Mrs. Vitali: Exactly, all of my adult life. I know I've been drinking a little bit more since my husband died, but not all that much more. I mean, I never get drunk! I just don't understand what all the fuss is about.

T: You're really confused about why drinking might be a problem for you now, when you've been drinking all your adult life.

Mrs. Vitali: I know. I don't like it when doctors try to boss me around. I don't think that doctors respect women's opinions that much, especially older ones.

T: Well, in the end you're the only one who can make a decision about how much you drink and how you'd like to live your life.

Mrs. Vitali: That's right!

T: Looking at your life, what do you see as your goals?

Mrs. Vitali: Goals?

T: Yes, goals for the future.

Mrs. Vitali: Well, for right now I wish I could get out more. Since my husband died, I don't go out as much and it's kind of lonely. I don't want to rely on my children too much to be my social life.

T: Since your husband died your social life has shrunk, and you'd like to build that up without relying too much on your kids.

Mrs. Vitali: Yes, that really is important to me. I know I need to work on that—to get involved in something. I do want to have friends and interests as I get older and to stay as healthy and independent as possible.

T: So, on one hand, you've been lonely since your husband died and have been drinking a bit more. On the other hand, you really want to increase your social life, stay healthy and in control of your own life.

Mrs. Vitali: Yes, I guess all of that's true.

T: When looking at your life and the quality of life you want for yourself, which of these do you think is most important?

Mrs. Vitali: They're all important. I know they are. I've just kind of let them slide. I think I spent so much emotional energy coping with my husband's death that, like I said, I just let things slide. I know that's not good.

T: Coping with your husband's death has been very tiring for you and you realize that in the midst of all of this, you've let go of some life goals that are really important to you.

Mrs. Vitali: Well, I know I certainly haven't been exercising at all. I used to do yoga two times a week, and tai chi on Saturday mornings. They're both really good for "older folks" like me (small smile) because they help with strength and balance, and I really don't want to fall.

T: You're really committed to keeping yourself healthy! How did you get yourself to exercise three times a week?

Mrs. Vitali: Well, first I like it. Sometimes it was hard to get out of bed in the mornings, though, especially when I first started going. But I just made up my mind to do it, and I did.

T: You're a very determined woman when you set your mind to something!

Mrs. Vitali: I guess I am. My husband would have said "stubborn" (laughs).

T: You've said that getting back to exercising is important to you right now. I'm going to show you a card I have here with a scale on it from 1 to 10. At the top there is a question "How important is (blank) to you right now. I'm going to write in "exercising." On this card (showing card to the client) "1" means not important at all and "10" means extremely important. Think about this for a minute and then circle on this card the number that represents how important getting back to exercising is to you right now.

Mrs. Vitali: Pauses and thinks for a minute, circles "6" and hands the card back.

T: A "6." Wow that's pretty high. What made you circle a "6" instead of a "4" or "5"?

Mrs. Vitali: In thinking about it just now, I realized I not only miss doing yoga and tai chi but I miss the other folks in those classes.

T: The other folks in those classes are part of the social support you said you let go of and miss.

Mrs. Vitali: We're not extremely close friends; but we've gotten to know each other from class over the years. So, even though we'd only see one another in the mornings, maybe go out for coffee after class, they were—I guess—steady. If that makes sense.

T: They are people who know you, who were a steady presence in your life.

Mrs. Vitali: Yes, a steady presence, people who know me. I really do miss that.

T: Sounds like you have two very good reasons to get back to exercising. First, because it's good for your health and you enjoy it, and second, to be with your friends, people who know you, again.

Mrs. Vitali: That's true.

T: When do you think you might be able to start exercising again?

Mrs. Vitali: Well . . . the day after tomorrow is Saturday, that means tai chi. . . . I guess I'll go and get started then.

T: Is there anything that you can think of that might get in your way of going Saturday morning?

Mrs. Vitali: Not really. I'll just have to set my alarm clock and the coffee maker before I go to bed tomorrow night. That helps me get up.

T: Sounds like you have a plan.

Mrs. Vitali: I guess I do (nods).

T: I'd like to go back for a minute, if I can, to one of the things that we talked about in the beginning of this visit.

Mrs. Vitali: I know, the wine, right?

T: Right.

Mrs. Vitali: You know, I've drunk wine all of my life and I'm really not going to change that. My Italian grandparents drank until the day they died. And they lived long lives!

T: Your grandparents drank until their later years and, as far as you can tell, it didn't hurt them.

Mrs. Vitali: Right. I couldn't see anything. Maybe they were extra hardy!

T: Could be. Would you mind if I gave you a little information about alcohol and older adults? You can think about it and we can talk about it if you'd like.

Mrs. Vitali: I guess that's OK.

[Therapist provides Mrs. Vitali with a pamphlet on growing older and alcohol use and reviews the information. The two engage in a discussion about some of the major points discuss presented in the pamphlet.]

Mrs. Vitali: Humph. . . . Well, some of that is interesting. I'm still not going to stop drinking wine, but I guess I could cut back a bit. I've always had 2 glasses of wine with dinner. Then I started to have an extra glass later in the evening. I think I've just been feeling a little lonely and sorry for myself. I guess I can cut out that extra glass at night. If I want something to drink at night, I'll go back having coffee—decaffeinated. The doctor is going to have to live with that. Deal?

T: Deal. Let me make sure I have this right. You're going to cut back drinking the extra glass of wine at night. If you want something else to drink, you'll have decaffeinated coffee. And, Saturday morning you're going to start getting back to your exercise classes. I'll be I interested to hear how everything goes for you this week. I know you don't have to come back to the doctor's for a while. How about I give you a call next Friday to see how you're doing? Would 3:00 p.m. work for you?

C: Yes, I should be home.

T: Great (hands the client a appointment card). I'll speak with you then.

CONCLUSIONS

Motivational interviewing is a brief, person-centered, directive counseling approach focused on helping people change by enhancing motivation to change through the resolution of ambivalence. Using techniques to work through ambivalence, therapists engage with clients to explore modifications in behavior, to take action, and to sustain positive change within their lives. MI is a widely used and flexible psychotherapeutic method that is employed in a variety of settings and with diverse populations.

Few adaptations are required for the use of MI with older adults. However, MI practitioners working with older clients should be knowledgeable of the medical issues and comorbid conditions faced by older adults that often necessitate behavioral adaptations and of common factors that frequently motivate older individuals toward change. In addition, minor modifications that enhance the older client's ability to comprehend and integrate the major aspects of the counseling session are recommended. As the number and longevity of older adults grows, an increased number of individuals will be challenged with the need to adapt in order to enhance their physical and psychological well-being. Medical and behavioral health practitioners who are familiar with and able to apply MI-based approaches will have skills needed to help advance their clients' ability to enrich their lives by engaging in behavioral change.

REFERENCES

Beck, J. S. (2011). *Cognitive therapy: basics and beyond*. New York: Guilford Press.

Bugelli, T., & Crowther, T. R. (2008). Motivational interviewing with the older population in psychiatry. *Psychiatric Bulletin, 32*, 23–25.

Center for Substance Abuse Treatment. (1999). *Enhancing Motivation for Change in Substance Abuse Treatment*. Treatment Improvement Protocol (TIP) Series, No. 35. HHS Publication No. (SMA) 13-4212. Rockville, MD: Substance Abuse and Mental Health Services Administration.

Chand, S., & Grossberg, G. T. (2013). How to adapt cognitive-behavioral therapy for older adults. *Current Psychiatry, 12*, 10–15.

Cooper, L. (2012). Combined motivational interviewing and cognitive-behavioral therapy with older adult alcohol and drug abusers. *Health & Social Work, 37*, 173–179.

Cummings, S. M., Cooper, R. L., & Cassie, K. M. (2009). Motivational interviewing to affect behavioral change in older adults. *Journal of Research on Social Work Practice, 19*, 195–204.

Dozios, D. J. A., Westra, H., Collins, K. A., et al. (2004). Stages of change in anxiety: psychometric properties of the University of Rhode Island Change Assessment (URICA) scale. *Behaviour Research and Therapy, 42*, 711–729.

Festinger, L. (1957). *A theory of cognitive dissonance*. Stanford, CA: Stanford University Press.

Hanson, M., & Gutheil, I. A. (2004). Motivational strategies with alcohol-involved older adults: implications for social work practice. *Social Work, 49*, 364–372.

Hohman, M. (2012). *Motivational interviewing in social work practice*. New York: Guilford Press.

Lilienthal, K. R., Pignol, A. E., Holm, J. E., & Vogeltanz-Holm, N. (2014). Telephone based motivational interviewing to promote physical activity and stage of change progression in older adults. *Journal of Aging and Physical Activity, 22*, 527–535.

Miller, W. R., & Baca, L. M. (1983) Two-year follow-up of bibliotherapy and therapist-directed controlled drinking training for problem drinkers. *Behavior Therapy, 14*, 441–448.

Miller, W.R., & Rollnick, S. (1991). *Motivational interviewing: preparing people to change addictive behavior.* New York: Guilford Press.

Miller, W. R., & Rollnick, S. (2002). *Motivational interviewing: preparing people to change* (2nd ed.). New York: Guilford Press.

Miller, W. R., & Rollnick, S. (2013). *Motivational interviewing: helping people change* (3rd ed.). New York: Guilford Press.

Miller, W. R., & Rose, G. S. (2009). Toward a theory of motivational interviewing. *American Psychologist, 64,* 527–537.

Miller, W. R., Zweben, A., DiClemente, C. C., & Rychtarik, R. G. (1999). *Motivational enhancement therapy manual: a clinical research guide for therapists treating individuals with alcohol abuse and dependence.* Rockville, MD: National Institute of Alcohol Abuse and Alcoholism.

Motivational Interviewing Network of Trainers. (2008). *Training for new trainers manual.* Retrieved December 17, 2016 from http://www.motivationalinterviewing.org/sites/default/files/tnt_manual_2014_d10_20150205.pdf.

Moyers, T. B., & Rollnick, S. (2002). A motivational interviewing perspective on resistance. *Psychotherapy in Practice, 58,* 185–193.

Prochaska, J. O., and DiClemente, C. C. (1984). *The transtheoretical approach: towards a systematic eclectic framework.* Homewood, IL: Dow Jones Irwin.

Prochaska, J. O., and DiClemente, C. C., (1997). The transtheoretical model of health behavior change. *American Journal of Health Promotion, 12,* 38–48.

Rogers, C. R. (1951). *Client-centered therapy: its current practice, implications and theory.* Boston: Houghton Mifflin.

Rosengren, D. B. (2009). *Building motivational interviewing skills: a practitioner's handbook.* New York: Guilford Press.

Serdarevic, M., & Lemke, S. (2013). Motivational interviewing with the older adult. *International Journal of Mental Health Promotion, 15,* 240–249.

8

MOTIVATIONAL INTERVIEWING
EVIDENCE-BASED PRACTICE

Since the development of motivational interviewing (MI) in the early 1980s, there has been an exponential growth in published information on this therapeutic approach (Lundahl, Kunz, Brownell, Tollefson, & Burke 2010). The explosion of material concerning the practice of MI has been accompanied by a growing base of research supporting its efficacy. Multiple meta-analyses of MI interventions have been conducted that attest to the effectiveness of MI in reducing a range of problematic behaviors (Armstrong, Mottershead, Ronkley, Sigal, Campbell, & Hemmelgarn, 2011; Burke, Arkowitz, & Menchola, 2003; Heckman, & Egleston, 2010). All of these meta-analyses have focused on general, young adult, and adolescent populations. Thus far, no studies have concentrated specifically on older adults, although one meta-analysis did examine the moderating effect of age on MI outcomes (Lundahl, Kunz, Brownell, Tollefson, & Burke, 2010). Within the last decade, however, a growing number of randomized controlled studies (RCTs) have investigated the effectiveness of MI with older adults.

To examine the effectiveness of MI for effecting behavioral change in older adults, a comprehensive literature review was conducted. PubMed, PsychINFO, Web of Science, Academic Search Complete, Academic Search Premier, and Google Scholar were the databases searched. Search terms included the following: motivational interviewing, motivational enhanced therapy, and "older adult," elderly, senior, or geriatric. Only studies meeting the following criteria were included in this review: (1) MI or interventions derived from MI principles were specifically included as a target of study; (2) age of the participants or the mean age was 50 years or older; (3) study was a meta-analysis or RCT; and (4) study was published between 2000 and 2015.

Initially, 18 studies were identified that met the preceding criteria. However, two of these studies were later eliminated because the MI elements were very minor compared to the other therapeutic components of the interventions examined. One meta-analysis had also been originally identified. Although the moderating effect of age was examined, the age of "older" participants was never identified. In the end, 15 studies were included in this review, all RCTs. One category of research implemented MI with older substance misuers. That was the situation of Mrs. Vitali in Chapter 7, who was referred to a therapist by her physician because of concerns about her alcohol consumption. In addition, other MI research has focused on physical exercise and diet, and enhanced health/mental health outcomes.

SUBSTANCE MISUSE

Four studies examined the impact of MI-related interventions on older adults identified as misusing substances including alcohol, tobacco, and illegal drugs (see Table 8.1). Hansen, Becker, Nielsen, Grønbæk, and Tolstrup (2012) investigated the effectiveness of a very brief MI intervention (BMI) in reducing alcohol use among a non-clinical sample of older heavy drinkers. Older participants (aged 50–65 years) completed both an Internet-based questionnaire and an in-person health examination in nine municipalities in Denmark. Those identified as heavy drinkers (14 drinks/week for women and 21 drinks/week for men) were invited to participate in the study. In total, 747 older drinkers completed the study and remained through follow-up. Those randomly assigned to the BMI treatment group received a brief (10-minute) conversation based on MI principles concerning their drinking, two pamphlets on alcohol, an information sheet concerning local alcohol treatment programs, and a brief (5-minute) follow-up telephone booster session 4 weeks after the initial intervention. The control group received the same alcohol pamphlets and local alcohol treatment information sheet. The eight interventionists who carried out the treatment received 1 day of MI training prior to treatment implementation.

From baseline to 6- and 12-month follow-up, the number of alcoholic drinks consumed per week declined significantly for both the BMI and control groups. Although this decline favored the BMI intervention by one drink per week, this difference was not significant. The authors noted that MI treatment fidelity was suboptimal and suggested that more than 1 day of training may be required to effectively carry out such an MI intervention.

Older adults were the subjects of an RCT to investigate the impact of a multifaceted MI intervention on at-risk drinking behaviors among primary care patients (Moore et al., 2011). To be eligible, patients had to attend one of three primary care clinics in Southern California, be 55 years of age or older, speak either English or Spanish, and have consumed at least one alcoholic beverage in the past week. Eligible patients who agreed to participate were then administered a telephone-based screen using the CARET (Comorbidity Alcohol Risk Evaluation Tool) to assess past year drinking behaviors. Those who screened positive for at-risk drinking using this measure ($n = 631$) were randomized

TABLE 8.1 SUMMARY OF RCTS ON OLDER ADULT MI SUBSTANCE ABUSE TREATMENTS

Study	Inclusion/Exclusion Criteria	Description of Interventions	Number and Description of Participants	Outcomes	Findings
Hansen et al., 2012 RCT Brief motivational intervention (BMI) to reduce heavy drinking in non-treatment-seeking population	Participants ≥ 18 years. Screened positive for heavy drinking (14 drinks/week for women and 21 drinks/week for men) after completing an Internet-based health screening.	BMI group: 10-minute session based on MI principles; 2 pamphlets about alcohol and 1 sheet with local alcohol treatment information; brief telephone booster session 4 weeks later to maintain motivation to change. Control group: received same 2 leaflets about alcohol and information sheet about local alcohol treatment.	Total – n = 772. Men: M = 32 drinks per week. Women: M = 21 drinks per week. BMI Group: n = 391; men (49%): M age = 60 years; women (51%): M age = 58 years. Control group: n = 381; men (54%): M age = 59 years; women (46%): M age = 56 years.	From baseline to 6- and 12-month follow-up, alcohol consumption declined significantly in both the BMI group and the control group to about 7 drinks per week. No significant difference found between BMI and control group.	While short duration of the BMI makes it a realistic candidate for use in primary health care, duration of BMI may have been too brief to reduce alcohol consumption to a greater degree than the control group.
Moore et al., 2011 RCT Decrease drinking among older at-risk drinkers	Participants ≥ 55 years or older. Spoke English or Spanish. Had consumed at least one alcoholic drink in the past week.	MI-based treatment: personalized report and drinking diary to keep track of alcohol use; oral and written advice by PCP; follow-up MI-based telephone calls at 2, 4, and 8 weeks conducted by health educators. Control group: received booklet outlining recommended behaviors for alcohol use, nutrition, exercise, medication use, and smoking.	n = 631. Intervention group: n = 310; M age = 68.4 years; 71.6% male; 87.7% White. Control group: n = 321; M age = 68.1 years; 70.4% male; 86.9% White.	Both intervention and control groups: prevalence of at-risk drinking declined by 50%–60%; amount of drinking declined by 30%–40% prevalence of heavy; drinking days declined by 30%–70% from baseline to 3 months; persisted at 12 months. Intervention group: greater reductions in at-risk drinking, amount of drinking, and prevalence of heavy drinking days than control group at 3 months; at 12 months significant only for amount of drinking.	MI-based information and feedback regarding alcohol use are associated with reductions in at-risk drinking and amount of drinking in an older population in PCP settings.

(continued)

TABLE 8.1 (CONTINUED)

Study	Inclusion/Exclusion Criteria	Description of Interventions	Number and Description of Participants	Outcomes	Findings
D'Agostino, Barry, Blow, & Podgorski, 2006 RCT Increase participation in substance abuse treatment	Older adult with comorbid substance abuse disorders served by the Geriatrics Addiction Program	Multidimensional in-home motivational counseling to address barriers to treatment along with geriatric case management and linkages to aging services. Control group: usual referral approach. Average length of time from initial contact to completion of GAP program was 4 months.	n = 99. M age = 73.67 years; age range = 51–91 years; males = 41; females = 58. Diagnoses: alcohol: 89.9%; prescription drugs: 14.2%; depression: 36.4%; anxiety: 18.2%; dementia: 41.3%;	Multidimensional/MI group: 80% inpatient treatment completion rate; 40% outpatient completion rate. Traditional group: 57% inpatient treatment completion rate; 10% outpatient completion rate.	Those who received multidimensional motivational intervention approach had better inpatient and outpatient substance abuse treatment completion rates than traditional referral group.
Gordon et al., 2003 RCT Reduce hazardous drinking in community-dwelling individuals	Participants in current study: ≥ 65 years and older; for overall study: Received care at a study site; drinking hazardous alcohol levels at time of screening; no treatment for an alcohol problem in the previous year.	MET: initial 45–60-minute session focusing on feedback, consequences, and advice plus two 10–15-minute booster sessions at 2 and 6 months. Brief Advice (BA): initial 10–15 minute-session focusing on advice, feedback, and consequences. SC: alcohol assessment at baseline, 1, 3, 6, 9, and 12 months.	n = 45 older adults. Age 65 years and older; 66–75 years: 76%; 76 and older: 25%; 87% males; 69% White; 64% married.	ME, BA, and SC conditions all decreased alcohol consumption. MET and BA reduced alcohol consumption at 6 and 12 months after intervention. No significant differences between two treatment groups.	Both brief interventions were effective in reducing hazardous drinking. MET and BA are equally effective.

into an intervention or comparison group. The average age of participants in both arms of the study was 68 years. The majority were White, male, college-educated, and retired. Prior to seeing the physician, those in the intervention group received both printed feedback from the CARET screen that outlined their alcohol-related risk and potential consequences, and a drinking diary to keep track of their drinking behaviors. Using the CARET report, the physician then provided brief written and oral advice to the patient concerning alcohol consumption. Health educators followed up the baseline physician visit at 2, 4, and 8 weeks with telephone calls to provide MI-based feedback and counseling to further support participant reduction of alcohol consumption. Comparison group patients received a pamphlet concerning recommended health behaviors including alcohol consumption, diet, exercise, and smoking. They were then encouraged by research assistants to read the information and discuss it with their physician.

Results revealed that the percentage of at-risk drinkers, the amount of drinking, and the number of heavy drinking days declined sharply for both treatment and comparison group participants at 3 months. These results were sustained at 12 months. The MI group, however, contained significantly fewer at-risk drinkers at 3 months. Those in the MI group also had lower at-risk scores and fewer drinks per week during the same time period. At 12 months, MI participants maintained a significant decrease in number of drinks per week relative to the comparison group.

D'Agostino, Barry, Blow, and Podgorski (2006) conducted an RCT to examine the effectiveness of an MI-based intervention to enhance older clients' entry into the Geriatrics Addictions Program (GAP). The GAP, located in New York, focuses on harm reduction for older adults with comorbid substance abuse and mental health problems. One hundred and twenty older adults referred to the GAP were randomized into one of two groups. The treatment arm was a multidimensional MI group that combined in-home motivational counseling to address barriers to treatment with geriatric case management and linkages to aging services and chemical dependency programs. The control group received the usual referral approach that combined assessment and linkage to services. Of the 99 older clients who completed the study, the majority (58.6%) were women. Participant ages ranged from 51 to 91 years ($M = 73.7$ years). Over one-third (38.4%) of participants were referred by family, while 12.12% were referred by community agencies. Others were referred by primary care physicians (PCPs), hospitals, and mental health professionals. The presenting problem of the vast majority was an alcohol diagnosis (89.9%), while 14.2% presented with prescription medication abuse. Over one-third were also diagnosed with depression; slightly over 40% also had a dementia diagnosis.

At follow-up, those in the multidimensional MI group had an 80% inpatient treatment and a 40% outpatient completion rate. In contrast, those who received the traditional referral approach had a 57% inpatient treatment and a 10% outpatient completion rate. While this was a small study, it does support the utility of MI-based approaches as a pre-treatment approach to enhance older clients' participation in and completion of substance abuse and mental health interventions.

Older adults were included in a study to compare the effects of motivational enhancement therapy, brief advice, and standard care on the reduction of hazardous drinking behavior among community-dwelling adults (Gordon, Conigliaro, Maisto, McNeil, Kraemer, & Kelley, 2003). Patients were screened for hazardous drinking in waiting rooms of primary care physician (PCP) offices over a 2-year period. To be eligible for inclusion in the study, a patient had to be receiving care at a PCP study site, be over 21 years of age, be able to answer the screening survey and follow-up evaluations, and consume alcohol at hazardous levels as measured via the AUDIT or through frequency/quantity levels (16 or more drinks and 12 or more drinks per week for men and women, respectively). Exclusionary criteria included treatment for an alcohol problem in the previous year. Among the participants were 45 older patients (65 years of age and over) who screened positive for hazardous drinking. Of these, the vast majority were between the ages of 65 and 75 (76.0%), while an additional 23% were between 76 and 85 years of age. Compared to the younger participants, more older subjects (86.7%) were male and non-White (31.0%). Study subjects were randomly assigned to one of the three treatments and were assessed over 1 year for alcohol consumption. Those in the MET group received a 45–60 minute session that focused on feedback from the drinking screens, discussion of consequences, and goal-setting. The conversations between the participants and the interventionists were bidirectional and provided the clients with time to discuss their thoughts and select goals. The initial sessions were followed by two booster sessions (10–15 minutes each) at 2 and 6 weeks, during which the interventionist reinforced motivation and encouraged participants toward goal accomplishment. Those in the Brief Advice (BA) group received an initial 10–15 minute session that focused on feedback from the drinking screens, a discussion of possible consequences, and advice to stop or reduce consumption of alcoholic beverages. These discussions were unidirectional and consisted mainly of the interventionist providing information and advice. No follow-up sessions were conducted. Participants in the Standard Care group received whatever treatment their particular PCP typically provided for patients with a similar drinking profile, which may have included referral to treatment, a conversation concerning alcohol, medications, or nothing at all.

Older participants in all three arms of the study experienced significant decreases in alcohol consumption. No differences were found in drinking behaviors between those in the MET and BA conditions. Additionally, both older and non-older participants experienced similar effects from the treatments, indicating that brief treatment in PCP settings are equally applicable across age groups.

PHYSICAL EXERCISE AND DIET

Research indicates that older adults obtain significant health benefits from physical exercise and a wholesome diet. Older adults who are physically active have lower rates of high blood pressure, type II diabetes, stroke, coronary heart disease, and colon and breast cancer. In addition, exercise contributes to higher levels of physical and cognitive functioning (World Health Organization, 2015). Multiple medical conditions common in later life, such as diabetes and cardiovascular disease, require following dietary guidelines to maintain health and to deter the development of negative consequences. A healthy diet also reduces older adults' risk of obesity, high cholesterol and blood pressure, heart disease, cancer, and diabetes. As a result, physical exercise and diet are two behaviors that physicians often counsel older patients to modify in order to maintain optimal health. Consequently, a growing number of studies have examined the impact of MI on promoting exercise and diet among older adults (see Table 8.2).

Lilienthal, Pignol, Holm, and Vogeltanz-Holm (2014) investigated the efficacy of a telephone-based MI treatment for increasing physical activity in 86 older adults. Older adults were recruited for the study through senior centers located in Canada and then randomly assigned to either the MI or a control group condition. To be included in the study, participants had to be over 55 years of age, have expressed interest in increasing their levels of physical activity, and be approved for physical activity as indicated by the Physical Activities Readiness Questionnaire (PAR-Q). Two-thirds of the participants were women (66.3%) with a mean age of 64.5 years. All self-identified as Caucasian. No statistically significant differences were found for demographic characteristics between MI and control group members. The MI group (n = 43) received four telephone-based motivational interviews, lasting approximately 50 minutes, once per week for 4 weeks. The telephone sessions utilized the principle techniques of MI. Participants and the interventionist (a clinical psychology PhD candidate with previous MI training and experience) discussed the older adult's perceived importance of, and their ideas about and interest in, physical activity. The older participants' confidence in their ability to engage in physical activity, address perceived barriers, and achieve desired goals were also addressed. Those in the control group (n = 43) received information only about healthy living via a mailed copy of the "Canada's Physical Activity Guide to Healthy Active Living for Older Adults" pamphlet. The authors assessed participants' self-efficacy for physical activity, stage of change for physical activity, and total weekly caloric expenditure at baseline, after the 4-week intervention, and again at 6 months.

At the conclusion of the intervention, those in the MI group exhibited higher weekly caloric expenditures from physical activity than did control group members. In addition, those in the MI group evidenced higher self-efficacy and greater forward stage of change progression from baseline to 6-month follow-up. Caloric expenditures were not maintained at the 6-month follow-up assessment, however, prompting the researchers to conclude that regular and ongoing contact may be important in designing and developing MI interventions for older adults.

Tse, Vong, and Tang (2013) studied the effect of MI combined with physical exercise on chronic pain in 53 older adults and found promising results. Participants were recruited through two older adult community centers in Hong Kong. Eligibility criteria for participation in the study included (1) being age 65 or over; (2) suffering from

TABLE 8.2 SUMMARY OF RCTS ON OLDER ADULT MI TREATMENTS FOR PHYSICAL EXERCISE AND DIET

Study	Inclusion/Exclusion Criteria	Description of Interventions	Number and Description of Participants	Outcomes	Findings
Lilienthal, Pignol, Holm, & Vogeltanz-Holm, 2014 RCT MI for increasing physical activity in older adults.	Participants ≥ over 55 years; expressed interest in increasing physical activity; approved for physical activity as indicated by Physical Activity Readiness Questionnaire (PAR-Q).	Assessed for total weekly caloric expenditure, self-efficacy, and stage of change for physical activity, at baseline, post-treatment and 6 months. MI group: 4 weekly telephone-based MI sessions. Control group: Received physical activity guide to healthy active living for older adults.	n = 86. M age = 64.48 years; 100% White. MI group: n = 43; 67.4% women; 41.9% overweight. Control group: n = 43; 65.1% women; 36.9% overweight.	MI group: higher weekly caloric expenditures, self-efficacy, and forward stage progression from baseline to post-treatment, and baseline to 6-month follow-up compared to control. Effect of MI on caloric expenditures from physical was not maintained at 6-month follow-up.	Telephone-based MI sessions are effective for increasing physical activity in older adults. Additional or follow-up prompts may be needed to extend treatment outcomes.
Tse, Vong, & Tang, 2013—Hong Kong RCT Effect of MI on chronic pain.	Participants ≥ 65 yrs and older; suffering from chronic musculoskeletal pain for more than 3 months; ability to communicate in Cantonese; oriented to time and place.	MI group: 8-week integrated MI and physical exercise program; 1.5 hour per session. Control group: Regular activities in community center.	n = 53. 95.7% women; 63.8% widowed; 46.8% lived alone. MI group: n = 30; M age = 75.9 years. Control group: n = 23; M age = 77.2 years.	Significant improvements in pain intensity, self-efficacy, anxiety, mobility, and happiness for experimental group. Control group had significant improvement in happiness scale only.	MI and physical exercise program effective in improving pain, physical mobility, psychological well-being, and self-efficacy for community-dwelling older persons with chronic pain.
van Keulen et al., 2010 RCT TPC = tailored print communication	Inclusion = Age 45–70; diagnosed by GP as hypertensive; not participating in other studies;	TPC group: 4 printed letters about physical activity and fruit and vegetable consumption. TMI group:	n = 1,629 M age = 57.15 years; 52% hypertensive; 55% male. TPC group: n = 405.	All intervention groups improved physical activity and fruit and vegetable consumption significantly more than did the control group.	Telephone MI, tailored print interventions, and a combination of the two were all effective. However, tailored print was more cost-effective.

TMI = telephone motivational interviewing.	Exclusion = Physically not able to comply with healthy lifestyle; cerebral vascular or cardiac event in last 6 months; suffering from disorders whereby a change in lifestyle might harm health; "other."	4 MI telephone calls addressing physical activity and fruit and vegetable consumption. Combo group: 2 tailored print letters and 2 MI telephone calls. Control group: One print letter after last follow-up.	TMI group: n = 407. Combo group: n = 408. Control group: n = 409.	No difference in outcomes found among 3 treatment groups.	
Campbell et al., 2009 USRCT Increase vegetable and fruit consumption among colorectal cancer (CRC) survivors and non-colorectal-cancer-affected (N-CRC) individuals.	Participants from North Carolina Colon Cancer Study; ages 40–79; of African-American or European-American ethnicity; being treated in one of 38 non-federal hospitals; reported being healthy enough to make lifestyle changes and participate over a 1-year period.	TMI only: four 20 min. telephone motivational calls. TPC only: four individually tailored, printed newsletters. Combined group: four print newsletters and 4 MI calls. Control group: 2 "generic" health mailings during intervention period and 4 print newsletters after final survey.	n= 735. TPC: n = 181; M age = 66.2 years; 45.9% male; Black - 29.3% Black; TMI: n = 185; M age = 67.1 years; 56.8% male; 42.2% Black; 45.9% income of < $30,000 Combo: n = 181; M age = 65.9 years; 49.1% male; 35.9% Black. Control group: n = 188; M age = 66.6 years; 50.5% male; 34% Black.	Combined group more efficacious (e.g., had greater fruit and vegetable consumption) and more cost-effective. No substantial evidence of differential effectiveness of interventions among demographic subgroups.	Combining tailoring and motivational interviewing may be effective and cost-effective method for promoting dietary behavior change among older healthy adults.

(continued)

TABLE 8.2 (CONTINUED)

Study	Inclusion/ Exclusion Criteria	Description of Interventions	Number and Description of Participants	Outcomes	Findings
Bennett et al., 2007 RCT Increase physical activity in cancer survivors	Inclusion = Cancer survivors 18 or older; completed treatment at least 6 months prior to enrollment; were fatigued, underactive, willing to try to increase regular physical activity.	MI group: One in-person session followed by 2 MI phone calls over 6 months; initial session 30 minutes; 20-minute phone calls at 2 months and 4.5 months. Control group: 2 telephone calls without MI.	n = 56. Physically inactive adult cancer survivors; ages = 37–85 years. MI group: n = 28; M age = 55.5 years; 46.4% female; 96.4% White. Control group: n = 28; M age = 60.1 years; 42.9% female; 100% White.	Participants in MI intervention group increased self-reported regular physical activities. MI group participants more inactive than control group at beginning, but more active than the control group at the end of 6 months.	MI is effective in increasing choice-based physical activity in cancer survivors. Increase in activity was higher for those with greater self-efficacy.
Jackson, Asimakopoulou, & Scammell, 2007 RCT Increase levels of physical activity among persons with type 2 diabetes.	Participants: 34–75 years of age; diagnosed with type 2 diabetes.	MI group: 20–30-minute MI session and physical activity advice dietitian: standard exercise leaflet. Control group: Standard exercise.	n = 34. MI group: n = 17; M age = 58.4 years; 52.9% male; 47.1% female. Control group: n = 17; M age = 62.1 years; 52.9% male; 47.1% female.	Physical activities increased in both groups, but significant change in MI group alone. For MI group, 8 participants increased their stage of change compared with just 1 in control group.	Dietitian with MI training can successfully deliver a physical activity intervention to those with diabetes.

Study	Participants	Intervention	Sample	Results	Conclusion
Kolt et al., 2007 US RCT Improve physical activity and health-related quality of life in low-active older adults.	Participants: age ≥ 65 or older; participated in less than 30 minutes of activity on 5 or more days per week for 6 months or longer; no unstable major health problem Exclusion = physical activity contraindicated.	MI (TeleWalk): 8 telephone MI sessions over 12-week period (weekly for first 4 weeks and then every 2 weeks for remaining 8 weeks); walking logs and pamphlets included. Control group: No intervention but completed outcome assessment.	$n = 186$. MI group: $n = 93$; M age = 74.1 years; 62.4% female; 48.4% married; 84.9% retired. Control group: $n = 93$; M age = 74.3 years; 69.9% female; 50.5% married; 83.9% retired.	MI group had significantly greater increases in all measures of activity at 3 months, and spent significantly more time on moderate leisure activities than control group at 12 months. Physical functioning quality of life not sustained at 12 months.	TeleWalk MI intervention is effective at increasing physical activity in older adults, with low activity over 12-month period.
Brodie & Inoue, 2005 RCT Promote physical activity among those with chronic heart failure.	Participants ≥ 65 years; ability to walk; New York Heart Association functional class II, III and IV; diagnosed as having chronic heart failure. Exclusion = resided in or had a planned discharge to a residential home; had myocardial infarction or unstable angina within last 3 months; diagnosis of valvular heart disease that needed surgery.	MI + Exercise Program: Home-based MI plus physical activity information from nurse. Standard care: Information concerning physical activity and local activity options. MI Alone: Home-based MI with no input from nurse.	n= 60. Oldest person was 94. MI + Exercise: $n = 20$; M age = 79 years. Standard care: $n = 18$; M age = 76 years. MI Alone: $n = 22$; M age = 78 years.	MI group, and MI + Exercise group reported significant increase in level and type of activities; Standard Care group did not. All groups significantly increased 6-minute walk distance.	MI coupled with a flexible approach to promotion of activity increases reported physical activity in older patients with heart failure.

chronic musculoskeletal pain for more than 3 months; (3) ability to communicate in Cantonese; and (4) being oriented to time and place. The majority of the older adults were women (95.7%) who were widowed and lived alone. Participants experienced moderate levels of musculoskeletal pain. The mean age for the treatment and control group members was 75.9 and 77.2 years, respectively. The two community centers were randomly assigned to either treatment or control condition. The MI intervention condition consisted of 30 older adults who received weekly treatment over an 8-week period lasting 1.5 hours. The treatments consisted of MI sessions (30 minutes) in groups of 8–10 participants, and weekly physical exercise program (45 minutes) in groups of 15–20 participants. Intervention participants were also encouraged to perform exercises at home each day, a minimum of four times per week for 30 minutes. The MI interventionist was a psychologist trained in MI. The four MI sessions consisted of education concerning pain, pain assessment and methods of managing pain, the elicitation of self-motivating statements from the participants, and working with the participants to develop pain management contracts. The 23 control group participants (mean age 77.2 years) continued to perform their usual activities in the community centers.

Findings indicate that the MI group experienced significant improvements in pain intensity, pain self-efficacy, anxiety, happiness, and mobility compared to the control group. The control group showed significant improvements in only one area of assessment, the scale measuring happiness. Results of this study suggest that MI combined with a physical exercise program can be effective in improving pain, physical mobility, psychological well-being, and self-efficacy in this population, and that such programs can be effectively offered in community-based settings where older adults typically gather.

Research also supports the use of MI to increase physical activity in older adults who survived cancer. In a study composed of 56 physically inactive adult cancer survivors, Bennett et al. (2007) compared the outcomes of an MI intervention group with those of a control group at baseline, 3 months, and 6 months. Participants had to have completed cancer treatment at least 6 months prior to enrollment, be fatigued, underactive, and willing to try to increase regular physical activity. The majority of the participants were male and almost all were Caucasian. The treatment ($M = 55.5$ years of age) and control groups ($M = 60.1$ years of age) each contained 28 adults. Participants in the treatment condition received one in-person MI counseling session lasting 30 minutes that focused on the participants' perception of the pros and cons of exercise, barriers to physical activity, and their physical activity goals. The MI counselor provided affirmations and worked to build participants' self-efficacy concerning their ability to overcome barriers and engage in exercise. The initial session was followed by two 20-minute phone calls at 2 months and 4.5 months that focused on MI-based problem-solving strategies and reformulation of goals, as needed. Participants in the control group received two telephone calls without the MI component.

At the beginning of the study, those in the MI intervention group were more inactive than those in the control group. However, they were more active than the control group at the end of 6-month intervention period. In addition, participants in the MI intervention group reported engaging in an increased number of regular physical activities. In considering the self-efficacy of the MI participants, Bennett and colleagues found that cancer survivors with high exercise self-efficacy increased their number of regular physical activities more than did those with low self-efficacy. Physical activity modifications for the control group did not depend on self-efficacy. Thus, study results suggest that MI can increase regular physical activity in long-term cancer survivors and that promotion of self-efficacy is a critical element of intervention with this population.

Jackson, Asimakopoulou, and Scammell (2007) examined the potential use of MI to increase levels of physical activity among persons with type II diabetes. In a sample of 40 adults from the United Kingdom with type II diabetes, a treatment group of 17 participants (*M* = 58.4 years of age) was compared to a control group of the same number (*M* = 62.1 years of age). The majority in both groups (52.9%) was male. The participants were recruited during regular visits to the dietician. The MI treatment group received a 20- to 30-minute one-to-one discussion session, known as an exercise consultation interview, with a dietitian trained in counseling based on MI and the transtheoretical model of change (TTM). The dietician also provided advice related to physical activity to intervention subjects. The control group did not receive an exercise consultation interview. However, both groups were provided with a standard exercise leaflet.

While physical activities increased in both groups, a significant change was observed only in the MI group. Examination of stage of change among study subject also revealed that eight MI participants increased their stage of change, as compared to just one in the control group. The authors assert that a specialist dietitian with training in MI and behavioral change can successfully deliver an intervention for older diabetics that results in increased physical activity as well as increased stage of change.

In a 2007 study, Kolt et al. (2007) investigated the outcome of a telephone counseling intervention designed to improve physical activity and health-related quality of life in 186 older adults. Eligible participants were age 65 or older, participated in less than 30 minutes of activity on 5 or more days per week for 6 months or longer, and had no unstable major health problem contraindicating increased activity. Subjects were recruited for the study through three primary care offices in New Zealand. The majority of participants in both the treatment (*n* = 93) and control groups (*n* = 93) were women with an average age of 73 years. Known as "TeleWalk," the intervention consisted of eight MI telephone counseling sessions. The program was provided by a trained interventionist over a 12-week period—weekly calls for the first 4 weeks and then calls every 2 weeks for the remaining 8 weeks. The telephone counseling sessions employed MI-based strategies including (1) education concerning the benefits of physical activity, the consequences of a sedentary lifestyle, and opportunities for physical activity; (2) recognition and resolution of ambivalence; (3) identification of goal and behavior discrepancies; (4) enhancement of physical activity self-efficacy; and (5) problem-solving for the resolution of barriers. Phone calls ranged from 10 to 16.5 minutes in length. TeleWalk participants also received walking logs and pamphlets to support the counseling sessions. Control group participants received no intervention but did complete outcome assessments at the end of the study period.

The researchers found that MI group members showed significantly greater increases in all measures of physical activity when assessed at 3 months. The MI group also spent significantly more time (86.8 minutes) on moderate physical activities than did the control group at 12 months. Finally, the MI group displayed significantly greater improvements in the physical functioning domain of quality of life than did the control group at the 12-month assessment. In sum, the TeleWalk intervention was shown to be well suited to older adults and effective in increasing physical activity among participants who were previously less active. Notably, although participants were recruited from physicians' offices, this study revealed that physician participation is not needed in MI-based interventions to enhance physical activity.

Brodie and Inoue (2005) crafted a study to determine whether MI could be used to promote physical activity among adults age 65 and older diagnosed with chronic heart failure. Older patients who were able to walk and had stable cardiac conditions were randomized into three groups—standard care, MI combined with standard care, and MI alone. The 18 participants in the standard care group ($M = 76$ years of age) received information concerning physical activity and local options for engaging in such activity from a heart failure specialist nurse (HFSpN). The combined MI and exercise group members ($n = 20$; $M = 79$ years of age) participated in a home-based MI component focused on both resolving ambivalence and integrating exercise into the participants' daily routines. The MI component of the treatment was provided by the study researcher, while the HFSpN delivered physical activity information to combined treatment group members. The third group consisted of 22 participants ($M = 78$ years of age) who received MI from the researcher with no input from the nurse. The total length of the study was 5 months, and the 3 groups were assessed at baseline and, again, immediately following the end of the study.

Results showed that both the MI and the combined groups reported a significant increase in the level and type of physical activities in which they engaged, whereas the standard care group evidenced no improvement in either area. All groups, however, significantly increased their 6-minute walk distance. Study results indicate that MI, with its inherent behavior change principles and flexibility, can increase physical activity in older patients with heart failure, at least in the short term.

A Dutch study compared the behavioral outcomes and cost-effectiveness of four study conditions focused on physical activity and diet improvement (van Keulen et al., 2010). Participants were recruited through Dutch general medical practices based on the following inclusionary criteria: (1) between 45 and 70 years of age; (2) diagnosed by their general practitioner (GP) as hypertensive; and (3) not participating in other studies according to the GP database. A large sample of 1,629 participants was randomly assigned into the four separate study groups. Study subjects ranged from 45 to 70 years of age (M = 51.2 years). Fifty-two percent of the subjects were classified as hypertensive, and slightly over half (55%) were male. The tailored print education (TPC) group (n = 405) received four printed, tailored letters addressing physical activity and fruit and vegetable consumption. Telephone motivation interviewing (TMI) group members (n = 407) received four telephone calls, based on MI principles, on topics addressing physical activity and fruit and vegetable consumption. Members of the combined TPC and TMI group (n = 408) received two tailored print letters and two telephone motivational interviews, again addressing physical activity and fruit and vegetable consumption. Control group subjects (n = 409) received no intervention but were sent one tailored letter based on the follow-up questionnaire after the conclusion of the study.

Participants in all intervention groups increased their level of physical activity and intake of fruit and vegetables significantly more than did control group members. No differences in effectiveness were found among the three intervention groups. While TMI intervention participants reported greater overall satisfaction than did TPC participants, the TPC intervention was found to be more cost-effective.

In studying interventions to increase vegetable and fruit consumption among colorectal cancer survivors and non-colorectal-cancer-affected individuals, Campbell et al. (2009) also compared TPC, TMI, and combined (TPC+TMI) groups. To be eligible for inclusion in the study, participants were required to be (1) participants in the North Carolina Colon Cancer Study; (2) between the ages of 40 and 79 years; (3) of African-American or European-American ethnicity; (4) treated in one of 38 non-federal hospitals; and (5) healthy enough to make lifestyle changes. The average age of participants (n = 735) was 66.5 years; 55% were male, 35% were African-American, and 37% were colorectal cancer survivors.

Study participants were stratified by cancer or non-cancer status. Almost one-quarter of the participants (n = 181) were randomized into a TPC group that received four individually tailored printed newsletters, while 185 were randomized to a TMI group that received four 20-minute MI phone calls. Combined TMI +TPC group members (n = 181) received four individually tailored printed newsletters as well as four MI phone calls. Finally, the control group (n = 188) received two generic health education mailings during the intervention period and four individually tailored print newsletters after the final survey was conducted. Interviewers conducting the MI sessions used a client-centered approach, allowed for resistance, employed reflective listening and open-ended questions to elicit desires and goals, and encouraged participants to make arguments for change. Interviewers received extensive training in MI prior to study implementation. Assessments of treatment fidelity revealed that the interviewers scored in the higher range of consistent use of MI principles and techniques.

Unlike van Keulen et al. (2010), Campbell and colleagues (2009) found that the combined group participants exhibited greater fruit and vegetable consumption at the 1-year follow up than did control group members. Although the combined TPC+TMI intervention was the most expensive, it was also the most effective. No strong evidence, however, was found for differential dietary changes according to treatment condition in the cancer survivor subgroup. These results led Campbell et al. to conclude that a combined print tailoring and motivational interviewing approach is an effective intervention in terms of both cost and promoting dietary behavior change among healthy older adults.

HEALTH/MENTAL HEALTH BEHAVIORS

In addition to substance use, physical activity, and diet, MI has also been used to promote various other types of health and mental health behavior changes among older adults. While the evidence supporting these interventions is still in the nascent stage, some random controlled trails do exist that support the further application of MI-based interventions in older populations (see Table 8.3).

Hawkins (2010) employed a motivational interviewing intervention to enhance diabetes knowledge and diabetes self-efficacy among older diabetics, with the goal of reducing blood glucose levels. Convenience sampling was employed to obtain a sample of 66 rural older adults from three primary care offices who (1) were 60 years of age and older; (2) had uncontrolled blood glucose levels; and (3) were interested in improving their control. Participants were randomly assigned to either an MI-diabetes self-management education protocol ($n = 34$) or to a comparison group ($n = 32$). The majority of subjects in each arm of the study were African-American women with a high school education and an average age of 64.9 years.

Utilizing a videophone system for delivering MI for diabetes self-management education (DSME), two nurse practitioners, who had taken a self-instructional MI course, provided 15-minute weekly videophone calls for 3 months, followed by 15-minute monthly DSME calls for an additional 3 months. During each of these calls the nurse practitioners used MI techniques and DSME information to facilitate knowledge gain and behavioral change among study participants. Initial and subsequent videophone calls averaged 28 minutes and 14 minutes, respectively. The 32 control group participants were contacted monthly via videophone for 4–5 minutes to discuss one of six handouts from a healthy lifestyle packet that reviewed good health habits related to skin care, sleep habits, dental care, adult immunizations, home safety, and sensory changes with aging.

Study results indicate that the blood glucose levels of the MI-DSME intervention group members significantly declined during the course of the study. Those in the intervention group also experienced a significant increase in diabetic knowledge and self-efficacy, both of which have been shown to be key in improving glycemic control in older adult diabetics. Once again, no significant change was found among control group members in either of these areas. This study suggests that the videophone MI care may be a viable alternative to traditional home-based care for rural older adults suffering from diabetes.

TABLE 8.3 SUMMARY OF RCTs ON OLDER ADULT MI TREATMENTS: OTHER

Study	Inclusion / Exclusion Criteria	Description of Interventions	Number and Description of Participants	Outcomes	Findings

Watkins et al., 2011
 	
RCT
 	
Increase in mood and mortality at 12 months post-stroke.
	On stroke register; ≥ 18 years old; no severe cognitive and communication problems; not already receiving psychiatric or clinical psychology treatment.	MI group:
		4 individual MI weekly sessions plus usual stroke care lasting 30–60 minutes.
		
		Control group:
		Received usual stroke care.
			n = 411.
			
			MI group:
			n = 167;
			median age = 70 years;
			age = 61–78 years;
			57.8% male.
			
			Control group:
			n = 163;
			age = 61–77 years;
			58.9% male.
				The significant benefit of MI on mood at 3 months remained at 12 months.
				
				Reduced mortality at 12 months after stroke for MI participants.
				
				No demonstrable impact of MI on functional ability or beliefs and expectations of recovery.
					MI improves patients' mood and reduces mortality at 12 months post-stroke.
					
					Protective effect of MI on survival suggests that improving mood could increase post-stroke survival.

Hawkins, 2010
 	
RCT
 	
HbA1c = glycosolated hemoglobin values (similar to blood glucose levels).
	Participants ≥ 60 years of age; uncontrolled diabetes (HbA1c > 7.0 mg/dl); interested in improving blood glucose control; passed Short Portable Mental Status Questionnaire.	MI group:
		15-minute weekly videophone calls for 3 months, followed by 15-minute monthly DSME calls for 3 months; educational handouts.
		
		Control group: Monthly 5-minute videophone calls to discuss 1 of 6 handouts from the healthy lifestyle packet.
			n = 66.
			M age = 64.9 years;
			
			MI group:
			n = 34;
			M age = 64 years;
			85.3% female;
			17.6% White;
			73.5% Black.
			8.9% Hispanic.
			
			Control group:
			n = 32;
			M age = 65.8 years;
			87.5% female;
			15.6% White;
			71.9% Black;
			12.5% Hispanic.
				MI group: significant decrease in blood glucose values, increase in diabetes knowledge and diabetes self-efficacy.
				
				Control group: no significant change in blood glucose levels.
					MI Telehomecare is a potentially viable option to help older adults deal with chronic illnesses such as diabetes.

(continued)

TABLE 8.3 (CONTINUED)

Study	Inclusion / Exclusion Criteria	Description of Interventions	Number and Description of Participants	Outcomes	Findings
Watkins et al., 2007 RCT Improve mood in post-stroke patients.	Same as Watkins et al., 2011	Same as Watkins et al., 2011	Same as Watkins et al., 2011	Significant improvement in mood for MI group usual care on mood at 3 months. No demonstrable effect of MI on either function or expectations of recovery.	MI leads to improvement in patients' mood 3 months after stroke. MI was effective with up to just 4 sessions, which would facilitate its introduction as part of usual stroke care.

In 2007, Watkins et al. conducted a study in the United Kingdom to determine whether MI can benefit patients' mood 3 months after suffering from a stroke. Those eligible for the study were (1) on the stroke register; (2) 18 years of age or older; (3) free of severe cognitive and communication problems; and (4) not already receiving a psychiatric or clinical psychology intervention. With an initial sample of 411 adults, participants were divided into an MI intervention ($n = 204$) and a control group ($n = 207$). The overall age range for the patients was 61–77 years of age ($M = 70$ years). The majority of participants were male. All participants received usual stroke care. The MI group, however, also received up to four individual weekly sessions of MI. MI group members started the intervention between 2 and 4 weeks post-stroke, with 71.6% of the intervention participants receiving all four MI sessions. Sessions took place in a private area and lasted between 30 and 60 minutes. The treating therapists had received 4 days of MI training, followed by approximately 10 MI practice sessions.

At the conclusion of the 3-month study, the MI group participants' improvement in mood significantly surpassed that of usual care group members. The researchers also analyzed the impact of the MI intervention on subjects' functioning, expectations concerning recovery, and mortality. No significant improvement was found for the MI subjects in these areas over those in usual care.

Several years later (2011), Watkins et al. utilized the same sample of stroke patients to test whether the MI intervention described in the preceding had benefited study subjects' mood and mortality at 12 months post-stroke. Results revealed that the significant benefit of MI over usual care on stroke survivors' mood at 3 months remained at 12 months, demonstrating that MI had a long-term protective effect on the patients' psychological well-being. Of the subjects in the intervention group, 48.0% were found to have a normal mood compared to 37.7% of those in the control group. Although MI had no impact on the patients' completion of their activities of daily living or beliefs and expectations of recovery, MI was shown to reduce mortality at 12 months after stroke. Fewer deaths were seen in the intervention than in the control group during this time period. Study results suggest a longer-term protective effect of MI on survival, thus signaling that improvement in patients' mood may increase post-stroke survival.

CONCLUSION

Beginning research on the use of motivation interviewing with older adults suggests its efficacy for promoting behavioral change in this population. Results of randomized control trials reveal that MI is as effective as, or more effective than, other psychosocial interventions in fostering healthier behavior and improved mood. The strength of these studies includes the variety of populations utilized and the diversity of settings and formats in which they were conducted. Study samples were drawn from senior centers, primary care offices, and the general population, and included non-clinical samples as well as those diagnosed with specific illnesses such as diabetes, cancer, chronic health failure, and substance misuse problems. The majority of these studies focused on promoting increased physical activity and healthier diets and yielded consistent results suggesting the benefits of MI-based interventions. One study that examined the use of MI as a pre-treatment to encourage entry of older problem drinkers into a substance abuse program likewise yielded positive results (D'Agostino, Barry, Blow, & Podgorski, 2006).

The studies discussed in this review were also conducted in differing formats—face to face, telephone, and a combination of the two. The success of the telephone-based approach, as well as the face-to-face approach, extends the utility of MI interventions to homebound elders such as those who are functionally impaired or geographically isolated. These findings suggest that MI is a flexible intervention that can be used to help older adults overcome treatment barriers as well as engage in positive behavioral change in clinical and home venues.

While the studies discussed in this review do suggest the promise of MI for use with older clients, substantial limitations do exist. First, there was considerable variation in the way in which MI interventions were operationalized and implemented in these studies. As cited in the previous chapter, MI has been described as "any clinical strategy designed to enhance client motivation for change" (Center for Substance Abuse Treatment, 1999, p. xviii). MI is not a manualized intervention with prescribed clinical strategies that must be employed. Therefore, while the research studies in this review may have been faithful to the spirit and principles of MI, it is difficult to discern which aspects of MI were tested and, therefore, which are necessary for treatment efficacy. The MI interventions that were studied ranged from one brief (10-minute) conversation based on MI principles coupled with print materials (Hanson et al., 2012) to weekly treatments, lasting close to 30 minutes each for 3 months (Hawkins, 2010). Some of the studies included follow-up investigation of treatment efficacy at 3, 6 (Hansen et al., 2012), and 12 months (Moore et al., 2011), while others contained no post-treatment follow-up at all. The authors of at least one study (Lilienthal et al., 2014) suggested that regular and ongoing contact with MI participants may be important for maintaining the behavioral change that has been gained.

Another limitation is lack of information provided concerning MI treatment fidelity (see Chapter 13). The nature and extent of MI training received by research interventionists was not always noted. Some studies reported trainings that ranged from 1 day (Becker et al., 2012), an undefined "self-instructional MI course" (Hawkins, 2010), to 4 days of MI training followed by approximately 10 MI practice sessions (Watkins et al., 2007). Only two studies mentioned treatment fidelity. One of these, which found no significant difference between MI and the control group outcomes, reported sub-par adherence to MI techniques (Hansen et al., 2012).

While limitations do exist, the bulk of evidence supports the efficacy of MI for use with older adults. Additional studies focused on older populations are needed to confirm such findings. Future studies should ensure that interventionists are thoroughly trained, and should clearly describe the MI skills and techniques employed. Measurement of interventionists' adherence to treatment protocol is also critical, as is follow-up investigation to determine whether behavioral changes endure over time. Without such scrutiny, it is not possible to determine the true impact of MI interventions on older populations. As the number of older adults continues to grow, it is important to keep in mind quality of life as well as duration. Interventions such as MI that seek to enhance physical and mental health well-being through behavioral change hold great promise.

REFERENCES

Armstrong, M. J., Mottershead, T. A., Ronkley, P. E., Sigal, R. J., Campbell, T. S., & Hemmelgarn, B. R. (2011). Motivational interviewing to improve weight loss in overweight and/or obese patients: a systematic review and meta-analysis of randomized controlled trials. *Obesity Reviews, 12*, 709–723.

Bennett, J. A., Lyons, K. S., Winters-Stone, K., Nail, L. M., & Scherer, J. (2007). Motivational interviewing to increase physical activity in long-term cancer survivors: a randomized controlled trial. *Nursing Research, 56*, 18–27.

Brodie, D. A., & Inoue, A. (2005). Motivational interviewing to promote physical activity for people with chronic heart failure. *Journal of Advanced Nursing, 50*, 518–527.

Burke, B. L., Arkowitz, H., & Menchola, M. (2003). The efficacy of motivational interviewing: a meta-analysis of controlled clinical trials. *Journal of Consulting and Clinical Psychology, 71*, 843–861.

Campbell, M. K., Carr, C., DeVellis, B., Switzer, B., Biddle, A., Amamoo, M. A., . . . Sandler, R. (2009). A randomized trial of tailoring and motivational interviewing to promote fruit and vegetable consumption for cancer prevention and control. *Annals of Behavioral Medicine, 38*, 71–85.

Center for Substance Abuse Treatment. (1999). *Enhancing Motivation for Change in Substance Abuse Treatment.* Treatment Improvement Protocol (TIP) Series, No. 35. HHS Publication No. (SMA) 13-4212. Rockville, MD: Substance Abuse and Mental Health Services Administration.

D'Agostino, C. S., Barry, K. L., Blow, F. C., & Podgorski, C. (2006). Community interventions for older adults with comorbid substance abuse: The Geriatric Addictions Program (GAP). *Journal of Dual Diagnosis, 2*, 31–45.

Gordon, A. J., Conigliaro, J., Maisto, S. A., McNeil, M., Kraemer, K. L. & Kelley, M. E. (2003). Comparison of consumption effects of brief interventions for hazardous drinking elderly. *Substance Use & Misuse, 38*, 1017–1035.

Hansen, A. B. G., Becker, U., Nielsen, A. S., Grønbæk, M., & Tolstrup, J. S. (2012). Brief alcohol intervention by newly trained workers versus leaflets: comparison of effect in older heavy drinkers identified in a population health examination survey: a randomized controlled trial. *Alcohol and Alcoholism, 47*, 25–32.

Hawkins, S. Y. (2010). Improving glycemic control in older adults using a videophone motivational diabetes self-management intervention. *Research and Theory for Nursing Practice: An International Journal, 24*, 217–232.

Heckman, C. J. & Egleston, B. L. (2010). Efficacy of motivational interviewing for smoking cessation: a systematic review and meta-analysis. *Top Control, 19*, 410–416.

Jackson, R., Asimakopoulou, K., & Scammell, A. (2007). Assessment of the transtheoretical model as used by dietitians in promoting physical activity in people with type 2 diabetes. *Journal of Human Nutrition and Dietetics, 20*, 27–36.

Kolt, G. S., Schofield, G. M., Kerse, N., Garrett, N., & Oliver, M. (2007). Effect of telephone counseling on physical activity for low-active older people in primary care: a randomized, controlled trial. *Journal of the American Geriatrics Society*, 55, 986–992.

Lilienthal, K. R., Pignol, A. E., Holm, J. E., & Vogeltanz-Holm, N. (2014). Telephone-based motivational interviewing to promote physical activity and stage of change progression in older adults. *Journal of Aging and Physical Activity*, 22, 527–535.

Lundahl, B. W., Kunz, C., Brownell, C., Tollefson, D., & Burke, B. L. (2010). A meta-analysis of motivational interviewing: twenty-five years of empirical studies. *Research on Social Work Practice*, 20, 137–160.

Moore, A. A., Blow, F. C., Hoffing, M., Welgreen, S., Davis, J. W., Lin, J. C., . . . Barry, K. L. (2011). Primary care-based intervention to reduce at-risk drinking in older adults: a randomized controlled trial. *Addiction*, 106, 111–120.

Tse, M. M. Y., Vong, S. K. S., & Tang, S. K. (2013). Motivational interviewing and exercise programme for community-dwelling older persons with chronic pain: a randomized controlled study. *Journal of Clinical Nursing*, 22, 1843–1856.

van Keulen, H. M., Bosmans, J. E., van Tulder, M. W., Severens, J. L., de Vries, H., Brug, J., & Mesters, I. (2010). Cost-effectiveness of tailored print communication, telephone motivational interviewing, and a combination of the two: results of an economic evaluation alongside the Vitalum randomized controlled trial. *International Journal of Behavioral Nutrition and Physical Activity*, 7, 1–12.

Watkins, C. L., Auton, M. F., Deans, C. F., Dickinson, H. A., Jack, I. A., Lightbody, C. E., . . . Leathley, M. J. (2007). Motivational interviewing early after acute stroke: a randomized, controlled trial. *Stroke*, 38, 1004–1009.

Watkins, C. L., Wathan, J. V., Leathley, M. J., Auton, M. F., Deans, C. F., Dickinson, H. A., . . . Lightbody, C. E. (2011). The 12-month effects of early motivational interviewing after acute stroke: a randomized controlled trial. *Stroke*, 42, 1956–1961.

World Health Organization. Global strategy on diet, physical activity and health: physical activity and older adults. Retrieved September 23, 2015, from http://www.who.int/dietphysicalactivity/factsheet_olderadults/en/.

9

PSYCHOEDUCATIONAL AND SOCIAL SUPPORT INTERVENTIONS
THEORY AND PRACTICE

During later life, a number of changes occur that impact health and well-being. Regardless of the reason or whether they are normative or non-normative, the older adult experiencing these changes often needs to modify behaviors, learn new skills, or deal with the psychosocial consequences. Additionally, family members and care providers are also impacted by these changing conditions, which have significance for their own functioning. They also may have to develop coping skills, learn to handle situations in care provision, or deal with the new demands and responsibilities of care.

Two approaches that are used in these circumstances are psychoeducational and social support interventions. Within this chapter, theory and practice of both of these approaches are provided. While differences in structure and context exist, the underlying theoretical perspectives of these approaches are comparable, with goals and outcomes of enhanced coping, increased competence, and decreased stress. In the caregiving literature, for example, interventions are categorized into two overall types (Sörensen, Pinquart, & Duberstein, 2002). One is focused on reducing the *objective burden*, such as respite care. The second has the goal of decreasing the experience of care, or *subjective burden*. Psychoeducational and social support are primary interventions that center on reducing stress and enhancing competence in care provision. While these two approaches are discussed discretely in these chapters, they are often implemented jointly within practice situations.

Psychoeducational interventions are defined as those which provide opportunities to increase knowledge or skills and focus on imparting information and fostering skill development (Pinquart & Sörensen, 2001). Some examples are health promotion programs, preparation for retirement, or dealing with a particular life stressor such as chronic pain. Typically, these interventions are designed to enhance coping in a particular situation (e.g., caregiving for a person with dementia) or dealing with accompanying emotional states (e.g., anger management within the caregiving role) (Coon, Thompson, Steffen, Sorocco, & Gallagher-Thompson, 2003). Associated goals are educational and preventive in nature, and take precedent over self-awareness and self-understanding (Nokes, Chew, & Altman, 2003). These interventions are typically led by a professional facilitator, are often delivered within a group format, and employ a structured curriculum (Depp et al., 2003).

Social support interventions provide opportunities for members to share experiences and emotions, and foster connections with others in similar life circumstances. When facing challenges or difficulties, a person's established social network may lack the capability to provide the type of support that is needed; for example, family or friends who have not faced a life-threatening illness may not understand what a person who is having this experience needs. Social network members may need their own support, such as a safe environment for expressing fears, a sense of loss, or anger about their situation. A primary rationale for a social support intervention ". . . is that peers—people facing a similar stressor—are able to understand one another's situation in a way that naturally occurring network members may not" (Helgeson & Gottlieb, 2000, p. 224).

Social support groups are common interventions for those in care provision roles. Although caregiving for an older adult has become a normative part of the family life cycle (Brody, 1985), the accompanying experience can be a lonely and isolating one. Support interventions may be led by professionals; however, groups may also be led by peers or other non-professionals in the field (e.g., paraprofessional, self-help groups). Most typically, these programs do not use a structured format. Instead, the content is based upon the experiences and topics that the members share within the group.

The following case provides an example of a psychoeducational group that promotes healthy lifestyle changes. Although the group is based upon a curriculum to improve hypertension, there is also time for participants to discuss issues and challenges that they face. As a result, connections and social bonds can be established between members, as in the case of Mrs. Melvin.

Mrs. Bernita Melvin is a 73-year-old widow who is overweight and suffers from hypertension. Recently, she had a "black out," which was a result of her uncontrolled blood pressure. As a result, she fell and injured her wrist and ankle. Although the injuries were not serious, the incident was a "wake-up call," and her daughters have become more concerned about her ability to live alone. They had a serious discussion with her about her health, and as a result, she has agreed to make some important lifestyle changes.

In several ways, Mrs. Melvin was uncommitted to her health-care needs. As a Southerner, Mrs. Melvin learned to cook from her grandmother and was known for her traditional dishes and baked goods. Although she believed that her diet was healthy, her method of cooking was high in sodium, fat, and sugar. In addition, she was erratic with her medication, and was unmotivated to be physically active.

After the latest health scare, her daughters enrolled her in a class at the local hospital and attended along with her. The class used a standard curriculum that incorporated health, nutrition, and psychological aspects of managing hypertension. This psychoeducational group had several components, including information about hypertension and its impact on the body, medication management, and lifestyle changes to manage this condition. In addition, a kinesiologist provided information and instruction on exercise, and a nutritionist demonstrated several ways to prepare healthy food.

There were a total of eight sessions, and each lasted 90 minutes. Each class included handouts and resources that the participants could keep for future reference. All sessions included a brief lecture about the topic, and either an experiential activity or demonstration. Additionally, the participants were encouraged to ask questions and share their experiences.

Though Mrs. Melvin was initially reluctant to attend, she found the sessions very enjoyable. She became friends with another member of the class who was also struggling with her weight. Since they lived near each other, they started to walk around the neighborhood together, which neither would do independently. Some days, they would have lunch together, which provided support and motivation to continue with their healthy diet. This experience was pleasant for Mrs. Melvin and her new friend, and it also provided relief for her daughters, who felt that their mother had a strategy to take better care of herself.

HISTORY AND BACKGROUND

To manage changes that occur in later life, psychoeducational and social support interventions enhance competence and connection to improve outcomes in functioning. As discussed in Chapter 1, aging can lead to attenuated networks as older adults have less ability and access to social ties. Role changes, such as retirement and widowhood, limit the opportunity for involvement with others. In addition, members of the individual's social network may lack the skills and abilities that are needed for later life changes, such as managing a health problem. The two intervention approaches in this chapter focus on increasing the capabilities of older adults and their informal support systems.

During times of challenge and transition, members of a person's social network can provide information and support to deal with the associated situation. With advancing years, coping skills and capacities diminish, which can lead to a loss of social functioning. The interaction of low levels of coping with low social support is an at-risk situation for older adults (Biegel, Shore, & Gordon, 1984). Social relationships are crucial for health and functioning, especially in later life. In fact, the lack of social support can have dire consequences for older adults. The risk of death in those with low levels of support are comparable to smoking and alcohol consumption, and are greater than obesity or physical inactivity regardless of age, gender, initial health status, and ultimate cause of death (Holt-Lunstad, Smith, & Layton, 2010).

An interest in social networks and their importance in health and mental health outcomes started to emerge in the 1970s and 1980s. During this time, attention to informal supports increased with the realization that formalized services were insufficient to meet the needs of older clients (Biegel et al. 1984; Sauer & Coward, 1985). Instead, intervention approaches were refocused on those who were connected to the older adult—family, friends, neighbors, and other systems of natural helpers—to provide support and care. Formal service providers considered ways they could assist those in care roles to be effective and competent, even with some challenging conditions such as dementia care.

Through social connections, older adults receive aid and assistance during times of need. However, social networks also buffer adverse circumstances and reduce the negative outcomes for individuals. Maguire (1980) conceptualized social networks as "preventive forces or buffers" to assist individuals in coping with "transitions, stress, physical problems, and social emotional problems" (p. 42). Connecting older adults and their care providers to others who can provide information, support, and mutual aid can buffer stress and decrease isolation and loneliness during this life phase.

THEORETICAL FOUNDATION

Various theoretical perspectives provide the foundation for both psychoeducational and social support approaches. *Social learning theory* is based on the premise that individuals learn new behaviors by observing others and witnessing how these actions are reinforced (Bandura, 1977, 2001). This perspective views behavior as influenced by both the individual and the environment, that is, as a combination of past experiences, sense of mastery, and current social contexts and conditions. Appraisal is an aspect of the learning process where individuals evaluate observed actions and determine the benefit for their own lives. This is easily seen in young children who imitate behaviors of their older siblings with hopes of receiving attention, praise, or some other rewards. This process happens across the life course, as individuals adopt behaviors that are rewarded or positively regarded by others.

Appraisal is also a concept that is embedded within the stress and coping literature. The buffering hypothesis suggests that social support can protect individuals from stress as they perceive it less negatively (Cohen & Hoberman, 1983). How individuals evaluate a situation is critical to their perception of magnitude or level of stress. Lazarus and Folkman (1984) describe two different types. *Primary appraisal* is how the person perceives a circumstance, especially a potentially stressful situation. Corresponding questions are "Is this a threat?" "Is this a good opportunity?" "Am I in trouble?" "Is something terrible happening?" *Secondary appraisal* involves the evaluation of the resources and coping abilities that the individual has to meet the challenge—for example, "What can I do about it?" "How can I get through this situation?"

If an individual believes that support is available, the negative effects of stress may be reduced and the person appraises the situation in a more balanced way. Lakey and Cohen

(2000) provide the example of a recent widow. Her primary appraisal of her husband's death might be that she is all alone now, with the secondary appraisal being that she cannot take care of herself. However, if she perceives that she is embedded within a network of caring people (e.g., her family, faith community, neighborhood), her primary appraisal might be "I have lost my husband, but there are many dear people I am close to." The secondary appraisal might be modified to "I can count on others to help me with shopping and home maintenance" (pp. 34–35). According to the stress and coping theory, the modified appraisals should lead to a less severe reaction to her recent bereavement.

Bandura (1977) also promoted the concept of *self-efficacy*, which is an individual's perception of the ability to perform particular tasks or actions. This perception is context specific; that is, a person may feel more effective in one situation and less effective in another. Within gerontology, self-efficacy has been extensively studied in terms of adjustments in health status and functioning (e.g., Jones & Riazi, 2011; Paukert et al., 2010; Turner, Ersek, & Kemp, 2005), as well as mental health functioning and social engagement (e.g., Gilliam & Steffen, 2006; Orsega-Smith, Payne, Mowen, Ho, & Godbey, 2007).

Self-efficacy is directly connected to an individual's sense of competence. Someone is more likely to carry out an action if she or he believes that it can be accomplished with success (Greene & Kropf, 2011). Within care provision, self-efficacy relates to the caregivers' perceptions of their abilities to successfully complete care tasks and responsibilities. Research indicates that psychoeducational interventions have positive outcomes on the self-efficacy of caregivers, including managing challenging behaviors, increasing self-care, and stress management (Rabinowitz et al., 2006; Savundranayagam & Brintnall-Peterson, 2010).

Psychoeducational and social support interventions improve functioning by enhancing coping and offering information that can help relieve challenges. Baltes and Baltes's (1990) selection, optimization, and compensation model provides a framework for understanding ways that older adults cope with life changes to retain resilience and functioning (see Figure 9.1). As an individual faces age-related declines, such as decreased physical abilities or fewer social ties, she or he is able to use resources to devise alternate strategies (Freund & Baltes, 1998). In this model, *selection* is the individual's decision about alternatives to pursue in light of changes (often losses) that are experienced. *Optimization* is the individual's use of internal and external resources to achieve a higher level of functioning. From an intervention perspective, this process could include taking a health promotion class to deal with a health challenge, as in the case of Mrs. Melvin presented earlier in the chapter. In the class, she gained information, skills, and relationships to manage her hypertension. *Compensation* involves substituting new behaviors or abilities that promote or maintain functioning in spite of the initial challenges. Using the example of Mrs. Melvin, she started to incorporate exercise, adhere to her medication regime, and consume a healthier diet. As her health stabilized, she was able to remain in her own home and reduce the possibility of relocating to a long-term care setting.

Within the following sections, an overview of psychoeducational and social support interventions are discussed. Differing from previous chapters, these two types of

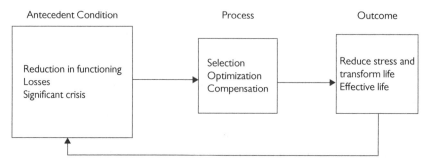

FIGURE 9.1. Selection, optimization, and compensation.

approaches are discussed separately to make distinctions about the implementation, process, and outcomes of each. While these are distinguished for learning purposes, in reality these approaches may be integrated with interventions providing both education and support together. In fact, some evidence exists that interventions are more effective if both approaches are included (Thompson, Spilsbury, Hall, Birks, Barnes, & Adamson, 2007).

PSYCHOEDUCATIONAL PRACTICE APPROACHES AND APPLICATION

Psychoeducational interventions focus on assisting individuals and families to adapt and manage challenges and transitions. The typical method of psychoeducation is to provide information that educates the participants about the situation, offers resources and support to address the issues, and helps develop coping skills (Walsh, 2010). This type of intervention is used across a variety of client populations and problem situations with high levels of efficacy (Lukens & McFarlane, 2006).

Although psychoeducational interventions vary across populations and issues, there are common elements. The learning process is most compatible to a group format, and the typical method of delivery is within a group structure. The target for change may be the individual (e.g., health promotion or managing disease), the family or other relationship (e.g., caregiving for a person with dementia, grandparents raising a grandchild), or community (e.g., learning about HIV risks, driving safety). Walsh (2010) provides a summary of the major elements within a psychoeducational approach (see Box 9.1).

A central component of a psychoeducational model is the facilitator, who typically is a professional who has expertise in the area or topic. Since psychoeducational programs are typically held in groups, the facilitator needs to have basic assessment information about the participants, including their learning styles and an understanding of group dynamics (Brown, 2004). While the focus on psychoeducational groups is more on the content than interaction among members, the context needs to be safe and pleasant enough that participants feel comfortable with one another.

BOX 9.1 DEFINITION OF PSYCHOEDUCATIONAL APPROACHES

A range of programs that focus on the following:

- Educating participants about a challenge in living
- Helping participants develop social and resource supports in managing the challenge
- Developing coping skills to deal with the challenge
- Developing emotional support
- Reducing participants' sense of stigma
- Changing participants' attitudes and beliefs about a situation or experience
- Identifying and exploring feelings about the issue
- Developing problem-solving skills
- Developing crisis-intervention skills

Source: Adopted from Walsh (2010). *Psychoeducation in Mental Health* (p. 4). Chicago: Lyceum.

While multiple models of psychoeducational interventions exist, these programs tend to include common elements. First there is *knowledge* about the topic that might be provided in a mini-lecture format, through reading materials or media. Information might include incidence and prevalence statistics; progression of an illness, disease, or caregiving trajectory; normative and non-normative situations; and emotional correlates such as grief and loss. The purpose of this content is to enable participants to increase their proficiency about their situation and to place their experience within a broader context. A second component is *skill development*, which is typically done through activities or experiential learning. Examples of techniques include role playing, modeling and simulations, and demonstrations. A third component is *application*, which enables participants to generalize learning beyond the group setting. How can they take materials learned and apply them within their own lives? Participants may have homework assignments such as journaling about their experiences, or trying out skills within their own home. Additionally, discussions are often included within the sessions such as identifying the rewards and challenges participants' experience from their new behaviors.

A few examples of psychoeducational interventions are presented for those in caregiving roles. An example of a psychoeducational intervention that has been implemented across multiple sites is the Coping with Caregiving Class. This intervention approach is part of the Resources of Enhancing Alzheimer's Caregivers' Health (REACH), which is a federally funded project to evaluate multiple types of intervention approaches for caregivers of individuals with dementia (Schulz et al., 2003). A major advantage of this intervention is the application and implementation with diverse groups of care providers using diverse administration methods (Au et al., 2010; Gallagher-Thompson et al., 2003; Kajiyama et al., 2013). A second example of a psychoeducational course is an

TABLE 9.1 SAMPLE PSYCHOEDUCATIONAL GROUPS FOR CAREGIVERS

Group	Authors	Theoretical Foundation	Skills
Powerful Tools for Caregivers (PTC)	Savundranayagam, Montgomery, Kosloski, & Little (2010)	Self-efficacy	• Caregiving challenges and self-care • Effective stress management • Effective communication skills • Assertive communication • Dealing with emotions • Managing difficult decisions
Coping with Caregiving	Gallagher-Thompson et al. (2003)	Stress and appraisal	• How to relax in a stressful situation • How to appraise the care recipient's behavior more realistically • How to communicate more assertively • Learning to see the contingency between mood and activities • Learning to set self-change goals and reward oneself for accomplishments
Increasing Life Satisfaction	Gallagher-Thompson et al. (2000)	Cognitive behavioral	• How to monitor daily mood rate of engagement in pleasant events • How to identify potentially powerful pleasant events • How to develop a self-change plan targeting pleasant events • Identify barriers • Set weekly goals • Reward oneself to maintain new activity levels
Increasing Problem Solving	Gallagher-Thompson et al. (2000)	Problem-solving	• How to achieve a calm state of mind before problem solving • How to define a problem as specifically as possible • How to generate multiple solutions to a problem • Evaluating negative and positive aspects of each option • Choosing one solution for implementation • Evaluating implementation, and modifying as necessary

Adapted from: Depp et al. (2003).

intervention for spousal care providers: "Powerful Tools for Caregivers" (PTC) is a six-session course of 2.5-hour sessions and is led by two class facilitators (Savundranayagam, Montgomery, Kosloski, & Little, 2010). In this curriculum, the first session deals with caregiving challenges and self-care. As part of each topic, a "powerful tool or skill" is taught, and participants use these skills within action plans for their own life. In this way, they take the content and apply it to their own caregiving situations. A summary of four psychoeducational groups for caregivers is provided in Table 9.1.

CONTEXTS AND SETTINGS

As psychoeducational approaches are focused on promoting knowledge and skill development, these interventions are offered in a variety of different contexts. Health-care settings are common sites, with the focus on helping older adults and their care providers with preserving function and managing health conditions. In addition, programs also address comorbid conditions such as depression and anxiety that are experienced with health-care challenges. Hospitals and primary health-care offices/clinics are a common setting for these types of programs (e.g., Paulo & Yassuda, 2012).

Various organizations that offer resources and support for specific conditions also offer psychoeducational courses. Conditions such as diabetes or dementia have national and state associations or organizations that offer specific programs on these diseases. For example, a psychoeducational program to assist caregivers of adults with a recent dementia diagnosis was offered to facilitate the transition into a caregiving role (Ducharme et al., 2011).

Psychoeducational programs can also be provided within community-based settings, such as senior centers and congregate meal programs. In these sites where participants naturally congregate, there is a great opportunity to introduce an intervention to enhance skill development and impart information.

Although used less frequently, psychoeducational groups may also be included in long-term care settings. An example is a stress-reduction group that was offered to help nursing home residents manage chronic pain (McBee, Westreich, & Likourezos, 2004). The group had 10 sessions, which included relaxation and pain management techniques such as guided meditation, breathing exercises, and simple yoga and stretching. After the intervention, group members reported greater satisfaction and a reduced sense of sadness.

CASE EXAMPLE

The following example is a psychoeducational group with care providers of persons with dementia. The setting for the group was a local Alzheimer's Association chapter in a medium-size city. The course was available to any informal caregiver who had care responsibility for a person with this disease. A total of 15 participants took the course, with most of those in attendance being spouses, but some were adult children as well. The majority of participants lived in the same household as the care recipient, but a minority of adult children were providing care to a parent who continued to live with a spouse or was in a long-term care residence. Advertising for the group was through the Alzheimer's Association's newsletters, local churches, public service announcements, and hospitals/clinics.

The group sessions lasted for 2 hours, and respite care was offered for the person with dementia, if caregivers wanted to use that service. A total of eight sessions were provided over a 2-month time period. The group was a closed one, meaning that the participants went through the curriculum as a cohort. Those who missed the initial session could join a subsequent group, as the course was offered several times per year. The location of the group was purposeful, to promote the Alzheimer's Association as a place for caregivers to find resources and information. They were encouraged to check out books, videos, and audio programs, and to attend other informational programs that were sponsored by the association.

The REACH curriculum, Coping with Caregiving, was used as the basis for the sessions. Care providers started with introductions, which fostered familiarity and normalcy within the group. This session was devoted to relaxation, and helping care providers reconnect with their bodies and let go of physical stress. The facilitator modeled breathing and other stress-reducing techniques, and the group practiced together. These techniques were re-employed throughout the sessions as a way to help the caregivers learn positive stress-reduction methods. Each session ended with a stress-reduction exercise that the group did together.

In the second session, information about dementia was presented. A social worker described the neurobiological and behavioral changes in the individual with Alzheimer's disease. Brain images were shown so that participants could see the areas that were affected by the disease. Discussions about the experience of caregiving for a loved one with those conditions ensued in small groups and then in the class as a whole.

In the next two sessions, caregivers learned various behavioral management techniques for challenging situations. Examples included dealing with verbal repetitions, wandering, hostility, disorientation, and memory loss. Each of these difficult behaviors was described, along with ineffective ways to deal with them (e.g., correcting the person or becoming agitated with multiple questions). Alternate methods were employed, and participants role-played these new techniques. A homework assignment was to introduce the new method within the caregiving situation, and journal about its effectiveness.

The following session discussed caregivers' thoughts and reactions to situations that they experienced in their role. Using their journal entries, they discussed how they felt in various situations and the messages that they told themselves about their experiences. The facilitator provided a brief summary about the relationship between cognition and behavior and presented alternate ways of "storying" their caregiving experiences—especially their challenges.

Communication between the caregiver and care recipient was the topic of the next session. The primary goal was to help the caregiver connect to the person with dementia. A film was played that showed examples of how to move from a "here and now" conversation to meet the care recipient wherever he is in his thought process. The facilitator gave "permission" to engage the individual in his or her stories and reminiscences without trying to correct or orient. The homework was to try these new communication strategies and journal about them.

The seventh session was on resources to help caregivers. A panel of agency and organizational representatives attended and discussed the services that they provided that might be useful. Informational material was distributed, and time was allotted for informal conversations between participants and panel members.

The final session was a celebration for making positive memories with the care recipient. If possible, the caregivers attended with the care recipient and had a "celebration." Often there are few opportunities for care providers to have joyful gatherings; this time promoted a shared experience of lightness and fun. Refreshments were served, music was played, and each caregiver was presented with a token for completing the class. Additionally, a master list was distributed of email addresses, as many of the members requested contact information so they could stay in touch after the conclusion of the course.

SOCIAL SUPPORT PRACTICE APPROACHES AND APPLICATION

Similar to psychoeducational interventions, social support is often a group intervention. The goal of a social support group is to provide a safe environment for individuals to share their experiences, especially with others who face comparable situations. ". . . Support groups are called for when people find themselves in relatively novel stressful circumstances . . . the support group serves as a temporary, personal community that supplements or compensates for deficiencies in the participant's natural network" (Helgeson & Gottlieb, 2000, p. 223). In this way, individuals can find connection, involvement, and compassion for those aspects of their lives that feel overwhelming or isolating. While support groups can have various structures (e.g., open or closed membership, ongoing or time limited), a common element is the attention to the emotional needs of the participants as related to life events or challenges (Ruffin & Kaye, 2006). While a group may be led by a facilitator, peer support (or self-help) groups can be led by someone who has a background or experience in the issue. Unlike a psychoeducational group, the agenda is more typically decided by the participants themselves, who bring their experiences to the group format. Additionally, the structure is often more fluid, as the topics are brought to the sessions by the participants. As part of this process, the members use their own experiences to provide aid and assistance to each other.

In a meta-synthesis of the literature on social support, Finfgeld-Connett (2005) organized conceptual definitions of social support into either emotional or instrumental

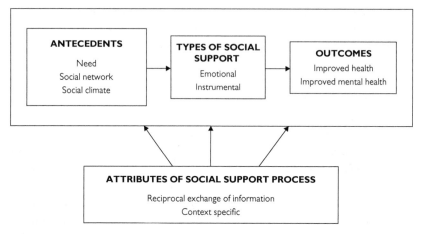

FIGURE 9.2. Process of social support. Source: Adapted from D. Finfgeld-Connett (2005). Clarification of social support. *Journal of Nursing Scholarship*, *37*(1), 4–9.

types. *Emotional support* consists of various behaviors that provide individuals with comfort and aid through information exchange, listening, physical presence, and normalizing situations. A second type, *instrumental support,* involves tangible resources such as services, assistance, goods, or materials. The benefit of support is the link to the need of the individual; that is, emotional support is not helpful if someone needs a particular resource. A diagram outlining the flow of the social support process is presented in Figure 9.2.

Since support interventions rely on the connection between individuals, technology has been used to foster engagement among those who are unable or unwilling to participate in a face-to-face session. Telephone and Internet-based support programs have been implemented with caregivers and individuals with chronic health conditions, among other situations (Boots, Vugt, Knippenberg, Kempen, & Verhey, 2014; Mahoney, Tarlow, & Jones, 2003; Nokes et al., 2003; Strozier, Elrod, Beiler, Smith, & Carter, 2004). These technology-based interventions allow participants to connect and engage with others without attending a place-based program. For those who are frail, live in remote areas, or feel a level of stigma about their situation, this alternative provides another way to connect with others.

CONTEXTS AND IMPLEMENTATION

Social support interventions are offered in a wide array of settings and contexts. Similar to psychoeducational groups, they may be held in settings where there is a connection to the particular life circumstance that is paramount in participants' lives (e.g., hospital, mental health center). Participants may feel a connection to the settings where they receive services and may be likely to perceive it as a safe environment to share their experiences.

Faith-based communities can also sponsor support interventions for those who are part of their congregations. Especially in communities of color, older participants may feel strong connections to their faith family as a primary social tie (Iris, Berman, & Stein, 2014). Partnering with faith communities can provide access for older adults to support services since a primary connection is to clergy (Bergman & Haley, 2009). Typical support groups offered under the auspices of a religious congregation are bereavement, addiction recovery, and caregiver support groups.

Because support groups serve a function of linking people with others who have similar life circumstances, this connection may be even more critical for individuals who live in areas with lower population density. In a study of support group use for individuals with multiple sclerosis, those who lived in small towns or rural areas were more likely to participate in support groups than those in more urban areas (Finlayson & Cho, 2011). The authors discuss the importance of the groups in these settings, through not only promoting a network of individuals who face the same disease process, but also fostering a stronger sense of identity within their community.

CASE EXAMPLE

Ms. Audrey Barnes is a 66-year-old woman who has been caring for her 14-year-old grandson for 4 years. Her daughter has a drug addiction and spent 3 years in prison for possession. Although she is no longer incarcerated, the daughter has started abusing drugs again and has not re-entered the family. Ms. Barnes's grandson, Travis, has no relationship with his father either.

Now that Travis has entered his teenage years, Ms. Barnes is starting to have some difficulties with him. Recently, he was expelled from school for smoking marijuana and has started failing some of his classes. Although Ms. Barnes never finished high school herself, she is intent that Travis will not "fall into trouble" like her daughter did when she was a teenager. She has been very worried and anxious about Travis's situation, and his teacher suggested that she become involved with a grandparent support group. Since about 10% of grandparents are in custodial parenting roles (Ellis & Simmons, 2014), these groups have become available in many locations and communities.

Although initially reluctant, Ms. Barnes attended a session that was held at a community mental health center. The group was co-facilitated by a grandmother caregiver and one of the therapists on staff. At the first session that Ms. Barnes attended, she was invited to tell a bit about her situation and her background in caring for Travis. While she started out slowly, the positive reaction from the other grandparents was very assuring, and she began to describe the difficulty that she was experiencing with Travis's challenging behaviors. Several of the grandparents told their own stories about their grandchildren acting out and experimenting with cigarettes, alcohol, and marijuana. The therapist asked any grandparents if they talked with their grandchildren about drugs. A few had done that, and they described how the conversations went and the way to deal with some of these behaviors.

At the conclusion of the meeting, Ms. Barnes felt like she had a group that understood her situation. Although she had been raising Travis for several years, she didn't know any other grandparents in this situation. As a result, she felt alone in her role. She found that she was looking forward to going back to the group when it was held again in 2 weeks.

Ms. Barnes continued to attend the group sessions. As she became a more regular member, she started to help some of the other grandparents with their issues as a source of information and aid as well. In particular, one of the grandmothers was struggling with a younger grandson and how to deal with some of his bossy attitudes. Ms. Barnes was able to provide some helpful information about how she dealt with this situation in her own life. As a result, she felt like she was contributing to the group in a way that increased her own self-esteem and confidence.

Although the support group provided a safe place for the grandparents to share experience, there were times that the members provided instrumental support to each other as well. Every season, the grandparents would have a clothing swap, where they would bring in the clothes that their grandchildren had outgrown. This exchange became a favorite session for the grandparents, as they would swap stories as well as articles of clothing.

The group also became a source of mutual aid during times of crises for the members. Sadly, the daughter of one of the grandmothers (the mother of the two grandchildren whom she was raising) was murdered and found in an abandoned house in the community. During this tragic time, the members of the support group provided a number of resources to the family, including attending the funeral together, cooking meals for the family, and taking the grandchildren into their homes as a form of respite for the grandmother. The support and caring that transpired during this time was a tribute to the connection and bonds that had developed among the members.

PSYCHOEDUCATION AND SOCIAL SUPPORT INTERVENTIONS WITH OLDER ADULTS

With older adults, some additional considerations are necessary to ensure that participants gain the most from the psychoeducational and social support interventions. Since these interventions are frequently provided within a group format, attention to the dynamics and context of the group setting in important. Groups held in congregate living places (e.g., long-term care, nursing home), for example, need to be sensitive that treatment is offered where the participants also live. Practitioners need to respect the privacy and dignity of the participants in designing the treatment.

Additionally, cognitive speed and memory abilities need to be considered, as changes in fluid intelligence are a normal part of aging (Chand & Grossberg, 2013). As a result, content may need to be presented more slowly, and the sessions may need to include opening and closing summaries as well as learning aids (e.g., visuals, bullet points) that help retention. These strategies may include shortening session lengths as appropriate, considering the environmental setting as conducive to interaction, and taking into account any physical conditions that can impede engagement (e.g., hearing or vision loss).

Sociodemographic factors need to be considered as well. In the current population of older adults, for example, educational attainment is not as high as in younger cohorts. Information needs to be presented in ways that are grasped by the participants. In addition, cultural considerations, which are important in any intervention method, should be carefully considered in presenting psychoeducational programs with older participants. Similarly, social support groups invite participants to discuss experiences and feelings, which may feel unfamiliar to some older adults. These aspects need to be considered when designing and implementing psychoeducational and social support interventions with the older population.

CONCLUSION

To deal with the transitions and changes that occur in later life, psychoeducational and social support are evidence-based interventions that provide individuals and care providers with information, skill development, coping, and connections to others. While there are similar elements in these two intervention approaches, psychoeducational interventions have stronger knowledge- and skill-based components and are typically delivered within a structured curriculum format. Conversely, social support interventions are founded upon exchanges and mutual aid between participants and often have a more unstructured approach. The following chapter summarizes various meta-analyses, systematic reviews, and individual research on both of these types of intervention approaches with the older population and their care providers.

REFERENCES

Au, A., Li, S., Lee, K., Leung, P., Pan, P. C., Thompson, L., & Gallagher-Thompson, D. (2010). The Coping with Caregiving Group Program for Chinese caregivers of patients with Alzheimer's disease in Hong Kong. *Patient Education and Counseling, 78*(2), 256–260.

Baltes, P. B., & Baltes, M. M. (1990). Psychological perspectives on successful aging: the model of selective optimization with compensation. *Successful Aging: Perspectives from the Behavioral Sciences, 1,* 1–34.

Bandura, A. (1977). Self-efficacy: toward a unifying theory of behavioral change. *Psychological Review, 84*(2), 191.

Bandura, A. (2001). Social cognitive theory: an agentic perspective. *Annual Review of Psychology, 52*(1), 1–26.

Bergman, E. J., & Haley, W. E. (2009). Depressive symptoms, social network, and bereavement service utilization and preferences among spouses of former hospice patients. *Journal of Palliative Medicine, 12*(2), 170–176.

Biegel, D. E., Shore, B. K., & Gordon, E. (1984). *Building support networks for the elderly: Theory and applications*. Beverly Hills, CA: Sage.

Boots, L. M. M., Vugt, M. E., Knippenberg, R. J. M., Kempen, G. I. J. M., & Verhey, F. R. J. (2014). A systematic review of Internet-based supportive interventions for caregivers of patients with dementia. *International Journal of Geriatric Psychiatry, 29*(4), 331–344.

Brody, E. M. (1985). Parent care as a normative family stress. *The Gerontologist, 25*(1), 19–29.

Brown, N. W. (2004). *Psychoeducational groups: process and practice* (2nd ed). New York: Brunner-Routledge.

Chand, S., & Grossberg, G. T. (2013). How to adapt cognitive-behavioral therapy for older adults. *Current Psychiatry, 12*, 10–15

Cohen, S., & Hoberman, H. M. (1983). Positive events and social supports as buffers of life change stress. *Journal of Applied Social Psychology, 13*, 99–125.

Coon, D. W., Thompson, L., Steffen, A., Sorocco, K., & Gallagher-Thompson, D. (2003). Anger and depression management: psychoeducational skill training interventions for women caregivers of a relative with dementia. *The Gerontologist, 43*(5), 678–689.

Depp, C., Krisztal, E., Cardenas, V., Oportot, M., Mausbach, B., Ambler, C., . . . Gallagher-Thompson, D. (2003). Treatment options for improving wellbeing in dementia family caregivers: the case for psychoeducational interventions. *Clinical Psychologist, 7*(1), 21–31.

Ducharme, F. C., Lévesque, L. L., Lachance, L. M., Kergoat, M. J., Legault, A. J., Beaudet, L. M., & Zarit, S. H. (2011). "Learning to become a family caregiver": efficacy of an intervention program for caregivers following diagnosis of dementia in a relative. *The Gerontologist, 51*(4), 484–494.

Ellis, R. R., & Simmons, T. (2014). *Coresident grandparents and their grandchildren: 2012 population characteristics*. Retrieved June 18, 2015, from http://www.census.gov/content/dam/Census/library/publications/2014/demo/p20-576.pdf.

Finfgeld-Connett, D. (2005). Clarification of social support. *Journal of Nursing Scholarship, 37*(1), 4–9.

Finlayson, M. L., & Cho, C. C. (2011). A profile of support group use and need among middle-aged and older adults with multiple sclerosis. *Journal of Gerontological Social Work, 54*(5), 475–493.

Freund, A. M., & Baltes, P. B. (1998). Selection, optimization, and compensation as strategies of life management: correlations with subjective indicators of successful aging. *Psychology and Aging, 13*(4), 531–543.

Gallagher-Thompson, D., Coon, D. W., Solano, N., Ambler, C., Rabinowitz, Y., & Thompson, L. W. (2003). Change in indices of distress among Latino and Anglo female caregivers of elderly relatives with dementia: site-specific results from the REACH national collaborative study. *The Gerontologist, 43*(4), 580–591.

Gallagher-Thompson, D., Lovett, S., Rose, J., McKibbin, C., Coon, D., Futterman, A., & Thompson, L.W. (2000). Impact of psychoeducational interventions on distressed family caregivers. *Journal of Clinical Geropsychology, 6*(2), 91–110.

Gilliam, C. M., & Steffen, A. M. (2006). The relationship between caregiving self-efficacy and depressive symptoms in dementia family caregivers. *Aging and Mental Health, 10*(2), 79–86.

Greene, R. R., & Kropf, N. P. (2011). *Competence: theoretical frameworks*. New Brunswick, NJ: Transaction.

Helgeson, V. S., & Gottlieb, B. H. (2000). Support groups. In S. Cohen, L G. Underwood, & B. H. Gottlieb (Eds.), *Social support measurement and intervention: a guide for health and social scientests* (pp. 221–245). New York: Oxford University Press.

Holt-Lunstad, J., Smith, T. B., & Layton, J. B. (2010). Social relationships and mortality risk: a meta-analytic review. *PLoS Medicine, 7*(7), e1000316.

Iris, M., Berman, R. L., & Stein, S. (2014). Developing a faith-based caregiver support partnership. *Journal of Gerontological Social Work*, 57(6–7), 728–774.

Jones, F., & Riazi, A. (2011). Self-efficacy and self-management after stroke: a systematic review. *Disability and Rehabilitation*, 33(10), 797–810.

Kajiyama, B., Thompson, L. W., Eto-Iwase, T., Yamashita, M., Di Mario, J., Marian Tzuang, Y., & Gallagher-Thompson, D. (2013). Exploring the effectiveness of an internet-based program for reducing caregiver distress using the iCare Stress Management e-Training Program. *Aging & Mental Health*, 17(5), 544–554.

Lakey, B., & Cohen, S. (2000). Social support theory and measurement. In S. Cohen, L G. Underwood, & B. H. Gottlieb (Eds.), *Social support measurement and intervention: a guide for health and social scientests* (pp. 29–52). New York: Oxford University Press.

Lazarus, R. S., & Folkman, S. (1984). *Stress, appraisal and coping*. New York: Springer.

Lukens, E. P., & McFarlane, W. R. (2006). Psychoeducation as evidence-based practice. In A. R. Roberts & K. R. Yeager (Eds.), *Foundations of evidence-based social work practice* (pp. 291–313). New York: Oxford University Press.

Maguire, L. (1980). The interface of social workers with personal networks. *Social Work with Groups*, 3, 39–49.

Mahoney, D. F., Tarlow, B. J., & Jones, R. N. (2003). Effects of an automated telephone support system on caregiver burden and anxiety: findings from the REACH for TLC intervention study. *The Gerontologist*, 43(4), 556–567.

McBee, L., Westreich, L., & Likourezos, A. (2004). A psychoeducational relaxation group for pain and stress management in the nursing home. *Journal of Social Work in Long-Term Care*, 3(1), 15–28.

Nokes, K. M., Chew, L., & Altman, C. (2003). Using a telephone support group for HIV-positive persons aged 50+ to increase social support and health-related knowledge. *AIDS Patient Care and STDs*, 17(7), 345–351.

Orsega-Smith, E. M., Payne, L. L., Mowen, A. J., Ho, C., & Godbey, G. C. (2007). The role of social support and self-efficacy in shaping the leisure time physical activity of older adults. *Journal of Leisure Research*, 39(4), 705.

Paukert, A. L., Pettit, J. W., Kunik, M. E., Wilson, N., Novy, D. M., Rhoades, H. M., . . . Stanley, M. A. (2010). The roles of social support and self-efficacy in physical health's impact on depressive and anxiety symptoms in older adults. *Journal of Clinical Psychology in Medical Settings*, 17(4), 387–400.

Paulo, D. V., & Yassuda, M. S. (2012). Elderly individuals with diabetes: adding cognitive training to psychoeducational intervention. *Educational Gerontology*, 38(4), 257–270.

Pinquart, M., & Sörensen, S. (2001). How effective are psychotherapeutic another psychosocial interventions with older adults? A meta-analysis. *Journal of Mental Health & Aging*, 7, 207–243.

Rabinowitz, Y. G., Mausbach, B. T., Coon, D. W., Depp, C., Thompson, L. W., & Gallagher-Thompson, D. (2006). The moderating effect of self-efficacy on intervention response in women family caregivers of older adults with dementia. *The American Journal of Geriatric Psychiatry*, 14(8), 642–649.

Ruffin, L., & Kaye, L.W. (2006). Counseling services and support groups. In B. Berkman (Ed.), *Handbook of social work in aging* (pp. 529–538). New York: Oxford University Press.

Sauer, W. J., & Coward, R. T. (Eds.) (1985). *Social support networks and the care of the elderly*. New York: Springer.

Savundranayagam, M. Y., & Brintnall-Peterson, M. (2010). Testing self-efficacy as a pathway that supports self-care among family caregivers in a psychoeducational intervention. *Journal of Family Social Work*, 13(2), 149–162.

Savundranayagam, M. Y., Montgomery, R. J. V., Kosloski, K., & Little, T. D. (2010). Impact of a psychoeducational program on three types of caregiver burden among spouses. *International Journal of Geriatric Psychiatry*, 26, 388–396.

Schulz, R., Burgio, L., Burns, R., Eisdorfer, C., Gallagher-Thompson, D., Gitlin, L. N., & Mahoney, D. F. (2003). Resources for Enhancing Alzheimer's Caregiver Health (REACH): overview, site-specific outcomes, and future directions. *The Gerontologist*, 43(4), 514–520.

Sörensen, S., Pinquart, M., & Duberstein, P. (2002). How effective are interventions with caregivers? An updated meta-analysis. *The Gerontologist*, 42(3), 356–372.

Strozier, A. L., Elrod, B., Beiler, P., Smith, A., & Carter, K. (2004). Developing a network of support for relative caregivers. *Children and Youth Services Review*, 26(7), 641–656.

Thompson, C. A., Spilsbury, K., Hall, J., Birks, Y., Barnes, C., & Adamson, J. (2007). Systematic review of information and support interventions for caregivers of people with dementia. *BMC Geriatrics*, 7(1), 18.

Turner, J. A., Ersek, M., & Kemp, C. (2005). Self-efficacy for managing pain is associated with disability, depression, and pain coping among retirement community residents with chronic pain. *The Journal of Pain*, 6(7), 471–479.

Walsh, J. F. (2010). *Psychoeducation in mental health*. Chicago: Lyceum Books.

10

PSYCHOEDUCATIONAL AND SOCIAL SUPPORT INTERVENTIONS
EVIDENCE-BASED PRACTICE

As discussed in the previous chapter, psychoeducational and social support interventions are common practices, to assist both care providers and older adults in adjusting to conditions of later life. With changes in health and functional abilities, for example, care provision roles deal with concomitant experiences of learning new skills (e.g., medication management, dietary changes, dealing with memory loss), and the emotional outcomes of care. Individual-focused interventions frequently deal with decreasing challenging conditions in later life, such as isolation and depression, as well as promoting positive health-sustaining practices.

The structure and content of this chapter are different from previous evidence-based practice chapters in two ways. First, two types of approaches are combined within this chapter. The rationale for discussing the two intervention types together is based on their similar theoretical foundation in social learning theory. In addition, group methods are often used to deliver the intervention, with the resulting connections that emerge among members. Goals of competence, coping, and empowerment are also shared within these approaches.

A second issue is the lack of manualization of the intervention. Although a curriculum is a part of psychoeducation groups, there often are open-ended segments to promote learning, integration, and practice within the the group. Within social support interventions, the goal is to provide an opportunity for the members to process issues that are being experienced, which is antithetical to a manualized process. Although these approaches are more fluid than some of the others discussed in other chapters of this volume, many of these interventions are successfully used in practice with older adults. For these reasons, the two approaches are included as evidence based treatment approaches.

In this chapter, meta-analyses, systematic reviews, and individual studies are reviewed. A literature review for the effectiveness of psychoeducational and social support interventions was conducted in several databases, which include PubMed, PsychoINFO, Social Science Abstracts, Social Service Abstracts, Cochrane Collaborative, and Ageline. The search terms were "older adult" or "elder" with "psychoeducational," "social support," or "supportive" interventions. Additional search terms of "caregiver" and "care provider" were also searched. Studies were included if they had participants who were 60 and older, were related to care provision for someone 60 and older, were published between 2000 and 2015, and included treatment outcomes of psychoeducational and/or social support interventions.

The literature is organized around either the care providers or older adults themselves. Typical outcomes in the caregiver studies are reduction of burden or stress, or increasing skills and coping abilities. Several of these studies specifically focus on dementia caregiving, which is demanding and complex. In the research with older adults, typical outcomes include increased social connections or quality of life, or decreased depression. Overall, the evidence from this research indicates that both psychoeducational and social support interventions are effective interventions with caregivers and older individuals.

META-ANALYSES AND SYSTEMATIC REVIEWS

Eleven meta analyses or systematic reviews report on psychoeducational and/or social support interventions. The majority of these reviews compare the effectiveness of interventions for various conditions (e.g., depression, care provision). Seven articles were reviews of interventions with care providers of older adults, such as the case example of the Alzheimer's Association chapter that sponsored the Coping with Caregiving class for care providers. Additionally, four focused on interventions with older adults themselves, such as the case example of Audrey Barnes in Chapter 9, who participated in a support group with others who were raising grandchildren.

INTERVENTIONS WITH CARE PROVIDERS

Of the seven articles on caregiving, four specifically focused on those who are providing care to older adults with dementia. The remaining three articles include samples that include caregivers for health-related or multi-causal conditions. Besides psychoeducational and support interventions, other treatment approaches that were compared included cognitive behavioral and other forms of psychotherapy, respite, education-based, and mutual aid. Psychoeducational interventions were more frequently represented than social support (see Table 10.1).

Dementia Caregiving
Of the four articles on dementia caregiving, one specifically focused on groups interventions (Chien et al., 2011). Thirty studies were included in the meta-analysis, with the

TABLE 10.1 META ANALYSES AND SYSTEMATIC REVIEWERS WITH CARE PROVIDERS

Study	Inclusion/Exclusion Criteria	Description of Interventions	Number and Description of Participants	Outcomes	Findings
Boots, de Vugt, van Knippenberg, Kempen & Verhey (2013) 12 studies Systematic review	Effects of Internet-based interventions; informal caregivers; care recipients with mild cognitive impairment or dementia.	Interventions included websites with information and support on caregiving, caring strategies, telephone support, caregiving exchanges, and email support.	Participants ranged from 11 to > 700. Typical number of participants was in the 20–40 range. The typical participant was a family caregiver; female, with an average age of 61 years.	Outcomes included caregiver self-efficacy, stress/burden, depressive symptoms, coping, social contact and support, knowledge, utilization of services, and general health and mental health.	Significant positive outcomes on well being, competence, decision-making confidence, self efficacy, and support. Inconclusive outcomes on burden.
Chien et al. (2011) 30 studies Meta-analysis	Informal caregivers of persons with dementia. Quantitative (not qualitative) methods. Groups format led by professionals. Quasi or experimental designs; included control or comparison groups.	Group interventions. Psychoeducational = 20; educational = 5, mutual aid = 5. 66% of participants were randomly assigned to groups. Group size was 6–10 members.	Majority of participants were wives. Average age ranges of caregivers was 44–72 years. Care recipients had moderate levels of dementia.	Outcomes were psychological well-being of the caregivers, caregiver depression or burden, or social isolation.	Positive outcomes were reported for all outcome measures. Caregivers had reduced depression, lower burden, and improved social connections. Greatest intervention effects were in the psychoeducational groups. Optimal: size of 6–10, randomized, and 8 or more sessions.
Gallagher-Thompson & Coon (2007) 19 studies Systematic review	Family caregivers of persons with dementia. Interventions derived from psychological theories of change (e.g. cognitive, behavioral or problem-solving); included a control or comparison group.	Psychoeducation/skill building (n = 14); the rest were psychotherapeutic/ counseling, or multicomponent.	Average age of participants was 62 years. Majority were White. Typically, wives or daughters.	Outcomes included behavior management training for caregivers (n = 4), depression management, skill training (n = 3), lowering caregiver stress threshold (n = 3), anger management (n = 2), and increasing support and family capacity (n = 2).	Psychoeducational and skill-building interventions are effective, with a large effect size across all studies (.81). Outcomes included decreased caregiver distress, enhanced coping and self-efficacy. Most effective interventions are those which include psychoeducational and skill-building components.

(continued)

TABLE 10.1 (CONTINUED)

Study	Inclusion/Exclusion Criteria	Description of Interventions	Number and Description of Participants	Outcomes	Findings
Thompson et al. (2007) 44 RCTs Systematic review	Informal caregivers of persons with dementia. Interventions were either supportive or informational.	Four interventions were technology based; 13 were group based; and 27 were individually based.	3,231 participants in psychoeducational interventions; 2,119 in social support interventions.	Outcomes were caregiver outcomes of quality of life, physical and mental health, burden. *Patient outcomes* were ADLs or behaviors. *Health utilization* outcomes were health-care contacts. *Economic* outcomes were time spent on caregiving.	Psychoeducation increased caregiver knowledge, caregiving role, and self-efficacy, and reduced negative outcomes of care such as depression. Social support interventions increased support and knowledge. Greatest benefits are the combination of these two intervention types.
Sörensen, Pinquart, & Duberstein (2002) 78 studies Meta-analysis	Care recipients 60 years or greater. Included a control group. Outcomes were either mental health or well-being. Peer-reviewed journals.	38 of the studies were psychoeducational interventions; 7 were supportive interventions. Median number of sessions was 8. Group administration (59%); individual sessions (22%); combined approach (18%). Dropout rate for psychoeducational interventions was 16.1% and 12.5% for supportive interventions.	Average age of the caregivers was 62.3 years; females (69%) and spouses (50%) or adult children (40%). The majority resided with the care recipient. More than half of the studies were care of persons with dementia (61%). Average length of care was 4 years. Majority were White (84%).	Six outcomes were identified—caregiver burden, caregiver depression, caregiver well-being, uplifts or rewards, ability and knowledge, or symptoms of care recipient.	Psychoeducation had significant and positive effects on all outcomes. Supportive interventions reduced caregiver burden and increased knowledge and abilities, but had no effect on other outcome variables. Group interventions were more effective in reducing care recipient symptoms but less effective in improving burden and well-being as compared to individual or mixed administrations.

Study	Inclusion criteria	Intervention characteristics	Participants	Outcomes	Findings
Yin, Zhou, & Bashford (2002) 26 studies Meta-analysis	Family caregivers of older adults. Burden as an outcome. Group or individual intervention; control group.	17 studies were randomized. 10 studies had group administration of 4–12 sessions, most offering 8 sessions. Session duration was most frequently 2 hours. Five groups were support interventions, and nine were psychoeducational. Eight studies had individual administrations that ranged from one session to 8 months. Session duration was 1–2.5 hours.	1,408 participants were in treatment conditions. Average sample size was 109. Mean age of the caregivers was 60.1 years, and 79% were women. Majority were White (86.4%). Most lived in the same household as the care recipient (80.3%). Care recipients' average age was 78.8 years; 54% had dementia.	Caregiver burden was the sole outcome evaluated.	All treatments had a positive impact on caregiver burden. In group studies, intervention effect was greater for caregivers who were not White.
Acton & Kang (2001) Meta-analysis 24 Studies	Caregivers of adults with dementia. Intervention was to lessen burden. Included a control group or was a pre–post test.	Interventions included support groups, education, psychoeducation, counseling, respite, or multi-component approaches.	Little information was provided about the participants.	Burden was the sole outcome reported.	Only two treatments resulted in significantly lowered burden scores.

following inclusion criteria: (1) included sample of caregivers for persons with dementia, (2) reported quantitative data, (3) had professionally led group interventions, (4) used quasi or experimental designs, and (5) included control or comparison groups. Twenty studies reported on psychoeducational groups, with the remainder being educational ($n = 5$), or mutual aid ($n = 5$). Sixty-six percent of the participants were randomized into groups, with the typical size being 6–10 members. The majority of the caregivers were female, with an average of 72.5% in the studies. The age range of participants was 43.6–71.8 years, with a caregiving duration of 20.8–70.2 months.

Results indicated that groups are beneficial for caregivers of patients with dementia. There were positive outcomes on caregivers' increased well-being, decreased depression, and increased social connection. There were inconsistent findings on caregiver burden, however, as two studies did not find significant changes after participation in treatment. The researchers conclude that psychoeducational groups are more effective at improving caregiver well-being and decreasing depression than achieving other outcomes.

One meta-analysis specifically focused on interventions to reduce the burden of caregivers for individuals with dementia (Acton & Kang, 2001). Twenty-four studies were included, with the following inclusion criteria: (1) the sample was of informal caregivers; (2) the care recipient had dementia; (3) the outcome measured caregiving burden; and (4) the study design included treatment/control groups or pre-post data. Six types of interventions were included: support ($n = 1$), psychoeducational ($n = 10$), counseling, respite, education, or multi-component approaches. The participants in the study samples ranged from 11 to 180, with a mean of 51.08. The most typical measure for burden was the Burden Interview (Zarit & Zarit, 1990), which was used in 18 studies, with the Burden Scale (Montgomery, Gonyea, & Hooyman, 1985) used in an additional four.

Results indicated that only two treatments had a statistically significant positive impact on burden: respite and a multicomponent intervention strategy. The researchers concluded that "burden" lacks conceptual clarity, making it difficult to measure, and that interventions have more success with increasing positive outcomes related to care provision, such as life satisfaction or meaning, than decreasing challenging aspects such as burden.

A systematic review of 44 RCTs also examined treatment outcomes for informal caregivers of persons with dementia. Intervention administration included individual ($n = 27$), group ($n = 13$), and technology-based ($n = 4$) approaches (Thompson et al., 2007). Inclusion criteria were the following: (1) being a caregiver of someone with dementia; (2) residing within the community; (3) interventions had either a support or educational focus; and (4) caregiver, health utilization, or economic outcomes were reported. Limited information was provided about the sociodemographics of the participants; however, 3,231 participants were involved in psychoeducational interventions, and 2,119 in social support treatments.

Group interventions that used a psychoeducational orientation were the only treatment to reduce caregiver depression. The authors conclude that greater evidence exists for the efficacy and effectiveness of psychoeducational models that provide caregivers information about their role, increase their self-efficacy, and reduce the negative outcomes of care (e.g., depression, anxiety, frustration). Social support interventions only resulted in increased knowledge about care. The authors further conclude that the combination of education and support is the most effective intervention. However, they question the validity of outcome data, as the studies all rely on self report (vs. observational or diagnostic) data.

A final systematic review focused on Internet-based supportive interventions for dementia caregivers (Boots, de Vugt, Knippenberg, Kempen & Verhey, 2014). Twelve studies were included in the analyses if they met the following criteria: (1) were Internet-based; (2) focused on informal (nonprofessional) caregivers; and (3) care recipients had mild cognitive impairment or dementia. Interventions included web-based information and support on caregiving, website + telephone support, website with discussion post shared by other caregivers, and a website with email support. Five studies contained a control group, which was either usual care or wait-list controls. The remaining studies used pre–post test data only. The most common topics of the websites were self-efficacy, stress and burden, depression symptoms, coping, social contact and support, knowledge, and utilization of health services.

Significant outcomes were reported in six of the 12 studies. These were improvement in caregiver depression, sense of competence, confidence in decision-making, and self-efficacy. Mixed results were obtained in caregiver burden, with multiple studies that reported no significant decrease. The researchers conclude that the most effective Internet-based interventions are multicomponent programs that include both informational and supportive aspects. Those programs increased caregiver knowledge, but also fostered connection to normalize the caregiving experience.

Health-Related or Multi-Causal Caregiving Situations
Three additional reviews included caregivers for individuals with health-related, unspecified, or multi-causal situations. Within these articles, dementia care may be included but is not an inclusionary criterion. However, these reviews all included informal caregivers of older adults.

Gallagher-Thompson and Coon (2007) reviewed interventions for reducing distress or improving well-being of family caregivers. While an inclusion criterion was care of an individual with a cognitive and/or physical impairment, dementia care was the predominant reason for care provision. Other criteria for inclusion were the following: (1) treatments were derived from a psychological theory of change; (2) studies were published between 1980 and 2005; and (3) studies reported on outcomes and impacts of treatment. Of the 19 studies included, 14 were psychoeducational or skill-building, with the remainder being counseling or psychotherapeutic, or multicomponent. The participants were mainly wives or daughters of the care recipient, were White, and had an average age of 62 years.

Psychoeducational and skill-building interventions had a large effect size across studies (.81), with the outcomes including decreased caregiver distress (e.g., burden, anger, anxiety, frustration), and enhanced coping and self-efficacy. The authors conclude that the most effective interventions overall are based upon a combined psychoeducational and skill-building format.

Sörensen, Pinquart, and Duberstein (2002) included 78 studies in a meta-analysis of interventions with care providers. The inclusion criteria were the following: (1) studies were of care recipients 60 years or older; (2) an intervention situation was compared to a control group; (3) mental health or well-being outcomes were reported; (4) results were published in a peer-reviewed journal; and (5) studies were written in English, German, French, or Russian. Thirty-eight studies were psychoeducational, and seven were social support interventions, with the remainder being respite, psychotherapy, interventions to increase caregiver competence, multicomponent, and miscellaneous. The most common administration was in a group (59%), followed by individual sessions (22%), or a combined approach (18%). Across the studies, the average age of the caregivers was 62.3 years, and most were female (69%). The majority were spouses (50%) or adult children (40%). The majority of care providers were caring for a person with dementia (61%), with the overall average length of care being 4 years. Only 14% of the caregivers were non-White. Six findings were identified: caregiving burden, caregiver depression, well-being, uplifts or rewards, ability and knowledge, and symptoms of the care recipient.

The results indicated that psychoeducation had the most significant positive effects on all outcomes. Supportive interventions reduced caregiver burden and increased knowledge and abilities, but had no effect on other outcome variables. Group interventions were more effective in reducing care recipient symptoms but less effective in improving burden and well-being as compared to individual or mixed administrations. The greatest changes in burden, well-being, ability/knowledge, and care recipient symptoms were in older (as compared to younger) caregivers.

The final meta-analysis for caregivers reviewed burden on family caregivers for frail older adults (Yin, Zhou, & Bashford, 2002). Twenty-six studies were included, with the following criteria: (1) included burden as an outcome; (2) employed a group or individual intervention; (3) included a control group; and (4) excluded unpublished reports. Seventeen studies randomized participants to a treatment or control condition. Ten studies had group administration, with range of 4–12 sessions, with the most frequent duration being 2 hours. Nine groups were psychoeducational and five were support groups. Eight studies had individual administrations that ranged from one session to 8 months, with session durations ranging from 1 to 2.5 hours. Other interventions included stress management and social skill training. Across studies, average sample size was 109. The mean age of the care providers was 60.1 years; 79% were women and 86.4% were White. Most lived in the same household as the care recipient

(80.3%). Care recipients had an average age of 78.8 years. Dementia was present in 54% of the care recipient sample.

Across the board, all treatments had a positive impact on burden. In the group studies, the intervention effect was greater for caregivers who were races other than White. In addition, RCTs had more robust outcomes than non-experimental designs.

The meta-analyses and systematic reviews in caregiving provide evidence that psychoeducational and support interventions are useful to reduce some of the challenges of this role. In these reviews, psychoeducational interventions were more prevalent than social support, and stronger evidence exists for the effectiveness of psychoeducational approaches. However, comparisons of multiple interventions conclude that both types have utility in practice with care providers.

Studies analyzed various outcomes for care providers. There is greater evidence that these interventions can reduce caregiver depression, and increase connection, well-being, and coping. However, inconclusive results were found on caregiver burden. Some reviews reported that interventions reduced burden, while others reported limited or no change on this outcome. These discrepancies may be a result of poor conceptual clarity about "burden" in caregiving situations, or the possibility that the demands of certain caregiving experiences are not amenable to change by either type of intervention (Acton & Kang, 2001). As a result, targeting interventions to realistic outcomes with caregivers is crucial.

There is support to combine psychoeducational and supportive approaches. Since these two methods target different outcomes for caregivers, the combined approach allows for the informational needs, as well as the opportunity for connection and engagement. A heartening outcome is that multiple methods can be used to provide the interventions, including Internet-based approaches, which can reach isolated care providers.

While there are positive conclusions, there are also areas where additional research is needed. No review specifically identified diverse care providers, including men or racial/ethnic variability. As the population in older adulthood becomes more diverse, approaches that can be applied to subpopulations are critical. In one review, a finding suggested that the intervention effects were higher for caregivers who were not White (Yin et al., 2002). Sorting out these differential outcomes across subpopulations is critical.

INTERVENTIONS WITH OLDER ADULTS

Four reviews focused on interventions for older adults themselves. These studies included interventions to reduce depression, increase well-being, or enhance social functioning. Various treatment conditions were compared, including cognitive behavioral interventions, insight-oriented therapies, interventions to enhance social connections, as well as

TABLE 10.2 META-ANALYSES AND SYSTEMATIC REVIEWERS WITH INDIVIDUAL OLDER ADULTS

Study	Inclusion/Exclusion Criteria	Description of Interventions	Number and Description of Participants	Outcomes	Findings
Leung, Orrell, & Orgeta (2015) 2 studies Systematic review	RCTs; included a control or comparison group. Participants with dementia or included data on those with dementia if mixed sample.	One multi-modal intervention, 20 weeks, 3 times per week, 1 hour. Social support group 90 minutes, weekly for 9 weeks.	Mean ages were 75 and 77 years. All participants were in early stages of dementia.	Primary outcome was depression. One study included quality of life and the second self-esteem.	All participants in had improved depression scores. Quality of life and self esteem scores also improved.
Pinquart, Duberstein, & Lyness, 2007 57 studies Meta-analysis	Mean or median age: ≥ 60 years. Subjects met criteria for major or minor depression or dysthymia according to ICD 10, DSM-III, III-R, or IV. Comparison group contained an untreated control.	CBT, psychoeducation, supportive, brief dynamic psychotherapy, exercise, reminiscence, and interpersonal therapy (IPT); 61.7% used a group format; 23.4% focused on inpatients; M # of sessions per treatment:15.2.	Studies included 1,956 treated participants. M age: 71.8 years (5.4); 67% were women and 43.3% were married.	All interventions, except IPT, significantly reduced depression. Effect sizes largest for CBT and reminiscence. CBT, reminiscence, and exercise had small to medium long-term effects. Smaller effect sizes found for those with major depression.	All treatment conditions were effective in reducing depressive symptoms in older adults. Psychoeducational and supportive interventions had medium effect sizes. No advantages were found for treatments of longer duration

Findlay (2003)	Sample defined as older adults.	Five studies were individual interventions.	Little information was provided about the participants.	Individual outcomes were social connection and contact, reduced suicide risk.	Interventions reduced isolation and enhanced social connection.
17 studies	Interventions targeted social isolation and/or loneliness.	Six were group interventions.		Group outcomes increased connection and social support.	Guidelines for offering effective programs include selecting and training effective facilitators and interventionists,
Systematic review	Studies were published in English between 1982 and 2002.	Two studies were service programs.		Service program outcomes decreased isolation.	
		Three studies were Internet support programs.		Internet outcomes were enhanced decision-making, decreased loneliness.	
		Six studies were RCTs.			
Pinquart & Sörensen, (2001)	Participants 55 years or older.	Nine treatments were compared, including supportive and psychoeducational.	Mean age ranged from 55 to 87, with a mean across studies of 71.4 years.	Outcomes were depression and/or subjective well-being.	Supportive and psychoeducational treatments significantly reduced depression.
122 studies	Control group.	1 to 250 sessions with a median of 9.	Female participants ranged from 0 to 100%, with a mean of 71%.		
Meta analysis	Outcomes were depression or subjective well-being.	Group treatments were examined in 65% of the studies, 28% used individual approaches, and 7% combined both.			
		Participants in the interventions ranged from 10 to 134, with a mean of 21.			

social support and psychoeducational approaches. These intervention approaches were compared to determine overall effectiveness (see Table 10.2).

Three of the four studies had depression as the sole or major outcome of the review. Pinquart, Duberstein, and Lyness (2007) reviewed 57 studies on the effect of psychotherapy and other behavioral interventions in depressed older adults. Inclusion criteria were (1) meeting diagnostic criteria for major or minor depressive disorder, or dysthymic disorder; (2) the mean age of the study was 60 years or more; (3) the intervention was psychological or behavioral; and (4) a control group was included. Eight programs were psychoeducational and three were classified as social support. Sixty-two percent of the studies had interventions provided in group formats, and 88% had random assignment to treatment or control conditions. Within these studies, the average age of participants was 71.1 years; 67% were female, and 43% were married.

The only outcome reviewed in the study was the change in depression of participants. The results indicated that all treatment conditions, expect for interpersonal psychotherapy, showed significant improvement post-intervention. Both psychoeducational and supportive interventions had a medium effect size. Changes in depression rates were also viewed by cohort groups. Improvements were found across all age groups, even those in the oldest group (> 76.2 years); however, the changes were more dramatic in those less than 68 years. The authors conclude that psychoeducational and supportive interventions are effective in reducing depression in the older population.

A second meta-analysis on depression examined 127 studies that examined nine types of psychosocial interventions, including supportive treatments and psychoeducational interventions (Pinquart & Sörensen 2001). Studies were included if (1) participants were 55 years or older, (2) the study had a treatment condition and a control group, (3) the study included outcomes of depression or subjective well-being, and (4) it was written in English, French, or German. The interventions were mostly offered in group formats (65%), with fewer having individual treatment (28%) or combined (7%) approaches. The number of participants in the interventions ranged from 10 to 134, with a mean of 21. Nine different treatments were compared, including social support and psychoeducational approaches. The number of sessions ranged from 1 to 250, with a median of 9. Group treatments were examined in 65% of the studies, 28% used individual approaches, and 7% combined both. The number of participants in the interventions ranged from 10 to 134, with a mean of 21. The average age of participants in the studies ranged from 55 to 87, with a mean across studies of 71.4 years. Female participants ranged from 0 to 100%, with a mean of 71%. Depression was measured by either self-reports (57 studies) or clinician ratings (12 studies). Measures of subjective well-being were self-reported (84 studies) and included happiness, life satisfaction, and self-esteem.

Results indicated that both intervention approaches were effective in reducing depression. Although not as strong as psychotherapeutic impacts, social support and psychoeducational treatments significantly reduced depression. For measures of subjective well-being, cognitive behavioral interventions were more effective than support or psychoeducational treatment.

In a final review on depression, this condition was measured in individuals who had mild dementia. Leung, Orrell, and Ortega (2015) conducted a systematic review of RCTs of social support groups in people with dementia and cognitive impairment. Only two studies met the inclusion criteria of (1) being an RCT, (2) having a comparison or control group, (3) providing separate data on participants with dementia or cognitive impairment if a mixed study, and (4) including older adults with a dementia or cognitive impairment diagnosis. One study was a multi-modal intervention including social support, CBT, and exercise. This class met for 3 times a week for 20 weeks. The second was a support group that included topics of medical causes and treatments, future planning, communication strategies, and daily living. This intervention was held in 90-minute sessions, weekly for 9 weeks. The mean ages in the studies were 77 and 75 years. All participants were in the early stages of dementia.

The findings indicated that participants in both studies had improved depression scores at post-tests. Quality of life, measured in one study, also improved, as did self-esteem, which was measured in the second study.

A final review with older adults was on social isolation or loneliness. Findlay (2003) reviewed studies that assessed effectiveness of interventions to reduce these conditions in the older population. Inclusion criteria were the following: (1) interventions targeted loneliness or social isolation; (2) interventions were intended to achieve health gain; (3) interventions had recorded outcome measures; and (4) results were published in English between 1982 and 2002. Seventeen studies were included, with five studies that focused on individual interventions to reduce suicide, increase support, and link to service networks; six were group interventions for older adults with disabilities, isolated caregivers, older women experiencing loneliness, and widows; two were service programs to increase support or contact with others; and four were Internet support programs for care providers or older adults. Six of the studies were RCTs. Unfortunately, no information was provided about the sociodemographic characteristics of the participants.

Results indicated that individual interventions had outcomes of increased social contact, reduced suicide rates, and increased referrals to social programs. Group interventions decreased loneliness, increased social connection, and enhanced social support. Outcomes of service programs were greater use of supports, decreased isolation, and decreased mortality rates. Finally, the Internet-based intervention outcomes decreased loneliness and enhanced decision-making. The author concludes that, despite the dearth of rigorous research in this area, existing studies suggest that there are multiple methods to decrease isolation and increase social connections within the older population.

Results from these reviews provide evidence that psychoeducational and support interventions are effective in decreasing problematic and challenging conditions of aging. Participants in the studies had lower depression rates, increased social connections, and enhanced well-being such as happiness and life satisfaction. As compared to other interventions, support and psychoeducational programs were more effective than several others. However, cognitive behavioral approaches had the strongest outcomes in decreasing depression.

CONCLUSION

Both psychoeducational and social support interventions have demonstrated efficacy with older adults and care providers. Research on psychoeducational approaches are more abundant in the literature, and when compared with social support, appear to yield better results. In particular, the combination of psychoeducational and support interventions as a multi-intervention approach can target knowledge, skills, coping, and social connection.

Meta-analyses and systematic reviews tended to compare psychoeducational and social support to other treatment conditions to evaluate effectiveness. In studies with caregivers or older adults, there is a clear need to target interventions to intended outcomes. Depending on the outcome variable (e.g., increased knowledge, decreased isolation), the intervention approach should be consistent with the available literature in that area. Unfortunately, decisions about the type and structure of interventions may not take these factors into account, with the misguided belief that similar outcomes are achieved. Distinctions between outcomes such as increasing well-being or decreasing depression, as compared to enhancing skill level, should lead to different types of intervention approaches.

Within group formats, evidence indicates that effectiveness differs by the duration of the group. For psychoeducational groups, 7–9 weeks is a sufficient duration for participants to gain increased competency (Sörensen et al., 2002). Emotional aspects, such as depression, that are the foundation of social support groups, take longer to change. Although no specific length was discussed, Chien et al. (2011) report that groups that last longer than 8 weeks have a higher treatment effect.

Like other interventions that have been reviewed, the study samples are homogeneous, which reflects a sample bias. Few studies have focused on diverse caregivers or populations of older adults, and as the population grows more diverse, this is a critical need. When specified, the typical focus is on caregivers of individuals with dementia. This is certainly a needed area of research, but research on care in other health or mental health situations is needed as well.

Compared to other interventions (e.g., reminiscence, life review, motivational interviewing), these approaches have fewer manualized approaches or constructed curricula. In fact, several studies evaluated individually constructed plans for helping with skill attainment or coping. While this approach is interesting, there is a lack of specificity in the intervention approach, which makes administration across multiple applications difficult. Questions about the fidelity of the interventions are warranted.

Future research needs to address some of the gaps. First, the inclusion of diverse populations within the interventions is necessary, as well as description about necessary changes in the implementation of the intervention. Additionally, the contexts for many of these interventions was in the community, or within acute care hospitals. There is limited application to residents in long-term care settings, or their care providers. As an example, family members struggle with issues of care and connection after the care recipient relocates to a more supported environment. How can these interventions help families deal with these difficult transitions? How can the new resident be assisted to cope with the changes and relocation? This context seems fertile for both psychoeducational and social support interventions.

Across the board, studies suffer from a lack of rigor in design and implementation. Numerous studies were excluded from the meta-analyses or systematic reviews because they did not meet inclusionary criteria of control or comparison groups, specificity about the intervention, or had limited sample size. Relatedly, samples tend to be homogeneous, mainly consisting of white female caregivers. Future studies that increase sample sizes, use multiple administrations, and include diverse care providers will strengthen knowledge about effective psychoeducational and social support interventions.

REFERENCES

Acton, G. J., & Kang, J. (2001). Interventions to reduce the burden of caregiving for an adult with dementia: a meta-analysis. *Research in Nursing & Health, 24*(5), 349–360.

Boots, L. M. M., Vugt, M. E., Knippenberg, R. J. M., Kempen, G. I. J. M., & Verhey, F. R. J. (2014). A systematic review of Internet-based supportive interventions for caregivers of patients with dementia. *International Journal of Geriatric Psychiatry, 29*(4), 331–344.

Chien, L. Y., Chu, H., Guo, J. L., Liao, Y. M., Chang, L. I., Chen, C. H., & Chou, K. R. (2011). Caregiver support groups in patients with dementia: a meta-analysis. *International Journal of Geriatric Psychiatry, 26*(10), 1089–1098.

Findlay, R. A. (2003). Interventions to reduce social isolation amongst older people: where is the evidence? *Ageing and Society, 23*(5), 647–658.

Gallagher-Thompson, D., & Coon, D. W. (2007). Evidence-based psychological treatments for distress in family caregivers of older adults. *Psychology and Aging, 22*(1), 37.

Lamdan., R. M., Taylor, K. L. & Siegel, J. E. (2000). *Treatment manual for support group interventions developed for African American women with non-metastatic breast cancer.* Unpublished manuscript.

Leung, P., Orrell, M., & Orgeta, V. (2015). Social support group interventions in people with dementia and mild cognitive impairment: a systematic review of the literature. *International Journal of Geriatric Psychiatry, 30*(1), 1–9.

Montgomery, R. J., Gonyea, J. G., & Hooyman, N. R. (1985). Caregiving and the experience of subjective and objective burden. *Family Relations, 34*(1), 19–26.

Pinquart, M., Duberstein, P. R., & Lyness, J. M. (2007). Effects of psychotherapy and other behavioral interventions on clinically depressed older adults: a meta-analysis. *Aging & Mental Health, 11*(6), 645–657.

Pinquart, M., & Sörensen, S. (2001). How effective are psychotherapeutic and other psychosocial interventions with older adults? A meta-analysis. *Journal of Mental Health and Aging*, 7, 207–243.

Sörensen, S., Pinquart, M., & Duberstein, P. (2002). How effective are interventions with caregivers? An updated meta-analysis. *The Gerontologist*, 42(3), 356–372.

Thompson, C. A., Spilsbury, K., Hall, J., Birks, Y., Barnes, C., & Adamson, J. (2007). Systematic review of information and support interventions for caregivers of people with dementia. *BMC Geriatrics*, 7(1), 18.

Yin, T., Zhou, Q., & Bashford, C. (2002). Burden on family members: caring for frail elderly: a meta-analysis of interventions. *Nursing Research*, 51(3), 199–208.

Zarit, S. H., & Zarit, J. M. (1990). *The memory and behavior problems checklist and the burden interview*. University Park: Gerontology Center, Pennsylvania State University.

11

REMINISCENCE AND LIFE REVIEW
THEORY AND PRACTICE

The act of reminiscing is a natural part of human interaction and takes place across the life course. For example, the allure of high school and family reunions is partially about retelling life experiences and recalling shared events. While reminiscing, people of all ages share the joys, pleasures, and sometimes pains of their previous selves with others who understand these experiences.

With age, older adults use event recall as a way to integrate their past with present-day functioning. Older adults' unique life stories are a mingling of their distinct and individual experiences. As Randall (2014) states, life is not only about *having* a story, but more important, about *being* a story. For example, being the oldest in the family, going off to war, getting married, and having children are unique experiences of an individual. While there are other oldest children, soldiers, married individuals, and parents, each of these experiences are distinct for *that* person.

The social era in which individuals developed also impacts their life story. Being an African American who lived during racial segregation, or being a gay man or lesbian when homosexuality was considered a sin or psychopathology, also influences development and sense of self. As older individuals, the unique aspects of their life course are combined with their experience of living during particular social times to become the story that they are (Randall, 2014).

Reminiscence can have particular functions for older adults. Reminiscence "is a phenomenological process of recalling the past that provides people with both pleasure and pain. It has healing qualities and provides a vehicle for socializing with others" (Haight et al., 2003, p. 165). With age, reminiscing becomes more prominent, as older adults use this process to create meaning and integration for events across their life course, have a heightened awareness of the finiteness of life, and work to create meaningful roles in a society that limits experiences in later adulthood (Westerhof, Bohlmeijer, & Valenkamp, 2004). For these reasons, reminiscence and life review have been used as therapeutic processes to address challenges experienced during late life.

A brief example will illustrate how reminiscence is a valuable approach for older adults. A social work intern was working at a senior center and noticed that the men rarely participated in any of the activities. In considering how to engage the men, she researched the history of the senior center building, which was an old railroad station. She used this situation as a way to design an activity that would engage the men, and help reduce their isolation at the center.

The intern constructed a history book about the railroad station and invited the men to look at the pictures with her. As a hub of the (then) small town, the railroad was a focal point for the community. As a result, the men began to weave their life stories with the various images and started the process of reminiscing together.

The stories that the men told were very poignant and established trusting relationships between them. Over the several weeks that the sessions were held, stories of "hellos" and "good-byes" at the train station were shared. A few men recalled being at the station with their families or sweethearts as they left as young soldiers. Another told about the joy of seeing his older brother return from war without harm. This facility was a pivotal structure that held a great deal of meaning for them, both individually and as a group.

In addition, the stories also provided a way to deepen understanding about how life circumstances differed among the group members. As a community in the South, this station was a segregated facility that separated spaces between Blacks and Whites. The two African-American men told emotional stories about walking through the "colored" door and seeing White families on the other side. While this experience was not shared by all group members, the recounting of this poignant example deepened the bonds between the men.

HISTORY AND BACKGROUND

Reminiscence and life review work have origins in several social gerontology theories. Reminiscence has different purposes and outcomes, depending on the theoretical lens and perspective. Wadensten and Hägglund (2006) review several social gerontology theories and link each one to positive outcomes of reminiscence work. Although there are ways of conceptualizing these processes based upon theoretical perspective, a unifying theme is that the past has significant implications for an individual's current life as an aging adult.

One of the early social gerontology theories was *social disengagement*, which was based upon a landmark book by Cummings and Henry (1961). This theoretical perspective cast older adults as disengaging from social interactions and networks as a way to prepare for death. Social withdrawal was also functional for society, as older adults would "move aside" to provide opportunities for younger generations. As part of the disengagement process, older individuals became more inwardly focused, that is, involved in their internal world. Neugarten (1968) termed this process "interiority." From a perspective of disengagement, older adults were turning inward to revisit their life experiences as they prepared for the ending period in the life course.

However, Robert Butler (1963) promoted a different viewpoint on the process of reminiscing in older adulthood. Butler is credited as an early proponent of the importance of reminiscence, and he redefined reminiscence as a naturally occurring and positive experience that was not totally associated with preparation for the end of life. Instead [it] "is a normal developmental task of the later years characterized by a return of memories and past conflicts" (Wadensten & Hägglund, 2006, p. 161). The review of past experiences, both pleasant and painful, can be therapeutic as older adults revisit and integrate their previous life experiences.

Partially in response to the negative characterization of aging that was promoted through disengagement theory, other theoretical perspectives were promulgated that had a more positive view of the aging process. *Activity theory* (c.f., Havighurst, 1961) is the opposite of disengagement theory, and this perspective argues that greater activity in later life is associated with a higher level of life satisfaction. For example, volunteering is a social role that is important to many older adults as a way to remain engaged within their communities. The opportunity provides structure, social connection, and feelings of purpose. In *continuity theory* (c.f., Atchley, 1989), life satisfaction is related to stable and continuing patterns that were present during early years. An adventurous person might choose to travel after retirement, while a "homebody" may take cooking lessons. The form of activity is aligned with the structure of their life during earlier years. For these perspectives, reminiscence has the function of retaining roles and identity of earlier times in later life. Revisiting aspects of their past selves provides a stable sense of who they are at this period of their life (Parker, 1995).

Another perspective on reminiscence is consistent with the *developmental perspective* of Erik Eriksen. Eriksen promoted an epigenetic view of human behavior, in which each period had foundations in an earlier phase (Greene & Kropf, 2009). The final stage, Integrity versus Despair, is the psychosocial crisis of "owning" one's life and coming to terms with mortality. Successful navigation of this stage involves integration of past, present, and future experiences. The "self story" or "autobiography" is part of this integrative process (Randall & Kenyon, 2001). A life review process, "according to Erikson, can help create an acceptance of one's one and only life cycle with few or no regrets. It does this by helping individuals integrate memories into a meaningful whole, and [providing] a harmonious view of past, present, and future" (Haber, 2006, p. 157).

Although the original focus of integrity was primarily on the individual's functioning, theoretical work has started to incorporate the place of the person within a social context. The social components involve consideration of the connection of the individual to future generations, and a desire to promote the development and well-being of those who are in younger cohorts (McAdams, 2006). Furthermore, older adults who do not feel connected to subsequent generations can feel dismissed, disengaged, or unvalued by others (Cheng, 2009). Reminiscence is a process that can facilitate the involvement of the older individual in establishing their connection and contributions to others, and establish these social bonds in later life.

A final theory base is *gerotranscendence*, which promotes the orientation that late life involves a transformation from the priorities of younger periods. In this theoretical perspective, "[o]ld age is not a mere continuation of the activity patterns and values of mid-life, but, rather, something different: a transformation characterized by new ways of understanding life, "activities," oneself and others" (Tornstam, 2005, p. 144). Gerotranscendence moves beyond the final stage of integrity in Erikson's development theory to the place in the life course where the individual introspectively examines his or her unique life course as a way to understand present and future functioning (Tornstam, 1999–2000). During this period, the individual focuses less on "superfluous social interactions" and spends more time on meditative and reflective solitude (Jewell, 2014, p. 118). In this way, revisiting one's previous life experiences through reminiscence is part of the identity formation at this place in life. At the final part of the life course, older adults have the task of knowing themselves as both unique and connected individuals.

THEORETICAL FOUNDATION

This section outlines some of the major tenets and principles of reminiscence and life review. A major function of these two approaches is to foster a sense of meaning within the lives of older adults. Various types of reminiscence and life review are highlighted with the connection to meaning-making activities of older individuals. Additionally, particular conditions, challenges, or problems where these approaches have been successfully implemented are highlighted within this section.

MEANING-MAKING FUNCTIONS

Regardless of the theoretical perspective, reminiscence and life review are related to meaning-making work for older adults. Dittmann-Kohli and Westerhof (2000) identify two different types of personal meaning systems. One involves understanding the significance of one's life and the ability to interpret the importance and uniqueness of experiences. This type of meaning system includes a search for a sense of *coherence* or *integration* that pulls together the components of one's life. A second type of meaning involves the goals and motives that are related to one's sense of personhood and life. This type of meaning is founded upon motivations to *find a purpose* in one's life. Therefore, "the term 'meaning of life' can thus be understood as the interpretation of what it means to live one's life on the one hand, and the goals and purposes one has in life on the other hand" (Westerhof, Bohlmeijer, & Valenkamp, 2004, p. 752).

Finding personal meaning is associated with positive outcomes for older adults. Life review and reminiscence interventions have been associated with improvements in meaning-making activities for older adults (Westerhof Bohlmeijer, van Beljouw, & Pot, 2010). Reker and Chamberlain (2000) examined meaning systems across different experiences in later life and suggest that meaning is important in dealing with challenges associated with later life, including illness, caregiving, and approaching death. In a meta-analysis of reminiscence research, Pinquart and Forstmeier (2012) discussed how this intervention approach has utility in assisting non-clinical older populations in achieving ego-integrity. These intervention approaches can be used to help older adults make meaning of their lives and integrate their experiences into a coherent sense of self. Research in this area demonstrates that there is utility in introducing these approaches not only with adults who are challenged by issues in later life, but also with those individuals who are doing well.

The terms "reminiscence" and "life review" have been used almost synonymously thus far; however, important distinctions exist. Even within the related literature, these two terms are used interchangeably and may be misunderstood (Shellman, Mokel, & Hewitt, 2009). In an early article, Burnside and Haight (1994) discuss the important differences in these two approaches. These authors describe *life review* as "a process of reviewing, organizing, and evaluating the overall picture of one's life with the purpose of achieving integrity by seeing one's own life as a unique story. The life review uses memory and reminiscence as tools to conduct the life review and achieve the aforementioned goal" (p. 56). Using a different lens, "life review is structured and evaluative, whereas the process of reminiscence can be more random and is not nearly as focused on integrating life's events" (Haight et al., 2003, p. 167). As described, life review has a therapeutic function that enables individuals to reconcile past experiences that have engendered hurts, pains, or feelings of incompleteness. Although these situations may have occurred years earlier, a lack of closure for these experiences may continue into late life.

Various types of life review have been identified, with different ways of incorporating one's past into the self-narrative. The two types that have received the most attention are integrative and instrumental reminiscence (Karimi et al., 2010; Korte, Westerhof, & Bolmeijer, 2012; Watt & Cappeliez, 2000). *Integrative reminiscence* involves the synthesis of both positive and negative memories in one's life. In addition, this type of reminiscence can be used to discover meaning in one's experiences—even through painful events or tragedies. For example, a parent who lost a son during a war may bring up the painful experiences of loss, anger, and sadness that resulted from his empty place in the family. However, the process may also bring up the joyful family times spent together during younger years, such as vacations and holidays. Even the experience of death can include emotions such as pride in a son's service to his country and appreciation of a community that embraced the family during their sadness.

A second type, *instrumental reminiscence*, uses past experiences to address situations or challenges that are part of present functioning. In this type of life review process, those places where memories evoke examples of strengths and resilience are incorporated into present narratives. As a result, an older adult who may be experiencing stresses or challenges of aging can access aspects of his or her past self to cope with present-day situations. An older man who emigrated during his young adult years, for example, may use that experience as he prepares to leave his home for an assisted living facility. Although he had to leave the familiarity of his homeland, culture, and language, he experienced many gains in his new country, including a good career, marriage, and opportunities for his children. Using these experiences as a foundation, he can reclaim a sense of resilience that is needed in his current situation of moving into an unfamiliar environment. Just as the previous journey yielded new opportunities, he may find that the new residence provides new friendships, a sense of safety, and engagement.

While life review has a more therapeutic focus, reminiscence has positive and pleasurable outcomes for older adults as well. Cappeliez, O'Rourke, & Chaudhury (2005) developed a model that synthesized research on reminiscence that outlines three primary functions (see Figure 11.1). The first category is *self functions*, which are intra-personal or private outcomes. Examples include reminiscence that promotes identity or continuity. For some older adults, especially the current cohort of older men, their work- or career-related identity has important meaning. Although retired, older men may relate their labor force roles to their sense of competence, being a provider, and productivity. Reminiscence that revisits these parts of their life can link their past self as a teacher, engineer, machinist, and so on, with their current sense of themselves. In addition, the

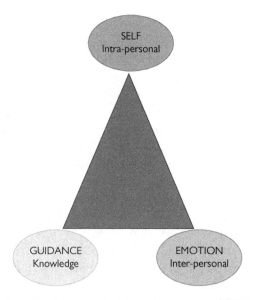

FIGURE 11.1 Functions of reminiscence. Adapted from Cappeliez et al. (2005). Functions of reminiscence and mental health in later life. *Aging and Mental Health*, 9(4), 296.

workplace may also be a site of connection, where friendships and respected relationships developed. These connections may also be a part of reminiscing about their jobs and careers. A second function is *guidance*, which can be in the form of a life lesson or important wisdom. In this type of reminiscence, older adults can revisit those experiences that have had sustained importance. For example, an older person may reminisce about the importance of forgiveness by recalling a time when he or she was forgiven for a hurtful action. This vital lesson can serve all of us well across the life course as we experience small, everyday assaults. A final type of reminiscence relates to *emotional functioning* and is linked to intimacy and the continuity of relationships. For example, some older adults have outlived many (or most) of their family members. Reminiscence that includes memories of times spent with others can provide a sense of connection to their family members, even if they are no longer alive. This type of outcome preserves their sense of family and relationships.

INDIVIDUAL AND COLLECTIVE FUNCTIONS

Life review and reminiscence have both individual and collective functions. Individually, this process can promote positive functioning for older adults by enhancing enjoyable, pleasant, and productive memories. For example, individuals can feel connected to others through remembering positive and socially engaged times in their past. Other memories can promote feelings of accomplishments, productivity, and worth that translate into positive feelings of self in the present. In addition, the experience of revisiting resilience in one's past can promote feelings of strength and coping in the present (Greene & Kropf, 2011).

The process of sharing one's memories is also functional as part of reminiscence and life review. In the course of remembering *life out loud*, an older adult and a listener create a "psychosocial legacy" (Kivnick, 1996, p. 49). Through sharing the experiences, the memories become part of the present-day exchange, which is meaningful its own right.

Reminiscing has a collective function as well. As the initial case vignette of the chapter exemplifies, shared experiences can produce a sense of bonds, relationship, or understanding. In life review with soldiers from World War II, the process promoted civic pride in these men who served their country together (Coleman, Hautamaki, & Podolskij, 2002). Through their shared storying, their narratives and remembering sparked gratification in their shared mission and accomplishments as young soldiers. In this way, the outcome of the reminiscence went beyond the individual outcomes to a collective sense of their importance in the history of their country.

THE PROCESS OF REMINISCENCE

How does reminiscence happen, and what facilitates the recall of past memories? Early research addressed the structure of reminiscence for older adults and the gateway to memory selection (Merriam, 1989). Initially, the individual *selects* certain memories; most often, this occurs through prompts such as "remember a family vacation." After the individual identifies particular instances that fit with the theme, she or he will select a particular vacation, such as a week at the beach. The next component is *immersion* within those memories; that is, the individual retrieves a holistic experience of that vacation. Typically, the individual will become aware of multiple sensory experiences, such as the sounds of the waves, the feel of the sand, or the smell of frying fish.

Upon retrieving and moving into the memory, the remaining phases are differentiating the experiences from later ones and present-day functioning. After retrieval, there is a process of *withdrawal*, which differentiates the past events from those in the individual's present life; that is, the individual is aware that this is a memory, and there is a contrast to the experience of his or her life today. In this process, the individual moves away from the telling of the historical experience to a statement of how that influenced subsequent life periods. For example, the person may describe the family vacation as a pivotal moment that influenced later life experiences, such as a love for travel and adventure. In addition, the person may also compare today—"I still love to travel, although now 'my trips' are outings organized through the activity director here. Although I can't drive anymore, I still get to visit new places!" Finally, there is *closure*, which involves a summation and provides an ending to the recall. Sometimes, this process involves learning or insight, for example, someone stating that "a family vacation meant that you had to be flexible. When it rained at the beach, you went inside and played cards. That was still fun! You have to be flexible with a lot of things in life—even learning to leave your home and move into assisted living like I did."

PRACTICE APPROACHES AND APPLICATION

The reminiscence process occurs naturally, so practitioners and clinicians can implement the interventions in a number of contexts, with various types of administration and different populations. One method to use reminiscence work is to have a structured approach, such as offering group sessions. This type is frequently used within congregate settings such as senior centers, or long-term care residences. As in the opening case example of the reminiscence group with older men, this type of intervention can facilitate bonding between members, can help them learn more about each other's experiences, and can provide a pleasant exchange for their life experiences.

Reminiscence groups can be powerful, pleasant, and poignant experiences for older adults. "Something occurs when people reminisce together, a spontaneous bond, a moment of shared recall, an eagerness to participate, as like memories push to the forefront of the mind" (Haight, et al., 2003, pp. 165–166). The process of reminiscing is a social condition, as the memories are shared from one person to others.

Several guides exist to help facilitators run reminiscence groups; they include topics and activities to help activate the reminiscence process (cf., Laurenhue, 2007). Different themes that can be introduced to facilitate reminiscence include music or arts, television or cultural events, historical experiences, holiday traditions, and special events. As part of this process, it is important to provide stimulation to help older adults retrieve memories. For example, music or pictures of the era when the participants were adolescents or young adults can be included.

Couples can also participate in reminiscence or life review work together. This intervention can be used when there is an impending juncture, such as deteriorating health or cognitive functioning. The process of reminiscence or life review can expand the range of memories that are shared within a couple or caregiving dyad, and can facilitate a richer and deeper relationship between the individuals (Haight et al., 2003). For example, The Couples Life Story Approach is an intervention with couples when one has dementia (Ingersoll-Dayton, Spencer, Kwak, Scherrer, Allen, & Campbell, 2013). Through a structured approach, couples create a storybook together, which provides a focus for their engagement. This process promotes interaction between the couple, allows them to revisit their history as a couple and family, and results in a tangible product that they can revisit after the program concludes.

Reminiscence and life review work can also be individual interventions. For example, transitions that occur in later life can be facilitated by these interventions as older adults access coping and resilience that can benefit their current life situation. In this way, structured approaches can be used by clinicians and practitioners to help with residential transitions, and health and social changes.

However, opportunities spontaneously arise with older adults in which reminiscence is therapeutic. As some older adults lose opportunities for social interactions through functional declines and social losses, their interactions may primarily be with formal supports. Families may feel uncomfortable witnessing feelings and emotions that accompany painful or sad reminiscences. Often, the formal caregiver (e.g., social worker, nurse, health aide) is the person who is engaged in reminiscence with older adults.

An example of a spontaneous life review with a formal provider is that between a care manager and an older woman who were reviewing family pictures together. The client, Mrs. Munday, lost a son to suicide several years before (Gillies & James, 1994). As she and the care manager were reviewing pictures, she described the relationships that she held with each of her three sons. When she discussed her youngest son, a soldier who was injured during service, she said, ". . . he had been unable to accept his life afterwards, and he had killed himself. She wept as she talked about him and seemed to relive her desperate wish to help him but 'I couldn't give him his legs back'" (p. 26). Furthermore, she described the close relationships that she shared with her other sons, and she was able to acknowledge all of the love and support that she provided them. Afterward, she discussed the importance of these memories, and how much she enjoyed sharing them with the care manager. She finished by stating that "she could not talk freely to her family: 'they don't like to see me upset, you see, but I can't just sort out the happy things, can I?'" (p. 26).

Other methods besides verbal interactions have been used to conduct life review and reminiscence. A life book is a tangible way to tell the story of one's life, typically including pictures or images that represent different aspects of the person's life, along with narrative that details the importance of these events. While these books cannot contain everything about an older adult's life, the older individual can be helped to sort out the events that have the most meaning to him or her and capture the associated story.

With technological advances, computerized life review versions have also been implemented. In an experiment using computerized modules, a life review intervention was conducted that had half in-person experience and half online (Preschl et al., 2012). Results indicated that the online intervention was effective in decreasing depression, suggesting that online interventions hold promise for work with older adults.

To facilitate reminiscence, the practitioner needs to be open to the experience with an older adult. Too frequently, contexts where reminiscence or life review takes place are settings where other tasks compete for time, for example, long-term care settings where staff assist residents with activities of daily living (ADLs), or hospitals where nurses are busy caring for other patients. However, listening for an entry into the recall of memories is an important step in facilitating reminiscence.

Even older adults who have cognitive decline can invite others into a reminiscence. For example, Gillies and James (1994) provide an example of a hospital nurse who was working with an older woman with a cognitive impairment. The patient continued to call the nurse Lily, although that was not her name. After trying to correct her, the nurse asked, "Do I remind you of Lily? Did Lily look like me? Was she Asian too?" (p. 30). With these prompts, the woman became animated and started to tell the story of Lily, who cared for her and her three siblings as her mother was widowed and had to work. After this exchange, the bond between the nurse and older patient developed, which allowed the nurse to help her adjust during her hospitalization.

Practitioners must also be aware of ways that they invite older adults into reminiscence or life review work. For example, a common reminiscence theme is recalling holiday celebrations, as these times typically spark positive and pleasant memories of family, cultural traditions, and connections. However, opening with a statement such as "Let's think about our favorite holiday when we were children" can be confusing. Most of us have several holidays that hold special meaning. Instead, some additional structure can help the older adult without engendering frustration. For example, the facilitator could state, "It's wintertime, and several holidays are part of the winter season—Thanksgiving, Hanukkah, Christmas, New Years. Think of one of these winter holidays that was special for you as a child." Starting with this type of reminiscence suggestion, older adults may have less difficulty selecting a time for recall.

REMINISCENCE AND LIFE REVIEW WITH DIVERSE OLDER ADULTS

Since life review and reminiscence are interventions that have been specifically designed for practice with older adults, there is no reason to discuss needed modifications for this age group. However, reminiscence and life review have been modified for greater utility with diverse segments of the older population. In this section, reminiscence and life review with diverse subgroups of older adults are presented. These include African-American older adults, people with dementia and psychiatric conditions, veterans, and the older LGBT population. As these studies demonstrate, older adults who have experienced marginalized or oppressed social status may benefit from these approaches to heal wounds as well as embrace the joy and resilience in their past.

AFRICAN AMERICAN OLDER ADULTS

The older population is becoming more racially and ethnically diverse, so application to minority elders is imperative. In particular, the use of interventions that are congruent with cultural traditions and practices are needed. There is evidence that African-American older adults use reminiscence for different purposes than their White counterparts. In a study of centenarians, African Americans were more likely to use reminiscence as a method for personal insight, to cope with changes that were occurring within their lives, and for transmission of information to younger cohorts (Merriam, 1993). Reminiscence, with the emphasis on telling one's life story, corresponds well with the strong oral tradition in the African-American culture. In addition, the non-stigmatizing approach is a sensitive intervention within the older African-American population (Gillies & James, 1994; Shellman, Mokel, & Wright, 2007).

Research on reminiscence with older African Americans indicates that this approach is effective in reducing depression symptomology. In research on three groups of African-American older adults, those who were in a reminiscence group had reduced depression scores as compared to older adults who participated in a health education or control group (Shellman, Mokel, & Hewitt, 2009). Asking older African Americans about their life history and story was interpreted as a form of caring and interest by these older adults (Shellman, 2004). While the participants discussed painful memories of discrimination and "otherness," they also described their resilience as "thrivers and survivors." As a result of this experience, "the elders gained insight into their coping mechanisms and strengths, realized accomplishments, and simply enjoyed the experience" (p. 315). Although African Americans had experienced significant hardship over their life course, the majority of the content in their life review was related to positive, adaptive, and resilient aspects of their past (Shellman, Ennis, & Bailey-Addison, 2011).

Another population for whom reminiscence and life review have specific relevance are those who have survived trauma during earlier periods of life. Even when the traumatic experience happened in early life, older adults may continue to struggle with the pain and suffering that was experienced. Military personnel and those who have served in war are one group that may bring trauma experiences to later years.

With the current cohort of older veterans, there is a tendency to keep silent about one's war experiences. In a project for Canadian veterans of World War II, a group inter-vention focused on autobiographical life review work (Shaw & Westwood, 2002). As a result, these older men had a greater appreciation of the service that they provided to their country and the world, greater integration of both their positive and painful memories of wartime, as well as validation of their courage, bravery, and honor. In addition, the group format provided an opportunity for solidarity and camaraderie with other veterans.

Reminiscence work with veterans in Northern Taiwan indicates that life review addresses some of the negative outcomes of wartime. In interventions with late-life single male veterans (mean age = 92 years; 90% unmarried), group life review sessions improved life satisfaction, cultivated new relationships, and dealt with the unique issues of displacement that these veterans had from serving in World War II and the Chinese Civil War (Chiang, Lu, Chu, Chang, & Chou, 2008; Chueh & Chang, 2013). After the group sessions, the veterans had greater connections to others in the group and were less depressed and lonely.

Other reminiscence work was conducted with European war veterans who served in World War II. Using a cross-national perspective, life stories of Finnish and Russian sol-diers were contrasted (Coleman et al, 2002). The Finnish soldiers had similar themes that had a collective emphasis on the liberation of Finland from Soviet invasion. As the authors state, "When asked how the war had influenced their lives, these men—many of whom had been disabled since the war—could answer affirmatively, integrating their losses with meaning for society as a whole" (p. 225). The Russians soldiers also spoke of pride in their service, but the amount of change and trauma experienced in this group was evident in their reminiscences. Within this group, there was a greater emphasis on the changes that took place in their country as a result of the war. The comparison of these narratives provides a sense of how collective meaning and shared social experiences can impact the themes and contents of reminiscence and life review.

The life reviews of those who have survived the Holocaust are also trauma-filled sto-ries. Listening to and bearing witness to the horrific events that many of these survivors have faced are often experiences of a different magnitude. For example, Klempner (2000) recounts his experience of listening to a life review of a woman whose entire family was murdered when she was 17 years old. With this magnitude of trauma, an aspect of the life review is bearing witness to the extent of the tragedy that took place. Even within the depths of these experiences, however, the life reviews of Holocaust survivors include stories of strength and resilience. "Life review may be stressful for Holocaust survivors as they may re-experience a sense of abandonment, isolation, and dehumanization. However, for those who are bearing witness, . . . survivors possess an ability to reconstruct memory in such a way that they feel a connection to the past and present, and establish the significance of their lives" (Greene, 2002, pp. 13–14).

GAY AND LESBIAN OLDER ADULTS

Older LGBT adults may also benefit from reminiscence and life review, as they lived during social eras that considered same-sex attraction to be a sin or a disease. In an early study on life review with the LGBT population, Galassi (1991) discusses the importance of both individual and collective reminiscence. The current population of LGBT older adults experienced critical developmental years prior to the advent of the gay rights movement started by the Stonewall Riots in 1969. Events such as the legality of marriage, adopting children, and non-discrimination in employment have been relatively recent phenomena. Although Galassi's (1991) work is dated, the importance of individually and collectively owning the experience of living a life as a gay man or lesbian woman continues to be relevant today.

The current cohort of older gay men also experienced the advent of the HIV/AIDS epidemic, which had considerable impact on their life course trajectory. Narratives of older gay men with HIV highlight themes of living past expected years, and surviving when others did not (Wright, Owen, & Catalan, 2012). Common themes from these men included feelings of uncertainty about the future, the need for independence within a sense of community, ageism within the gay community, and resilience and strength. Although these narratives were individually conducted, there is both an opportunity and need for a group life review format to connect the stories of these older men.

OLDER INDIVIDUALS WITH COGNITIVE/PSYCHIATRIC IMPAIRMENTS

Life review and reminiscence have also been used with populations that have cognitive or psychiatric conditions. Older adults with severe mental illness experience challenges in multiple areas of their biopsychosocial functioning (Cummings & Kropf, 2011; Palinkas et al., 2007). Willemse, Depla, and Bohlmeijer (2009) introduced a reminiscence program with older adults who had severe mental illness. Modifications included a focus on positive situations and experiences, a highly structured protocol, shortened length of sessions, and a small group size. Outcomes of this initial program were mainly positive, with increased life satisfaction and a more positive view of their aging process.

Life review has also been introduced with the population with dementia. Early studies reported that reminiscence with individuals having Alzheimer's disease can provide opportunities to return to preserved memories of earlier periods, which is enjoyable, promotes bonding, and reinforces their sense of worth as human beings (Gibson, 1994; Woods & McKiernan, 1995). Life review and reminiscence have also been introduced with couples in which one has a dementia diagnosis. When used in dyads, these approaches can promote positive memories about their life together, as they reminisce and tell the story of their relationship together, and can decrease a sense of stress and burden experienced by the care provider within the relationship (Haight et al., 2003; Ingersoll-Dayton et al., 2013).

CONTEXT AND IMPLEMENTATION

From a practice perspective, reminiscence and life review can be integrated into both community-based and longer care settings. While reminiscence is a natural and normal process for everyone, the use of these interventions may have special value for groups within the older population who have experienced social marginalization. Too often, they may not have had the opportunity to share their life stories, especially with others who have experienced similar circumstances. This section describes some of the contexts for conducting reminiscence and life review, as well as highlighting utility with subpopulations of older adults.

Since reminiscing is a naturally occurring process, reminiscence and life review interventions have been instituted in several contexts. Within the community, senior centers have been a common setting, and groups have been offered these interventions as part of the activities that take place (Perrotta & Meacham, 1981). However, these interventions have also been introduced with homebound older adults through programs such as Meals-on-Wheels, Visiting Nurses, or hospice (Haight, 1988, 1992; Jenko, Gonzalez, & Seymour, 2007; Sato, 2011). Congregate living situations, such as retirement communities, have also been sites for these interventions (Stevens-Ratchford, 1993).

Reminiscence and life review have also been used for older adults who are hospitalized. Depression can compromise treatment for other health challenges, and interventions such as life review and reminiscence therapy may be introduced within acute care settings (Gaggioli et al., 2014; Klausner et al., 1998). These interventions, as an adjunct to medical treatment, have the potential to address psychosocial functioning that is often a comorbid condition to the physiological challenges of later life.

Long-term care settings are frequent settings for these interventions (Gudex, Horsted, Jensen, Kjer, & Sørensen, 2010; Hsieh et al., 2010). Transitions to long-term care settings may be difficult for new residents, and these interventions can help with coping with the new environment and structure. Rates of geriatric depression are higher in these settings than in the community-dwelling population, with an estimate of up to 50% of residents suffering from depression (Kramer, Allgaier, Fejtkova, Mergl, & Hegerl, 2009). Interventions such as reminiscence and life review are treatments to deal with the high rates of geriatric depression within nursing homes. In addition, bonds between residents can be strengthened through these protocols, as reminiscence groups can bring together residents and increase interactions.

CASE EXAMPLE

The case of an aging parent whose son with Down's syndrome had died a few years earlier is presented as an example of a life review intervention. The outcome of the life review process allowed the mother to revisit pleasurable and rewarding times with her son, as well as deal with guilt and sadness from multiple painful experiences in her past. In addition, the process also promoted healing in her relationships with her living sons.

Mrs. Marva Jewell is a 79-year-old African-American woman who was the primary caregiver of her son, Elias, who had Down's syndrome. Her husband, Harold, died 12 years ago, and since then Marva and Elias lived together in their three-bedroom home. Two years ago, Elias died of heart failure at the age of 36. While he had ongoing health issues for most of his adulthood life, he was independent in his ADLs, and was able to assume responsibility for some household tasks (e.g., vacuuming, carrying in bags of groceries).

Marva is in good health, although she manages some chronic conditions. She is on hypertension medication, and suffers from arthritis. She was active in her church, and she and Elias would attend services together regularly. Since his death, however, she has been irregular in her attendance. Because he was not in any type of day program, she had few other social outlets, as most of the day was spent with Elias.

There are two other sons in the family, both of whom are in their forties. One son, Martin, lives in another state and is married with three adult children. The other son, Anthony, lives across town, is divorced, and has shared custody of his teenage daughter. Marva spends holidays with Anthony and her granddaughter, but has limited contact with them during other times of the year. She rarely sees Martin and his family.

Marva is comfortable financially, as her husband worked in an accounting office in city government. She receives a pension and Social Security, and the family also has some savings from investments that her husband had made. She no longer has a mortgage, and her home has retained value. Her assets are at the level where she is able to meet all her financial responsibilities without stress.

The reason for clinical interventions is Marva's depression since the death of Elias. She has been unable to change anything in his bedroom, and has stopped attending church services. Elias had been a client at community mental health, and protocol includes follow-up with the family for 1–2 years after a death has occurred. After the 2-year period ends, the case manager refers to other programs, as necessary. As Marva continued to exhibit grief reactions, the case manager referred her to aging services.

Aging services assigned one of their therapists, Edward Mack, to work with Marva. At the initial appointment, Marva started to cry as she described her life without Elias. As she discussed her current experiences, she used words such as "empty," "lonely," and "regretful." While she seemed sad about her husband's death, her discussion of Elias's death included much more sadness and pain.

Edward approached Marva's depression and grief by employing a life review protocol, as this approach is effective for working with grief and depression (Ando et al., 2010). Raising a child with a disability is a complex experience involving multiple emotions. Life review can explore the sources of reward and enjoyment, as well as the challenges and painful aspects, that are part of this parenting experience.

Edward introduced the topic of life review with Marva, and she agreed to participate as she acknowledged feeling sad, alone, and fatigued. Using a life review approach helped remove the stigma that Marva, as an older African-American woman, may have had about participating in mental health treatment (Shellman et al., 2007). The first session was introduced as "Marva's young life." During this session, Edward asked her to discuss her childhood and teenage years. She talked about her time as a child and adolescent, growing up in a strict religious family. Her father was a deacon at the church and her mother taught Sunday school. She and her brothers would sit through church service and Sunday school each week. In addition, they attended mid-week Bible classes. While she enjoyed being part of her religious family, she also discussed how she was not allowed to do many things that other children did (e.g., play popular music or sports). She discussed meeting Harold, and having him as her first and only boyfriend. Her parents were unhappy as he was not as religious, but Marva liked some of his adventurous ways. Before they had their first son, they would travel to other cities, listen to music, and go dancing. These were happy times—and Marva often smiled when she reminisced.

The second session had the theme of "beginning a family." For this session, Marva brought in some pictures of her wedding, and baby pictures of her sons. She also brought in a picture of her pregnant, and stated that "this was baby #3. He was stillborn. . . . I cried and cried—Harold cried too. We named him Harold Jr." Edward asked how Harold Jr. was part of the family. Marva stated that the hospital took a print of his little fingers, and she kept this image in her photo album, along with a few pictures of her during the pregnancy. She stated that her mother was not nurturing and seemed to blame Marva for the baby being stillborn. She stated, "I haven't talked about Harold Jr. in so many years." During this session, she discussed having Elias when she was 41 years of age. "We didn't plan for him—we didn't want another child after losing Harold Jr." But when he was born, my mother said, "God gave you this child to care for and love. He is a special gift—God gave you another chance after he called your other baby home." Further, Marva said, "She was right. . . . God did give me another chance for a baby. . . ." Although Elias was diagnosed with Down's syndrome early on, both Marva and Harold loved and doted on him.

A third session was organized around "the Jewell family" theme. Marva brought in some pictures of the boys, their vacations, and their school and sports pictures. Marva stated that there were many times that only one of them could go to the older boys' ball games . . . typically that was Harold and she would stay with Elias. The two of them would often go shopping, as Elias loved the grocery store and pushing the cart. This was a bonding time for the two of them, and these outings seemed happy and joyful for mother and son. Later in the session, however, she described the sadness when neighbors would have birthday parties and invite all the other children in the neighborhood except Elias. "On those days, I would take him someplace special—maybe for an ice cream cone—as it would break my heart to think about him sitting home while the other children were having fun."

The theme for the fourth session was "family changes." Marva started the conversation by describing how her older sons each left home, went to college, and got married. Edward asked, "What were these transitions like for you? For you, Harold and Elias who continued to live at home?" Marva got teary, and said that she missed a lot of the times in her other sons' lives. They were uncomfortable when they did things as a family, so Harold would take them to college and Marva would stay home. She said, "and it broke my heart to think about that . . . that their mother wasn't with them, but also, knowing how they felt about their own brother."

The final session was titled "our family puzzle." This was a bit confusing for Marva at first, so Edward introduced this session with more detail. He said that "our lives are like a jigsaw puzzle and sometimes you can fit pieces together right away. Other times, you try pieces that don't go together and have to start again to make good fits. Also, you don't always see the picture you are building right away—you might only see part of the picture before you can see the entire scene." Then he asked if she could identify some of the puzzle pieces from the sessions that they shared, and wondered how she saw them coming together.

Marva nodded when he explained it like that. She stated that she did see the puzzle pieces coming together from her early life—her life had been so strict as a child that she believed that the stillborn birth of Harold Jr. and the disability of Elias were punishments from God. She also said that she felt very protective of Elias as a result, and lost the chance to be present in the lives of her other boys. Then Edward asked, "Can you put those pieces together in a different way?" She was silent, then said, "Yes, two of my boys are still alive, and I am still strong enough to travel, which I've always enjoyed doing." At this point, she was suggesting that she could create a different relationship with her sons, even though she could not undo the past.

She also stated that she missed Elias—he was her son and her companion. She also stated that she grieved for Harold Jr., even though she only had him in her life a short time. At this point, she reflected that "it felt good to talk and cry about him. . . . It's been a long time and I felt tight inside if I thought of him. I miss Elias—and I miss Harold Jr. too."

At the close of the life review, there were several insights that Marva had as a result of the life review process. One was her grief over two dead sons—both Elias and Harold Jr. By untangling her experiences, she was able to give space for the grief that she had been carrying for her stillborn son. Elias's death was undoubtedly a sad occurrence, yet Marva had coupled responsibility for Elias and the loss of Harold Jr. The tangling of these two losses complicated the grief and bereavement process.

Marva also was able to recall happy times in the Jewell family that included her other sons. She also got in touch with her sadness about missing some of the important times in their lives. Through this process, Marva made the decision that she was going to call Martin and Anthony and invite them both home for a visit. In addition, she wanted to talk with Martin about a visit to his home to spend some time with his family.

Through this life review process, Marva revisited early experiences that might have seemed unconnected within her life. Through the life review framework, Edward guided her through various periods that not only had unique meaning for her, but also presented a mosaic for her to view in full. By the end of the sessions, she felt like she had reclaimed parts of her life that had been "off limits," as well as discovering some puzzle pieces that she had put together in ways that were not a good fit. During the intervention, she repositioned these pieces in a way to create a clearer picture for herself.

CONCLUSION

As a naturally occurring process, reminiscence work has several positive functions for older adults. For older adults who face mental health challenges, such as geriatric depression or anxiety, reminiscence and life review can help foster positive aspects such as coping and resilience. In addition, the therapeutic process of life review can address past wounds or unfinished issues that are brought into later life. However, these interventions can facilitate engagement among participants within group interventions and also promote pleasant memories that increase life satisfaction. In this way, the interventions have utility for multiple populations of older adults.

Reminiscence and life review have been used in multiple settings and contexts. Studies have reported effectiveness in community-dwelling populations, those in acute-care settings, as well as residents of long-term care facilities. These approaches have been used with individuals and in group formats, as well as through technology-based applications.

In the following chapter, studies are reviewed to provide an overview of evidence-based practice with older adults. As this body of research attests, reminiscence and life review have been used across a variety of client populations. Taken collectively, research indicates that these interventions are useful as practice approaches with older clients.

REFERENCES

Ando, M., Morita, T., Miyashita, M., Sanjo, M., Kira, H., & Shima, Y. (2010). Effects of bereavement life review on spiritual well-being and depression. *Journal of Pain and Symptom Management, 40*(3), 453–459.

Atchley, R. C. (1989). A continuity theory of normal aging. *The Gerontologist, 29*(2), 183–190.

Burnside, I., & Haight, B. (1994). Reminiscence and life review: therapeutic interventions for older people. *The Nurse Practitioner, 19*(4), 55–61.

Butler, R. N. (1963). The life review: an interpretation of reminiscence in the aged. *Psychiatry, 26,* 65–76.

Cappeliez P., O'Rourke, N., & Chaudhury, H. (2005). Functions of reminiscence and mental health in later life. *Aging and Mental Health, 9*(4), 296.

Cheng, S. T. (2009). Generativity in later life: perceived respect from younger generations as a determinant of goal disengagement and psychological well-being. *The Journals of Gerontology, 64B*(1), 45–55.

Chiang, K. J., Lu, R. B., Chu, H., Chang, Y. C., & Chou, K. R. (2008). Evaluation of the effect of a life review group program on self-esteem and life satisfaction in the elderly. *International Journal of Geriatric Psychiatry, 23*(1), 7–10.

Chueh, K. & Chang, T. (2013). Effectiveness of group reminiscence therapy for depressive symptoms in male veterans: 6-month follow up. *Geriatric Psychiatry, 29*, 377–383.

Coleman, P. G., Hautamaki, A., & Podolskij, A. (2002). Trauma, reconciliation, and generativity: the stories told by European war veterans. In J. D. Webster & B. K. Haight (Eds.), *Critical advances in reminiscence work: from theory to application* (pp. 218–232). New York: Springer.

Cumming, E., & Henry, W. (1961). *Growing old.* New York: Basic Books.

Cummings, S. M., & Kropf, N. P. (2011). Aging with a severe mental illness: challenges and treatments. *Journal of Gerontological Social Work, 54*(2), 175–188.

Dittmann-Kohli, F., & Westerhof, G. J. (2000). The personal meaning system in a life span perspective. In G. Reker & K. Chamberlain (Eds.), *Exploring existential meaning: optimizing human development across the life span* (pp. 107–123). Thousand Oaks, CA: Sage.

Gaggioli, A., Scaratti, C., Morganti, L., Stramba-Badiale, M., Agostoni, M., Spatola, C. A., & Riva, G. (2014). Effectiveness of group reminiscence for improving wellbeing of institutionalized elderly adults: study protocol for a randomized controlled trial. *Trials, 15*(1), 1–6.

Galassi, F. S. (1991). Life-review workshop for gay and lesbian elders. *Journal of Gerontological Social Work, 16*(1–2), 75–86.

Gibson, F. (1994). What can reminiscence contribute to people with dementia? In J. Bornat (Ed.), *Reminiscence reviewed: perspectives, evaluations, achievements* (pp. 46–60). Bristol, PA: Open University Press.

Gillies, C., & James, A. (1994). *Reminiscence work with old people.* London: Chapman & Hall.

Greene, R. R. (2002). Holocaust survivors: a study in resilience. *Journal of Gerontological Social Work, 37*(1), 3–18.

Greene, R. R., & Kropf, N. P. (2009). *Human behavior and the social environment.* New Brunswick, NJ: Transaction Press.

Greene, R. R., & Kropf, N. P. (2011). *Competence: theoretical frameworks.* New Brunswick, NJ: Transaction Press.

Gudex, C., Horsted, C., Jensen, A. M., Kjer, M., & Sørensen, J. (2010). Consequences from use of reminiscence: a randomised intervention study in ten Danish nursing homes. *BMC Geriatrics, 10*(1), 33.

Haber, D. (2006). Life review: implementation, theory, research and therapy. *International Journal of Aging & Human Development, 63*(2), 153–171.

Haight, B. K. (1992). Long-term effects of a structured life review process. *Journal of Gerontology, 47*(5), P312–P315.

Haight, B. K. (1988). The therapeutic role of a structured life review process in homebound elderly subjects. *Journal of Gerontology, 43*(2), P40–P44.

Haight, B. K., Bachman, D. L., Hendrix, S., Wagner, M. T., Meeks, A., & Johnson, J. (2003). Life review: treating the dyadic family unit with dementia. *Clinical Psychology & Psychotherapy, 10*(3), 165–174.

Havighurst, R. J. (1961). Successful aging. *Gerontologist, 1*(1), 8–13.

Hsieh, C. J., Chang, C., Su, S. F., Hsiao, Y. L., Shih, Y. W., Han, W. H., & Lin, C. C. (2010). Reminiscence group therapy on depression and apathy in nursing home residents with mild-to-moderate dementia. *Journal of Experimental & Clinical Medicine, 2*(2), 72–78.

Ingersoll-Dayton, B., Spencer, B., Kwak, M., Scherrer, K., Allen, R. S., & Campbell, R. (2013). The couples life story approach: a dyadic intervention for dementia. *Journal of Gerontological Social Work, 56*(3), 237–254.

Jenko, M., Gonzalez, L., & Seymour, M. J. (2007). Life review with the terminally ill. *Journal of Hospice & Palliative Nursing, 9*(3), 159–167.

Jewell, A. J. (2014). Tornstam's notion of gerotranscendence: re-examining and questioning the theory. *Journal of Aging Studies, 30,* 112–120.

Karimi, H., Dolatshahee, B., Momeni, K., Khodabakhshi, A., Rezaei, M., & Kamrani, A. (2010). Effectiveness of integrative and instrumental reminiscence therapies on depression symptoms reduction in institutionalized older adults: an empirical study. *Aging & Mental Health, 14*(7), 881–887.

Kivnick, H. Q. (1996). Remembering and being remembered: the reciprocity of psychosocial legacy. *Generations, 20*(3), 49–53.

Klausner, E. J., Clarkin, J. F., Spielman, L., Pupo, C., Abrams, R., & Alexopoulos, G. S. (1998). Late-life depression and functional disability: the role of goal-focused group psychotherapy. *International Journal of Geriatric Psychiatry, 13*(10), 707–716.

Klempner, M. (2000). Navigating life review interviews with survivors of trauma. *The Oral History Review, 27*(2), 67–83.

Korte, J., Westerhof, G. J., & Bohlmeijer, E. T. (2012). Mediating processes in an effective life-review intervention. *Psychology and Aging, 27*(4), 1172.

Kramer, D., Allgaier, A. K., Fejtkova, S., Mergl, R., & Hegerl, U. (2009). Depression in nursing homes: prevalence, recognition, and treatment. *International Journal of Psychiatry in Medicine, 39,* 345–358.

Laurenhue, K. (2007). *Getting to know the life stories of older adults: activities for building relationships.* Baltimore, MD: Health Professions Press.

McAdams, D. P. (2006). The redemptive self: generativity and the stories Americans live by. *Research in Human Development, 3*(2–3), 81–100.

Merriam, S. B. (1989). The structure of simple reminiscence. *The Gerontologist, 29*(6), 761–767.

Merriam, S. B. (1993). Race, sex, and age-group differences in the occurrence and uses of reminiscence. *Activities, Adaptation & Aging, 18*(1), 1–18.

Neugarten, B. (1968). *Middle age and aging.* Chicago: University of Chicago Press.

Palinkas, L. A., Criado, V., Fuentes, D., Shepherd, S., Milian, H., Folsom, D., & Jeste, D. V. (2007). Unmet needs for services for older adults with mental illness: comparison of views of different stakeholder groups. *The American Journal of Geriatric Psychiatry, 15*(6), 530–540.

Parker, R. G. (1995). Reminiscence: a continuity theory framework. *The Gerontologist, 35,* 515–525.

Perrotta, P., & Meacham, J. A. (1981). Can a reminiscing intervention alter depression and self-esteem? *The International Journal of Aging and Human Development, 14*(1), 23–30.

Pinquart, M., & Forstmeier, S. (2012). Effects of reminiscence interventions on psychosocial outcomes: a meta-analysis. *Aging & Mental Health, 16*(5), 541–558.

Preschl, B., Maercker, A., Wagner, B., Forstmeier, S., Baños, R. M., Alcañiz, M., Castilla, D., & Botella, C. (2012). Life-review therapy with computer supplements for depression in the elderly: a randomized controlled trial. *Aging & Mental Health, 16*(8), 964–974.

Randall, W. L. (2014). *The stories that we are: essays in self creation* (2nd ed.). Toronto: University of Toronto Press.

Randall, W. L., & Kenyon, G. M. (2001). *Ordinary wisdom: biographical aging and the journal of life.* Westport, CT: Praeger.

Reker, G., & Chamberlain, K. (Eds.). (2000). *Exploring existential meaning: optimizing human development across the life span.* Thousand Oaks, CA: Sage.

Sato, Y. (2011). Musical life review in hospice. *Music Therapy Perspectives, 29*(1), 31–38.

Shaw, M. E., & Westwood, M. J. (2002). Transformation in life stories: The Canadian War Veteran's Life Review Project. In J. D. Webster & B. K. Haight (Eds.), *Critical advances in reminiscence work: from theory to application* (pp. 257–274). New York: Springer.

Shellman, J. (2004). "Nobody ever asked me before": understanding life experiences of African American elders. *Journal of Transcultural Nursing, 15*(4), 308–316.

Shellman, J., Ennis, E., & Bailey-Addison, K. (2011). A contextual examination of reminiscence functions in older African-Americans. *Journal of Aging Studies, 25*(4), 348–354.

Shellman, J. M., Mokel, M., & Hewitt, N. (2009). The effects of integrative reminiscence on depressive symptoms in older African Americans. *Western Journal of Nursing Research, 31*(6), 772–786.

Shellman, J., Mokel, M., & Wright, B. (2007). "Keeping the bully out": understanding older African Americans' beliefs and attitudes toward depression. *Journal of the American Psychiatric Nurses Association, 13*(4), 230–236.

Stevens-Ratchford, R. G. (1993). The effect of life review reminiscence activities on depression and self-esteem in older adults. *American Journal of Occupational Therapy, 47*(5), 413–420.

Tornstam, L. (2005). *Gerotranscendence: a developmental theory of positive aging.* New York: Springer.

Tornstam, L. (1999–2000). Transcendence in later life. *Generations, 23*(4), 10–14.

Wadensten, B., & Hägglund, D. (2006). Older people's experience of participating in a reminiscence group with a gerotranscendental perspective: reminiscence group with a gerotranscendental perspective in practice. *International Journal of Older People Nursing, 1*(3), 159–167.

Watt, L. M., & Cappeliez, P. (2000). Integrative and instrumental reminiscence therapies for depression in older adults: intervention strategies and treatment effectiveness. *Aging & Mental Health, 4*(2), 166–177.

Westerhof, G. J., Bohlmeijer, E., & Valenkamp, M. W. (2004). In search of meaning: a reminiscence program for older persons. *Educational Gerontology, 30*(9), 751–766.

Westerhof, G. J., Bohlmeijer, E. T., van Beljouw, I. J., & Pot, A. M. (2010). Improvement in personal meaning mediates the effects of a life review intervention on depressive symptoms in a randomized controlled trial. *Gerontologist, 50*(4), 541–549.

Willemse, B. M., Depla, M. F., & Bohlmeijer, E. T. (2009). A creative reminiscence program for older adults with severe mental disorders: results of a pilot evaluation. *Aging & Mental Health, 13*(5), 736–743.

Woods, R. T., & McKiernan, F. (1995). Evaluating the impact of reminiscence on older people with dementia. In J. Webster, & B. Haight (Eds.), *The Art and Science of Reminiscing: Theory, Research, Methods, and Applications* (pp. 233–242). Taylor and Francis.

Wright, R., Owen, G., & Catalan, J. (2012). "I'm older than I ever thought that I would be": the lived experience of ageing in HIV-positive gay men. In R. Ward, I. Rivers, & M. Sutherland (Eds.), *Lesbian, gay, bisexual & transgendered ageing: biographical approaches for inclusive care and support* (pp. 85–101). London: Jessica Kingsley Publishers.

12

REMINISCENCE AND LIFE REVIEW
EVIDENCE-BASED PRACTICE

Reminiscence and life review are interventions that have been used to enhance well-being, promote cognitive functioning, and mitigate emotional difficulties of later life. Studies contained within this chapter review important research on these interventions. Since these are primarily used with older adults, the majority of participants in the studies are 60 years or older. However, a minority of studies introduced these intervention with younger cohorts to determine the effectiveness of reminiscence and life review at different times in the life course.

To compile the literature, a search was conducted using several databases. These included PubMed, PsychInfo, Ageline, Cochrane Collaborative, Social Science Abstracts, and Social Service Abstracts. The terms used were "older adults," "elderly," with "life review," "reminiscence," "life story." Studies were included if published in 2000 or later.

Ten studies that report on the effectiveness of reminiscence or life review are included. Six were reviews of the older population who participated in reminiscence or life review therapies for mental health issues or general well-being. Additionally, four were specifically for individuals with dementia.

MENTAL HEALTH AND WELL-BEING

In the six reviews that focused on mental health issues or well-being, four had depression as an outcome (see Table 12.1). In addition, well-being outcomes were part of the analyses and included life satisfaction, purpose in life, ego integrity, spirituality, and happiness. The studies included both group and individual administration of the interventions.

Study	Inclusion/Exclusion Criteria	Description of Interventions	Number and Description of Participants	Outcomes	Findings
Pinquart & Forstmeier (2012) 128 studies Meta-analysis	Reminiscence or life review intervention. Control condition; mental health or well-being outcomes. Published before November 2011.	82 studies were about reminiscence and 55 used life review. 90 = group formats. 95 randomized participants. Average number of sessions = 10.1. Average of 8.3 weeks duration.	4,067 in treatment conditions, 4,337 in control groups. Mean age = 73.1 years; 66% women; 28% married.	Significant improvements for all outcome variables. Order of greatest improvement = ego integrity, depression, purpose in life, death preparation, mastery, mental health, positive well-being, social integration, and cognitive performance.	Reminiscence interventions effective for multiple outcomes. Stronger outcomes for with the life review. No difference in group or individual administration.
Bohlmeijer, Roemer, Cuijpers, & Smit (2007) 15 studies Meta Analysis	Reminiscence or life review intervention. Pre-and post-test data. Control or comparison condition. Well-being or life satisfaction outcomes.	Reminiscence = 7 studies; life review = 8. Groups = 9 studies; individual treatment = 6; random assignment = 13 studies. 9 studies = < 6 sessions, 2 studies > 12. Session length ranged from 3 to 28 (M = 9.5)	426 in life review/reminiscence conditions; 135 in no treatment, and 309 in comparison conditions. Mean age = 76.9; 80% had samples that were mainly women9 = long-term care settings.	Outcomes were life satisfaction, well-being, and affect. Moderate effect for well-being and life satisfaction. No differences by age cohort.	Reminiscence and life review interventions produced moderately positive well-being outcomes. Greater effects for life review compared to reminiscence. Group and individual protocols were equally as effective.

(continued)

TABLE 12.1 (CONTINUED)

Study	Inclusion/Exclusion Criteria	Description of Interventions	Number and Description of Participants	Outcomes	Findings
Chin (2007) 15 studies Meta-analysis	Controlled trials. Prior to 2011. Outcomes on mental health. Pre–post design. Control group. > 5 participants in each condition.	Session length was 1–1.5 hours. Treatment duration = 12 sessions average. Only one study was not a group intervention.	220 participants in reminiscence, and 204 were in controls. Mean age = 75.2 years. Only 40 participants were men. Nine studies included were in residential facilities, six were community based.	Reminiscence = more positive happiness and depression scores. No differences on self-esteem and life satisfaction.	Reminiscence is effective with reducing depression and increasing happiness. No effect on measures of well-being.
Bohlmeijer, Smit, & Cuijpers (2003) 20 studies Meta-analysis	Interventions were reminiscence or life review. Report pre-test and post-test data. Control or comparison group. Measure depression as outcome.	Reminiscence = 15 studies; life review = 7 (two included both). Groups = 14; individual administration = 6. Duration < 6 weeks in nine studies. Duration > 12 weeks in two studies.	1,084 participants; 528 in treatment conditions. Mean age = 75.3 years. Community residents = 8 studies. Nursing home residents = 8 studies. Remainder were hospitalized or living in retirement communities.	A large significant effect was reported for reminiscence interventions. No differences between effectiveness of life review and reminiscence.	Reminiscence is effective to reduce geriatric depression. Trend in the direction of greater effectiveness for those in the community versus long-term care settings.

Study	Inclusion criteria	Methods/intervention	Sample	Results	Conclusions
Lin, Dai, & Hwang, (2003) 10 studies Systematic review	Aged > 65 years or older; nursing home residents. Outcomes included depression, quality of life, self-esteem, and well-being.	Group format in all studies. Three were pre-post only, three had comparison groups, two control, and two both control/comparison. Duration = 6–16 weeks. Group sizes = 6–22. Treatment length = 6–24 hours.	Nursing home residents = 7 studies. Community dwelling = 2 studies. Clinic patients = 1 study. All-female samples = 5. Age range = 57–95 years.	3 studies = significant decreases in reminiscence group. 2 studies = no difference on depression outcomes. Self-esteem outcomes: one study found a significant increase and a second found no difference between treatments. Life satisfaction: 3 studies = significant increase for those in reminiscence conditions. One study reported no difference.	Variation in length and duration of treatment makes effective comparisons difficult. Inconclusive whether reminiscence is effective with these outcomes.
Keall, Clayton, & Butow (2015) Systematic review 14 studies (9 RCTs)	Age > 18 years; palliative care patients, diagnosis of < 6 months to live; English; published in peer-reviewed journal.	1 group intervention, 1 patient-caregiver intervention; remainder were individual sessions with the patient. Individual sessions ranged from 2 to 7; dyadic approach = 4 sessions; group = 8 sessions. Session times 15–90 minutes. Interventionists were nurses or social workers.	Mean age across studies = 65.7 years. The majority of patients in the studies were female and had a cancer diagnosis. 8 interventions were delivered in patients' home, with the rest in clinics or outpatient settings.	Intervention yielded positive results in spiritual well-being (n = 6), quality of life/happiness (n = 5), mood (n = 3), symptom management/distress (n = 3).	Brief interventions had best outcomes. Caregivers had best outcome with legacy-leaving intervention (tangible outcome to remember patient after death).

One of the meta-analyses had a singular focus on the effects of reminiscence and life review on depression (Bohlmeijer, Smith, & Cuijpers, 2003). Studies were included if (1) the intervention was either reminiscence or life review, (2) both pre-and post-test data were reported, (3) a control or comparison group was included, and (4) depression was one of the outcomes. Fifteen studies were reminiscence, seven were life review, and two included both interventions. A total of 528 participants were involved in treatments. A group format was used in 14, and the remaining six were individual administrations. In nine studies, the interventions lasted 6 weeks or less, in another nine the sessions ranged from 7 to 12 weeks, and the other two had more than 12 weeks of sessions. The average age across studies reporting ages was 75.3 years. Eight studies involved those living in the community, eight were nursing home residents, and the remainder were hospitalized or living in retirement communities.

Across studies, a large significant effect (.84) was reported for reducing rates of depression. The authors conclude that reminiscence interventions are effective to reduce geriatric depression in older adults. In addition, no differences were found between effectiveness of life review and reminiscence interventions. Although not significant, there was a trend in the direction of greater effectiveness for those in the community versus long-term care settings.

The other reviews that included depression also contained outcomes that measured quality of life. Pinquart and Forstmeier (2012) conducted a meta-analysis that included 127 studies on reminiscence. Inclusion criteria were the following: (1) a control condition was included; (2) outcomes had variables that represented mental health or well-being; and (3) the study was published before November 2011. The review included 82 studies that were about reminiscence and 55 that used life review. Most studies ($n = 90$) used group formats. Ninety-five studies randomized participants to treatment/control conditions. The average number of sessions was 10.1, and the intervention lasted an average of 8.3 weeks. A total of 4,067 adults were in the treatment conditions, and 4,337 in control groups. The average age of participants was 73.1 years; 66% were women and 28% were married.

Significant improvements were found for all outcome variables. In order, the greatest improvements were in ego integrity, depression, purpose in life, death preparation, mastery, mental health, positive well-being, social integration, and cognitive performance. The authors conclude that reminiscence interventions have positive impacts on a broad range of outcome variables. Stronger outcomes were associated with the life review over reminiscence interventions. An analysis of intervention administration concluded that there were no differences between individual and group formats.

Chin (2007) conducted a systematic review on the clinical effects of reminiscence with older adults. Fifteen studies were included, based upon these criteria: studies (1) were designed as controlled trials; (2) were conducted prior to 2011; (3) included mental health outcomes; (4) had a pre–post design; and (5) had a minimum of five participants in each condition. All studies involved were of reminiscence interventions. Two hundred twenty participants were in reminiscence interventions, and 204 were in control conditions. The average length of sessions was 1–1.5 hours. The range of sessions was between 4 and 24, with the average being 12. All but one study reported on group interventions. Across studies, the average age of participants was 75.2 years. Only 40 of the total participants were men. Nine studies included participants from residential facilities, while the remaining six were community based.

Results indicated that happiness and depression scores were more positive for participants in reminiscence interventions. However, no differences between groups were found on either self-esteem or life satisfaction. The author concludes that a clear indication for the effectiveness of reminiscence is found for depression over measures of well-being.

The final analysis that included depression as an outcome was by Lin, Dai, and Hwang (2003). For this analysis, the inclusion criteria were the following: (1) participants were 65 and above or nursing home residents, and (2) outcomes included depression, quality of life, self-esteem, and well-being. Seven studies involved nursing home residents, while two focused on community-dwelling participants, and one drew from a clinic (residence was not specified). All interventions were administered in group formats. Three designs were pre–post only, three had comparison groups, two control, and two had both control and comparison groups. Interventions ranged from 6 to 16 weeks, and group sizes ranged from 6 to 22 members. Total duration of intervention ranged from 6 to 24 hours. For the participant characteristics, five studies employed all female samples. Ages were reported in only two studies and included participants aged 57–95 years.

Within this review, three studies found significant decreases for depression within reminiscence groups. In one of these, depression decreases were only significant in the under 75 age group. Two other studies found no difference on depression outcomes. Two studies had self-esteem outcomes. One study found significant increases in both a reminiscence and activity group as compared to controls. A second study, however, found no differences between treatment, comparison, and control groups. For the final outcome, life satisfaction, two of three studies reported a significant increase for those in reminiscence conditions. One study reported no difference between reminiscence and friendly visiting. The researchers discuss the difficulties in comparing outcomes because of a lack of distinctions in the types of reminiscence being implemented. Additionally, variation in length and duration of treatment makes effective comparisons difficult. As a result, researchers were inconclusive on whether reminiscence is effective for the outcomes.

Two additional meta-analyses focused on well-being outcomes. Bohlmeijer, Roemer, Cuijpers, and Smith (2007) reported the following inclusion criteria for their analysis: studies (1) reported pre-and post-test data, (2) included a control or comparison condition, and (3) measured well-being or life satisfaction. Fifteen studies were included; seven used a reminiscence intervention, and eight employed life review. Thirteen studies randomized participants into conditions. Of the 809 total participants, 426 participants were in treatment conditions, with 135 in no treatment and 309 in comparison conditions (e.g., current events, friendly visiting, standard care). The average age of participants was 76.9, and 80% of the participants were female. In nine studies, participants lived in a long-term care setting (e.g., nursing home, assisted living). Nine studies used a group format, and the remaining six were individual administrations. In nine studies, the number of sessions was six or fewer, and only two had more than 12 sessions. The number of sessions ranged from 3 to 28 ($M = 9.5$) and most lasted 1 hour.

Outcomes were reported for life satisfaction, psychological well-being, and affect. Across studies, a moderate effect was found for psychological well-being and life satisfaction. In examining cohort groups, no differences were found for those over and under 80 years of age. The authors conclude that reminiscence and life review interventions produced moderately positive well-being outcomes. However, life review interventions yielded significantly greater effects than reminiscence. No differences were found in types of administration of the intervention, as both group and individual protocols were equally as effective.

A systematic review reported on outcomes of life review in palliative care patients (Keall, Clayton, & Butow, 2015). Inclusion criteria were the following: (1) quantitative analysis of a manualized life review intervention with palliative care patients or those with a 6-month or less prognosis; (2) publication was in English; (3) publication was in a peer-reviewed journal. A final inclusion criterion was patient age over 18 years; however, about 72% of the studies had a mean age of > 60 years. Within the 14 articles of the review, 10 different types of life review protocols included both individual and group formats. All interventions were brief therapies, lasting from 2 to 8 sessions with the modal number being 2–4 sessions. Most typically, the interventionist was a nurse or social worker, and eight interventions were delivered in the patients' homes. The remainder with delivered in a clinic or outpatient setting.

The results suggest that life review is effective with end-of-life issues. In an analysis of the intervention structure, shorter interventions were associated with better outcomes. As the authors state, the shorter interventions appear to be more effective for those who are closer to death—a patient population that experiences high levels of fatigue and symptom severity. Additionally, there were positive outcomes for caregivers in the interventions that included patient and care provider. Although costly, interventions that provided the opportunity for the patient and caregiver to construct a legacy-leaving product (e.g., book, audiotape) were associated with less stress in the caregivers. This type of analysis is helpful in palliative care and hospice patient populations to determine goals for the interventions, as well as different life review approaches that lead to positive outcomes for patients and care providers.

DEMENTIA

One meta-analysis and three systematic reviews specifically focused on outcomes of reminiscence with individuals having dementia (see Table 12.2). All four included only reminiscence, not life review, treatment approaches.

TABLE 12.2 SYSTEMATIC REVIEWERS FOR PERSONS WITH DEMENTIA

Study	Inclusion/Exclusion Criteria	Description of Interventions	Number and Description of Participants	Outcomes	Findings
Kwon, Cho, & Lee (2013) Meta-analysis 10 RCTs	> 60 years; diagnosis of dementia. Pre–post experimental design using reminiscence therapy. Statistical analysis reported.	7 studies had outcomes of cognitive function; 6 studies had depression outcomes; 3 studies had behavioral outcomes; 3 studies had quality of life outcomes.	None given	Significant statistical change—great effect size for cognitive function increases, decreased depression, and increased quality of life. No support for changes in behavioral outcomes.	Reminiscence is effective with outcomes related to cognitive and emotional changes, no support for behavioral changes as a result of the intervention.
Cotelli, Manenti, & Zanetti (2012) 6 studies Systematic review	RCTs. Effects of reminiscence interventions on cognitive functions and/or mood. Individuals with dementia.	Comparison conditions or control. Session length = 30 minutes to 1 hour. Treatment duration = 1–5 weeks.	98 persons in treatment; 111 in controls/ comparison conditions.	Reminiscence increased cognitive functioning, decreased agitation, increased autobiographical memory.	Reminiscence effective for cognitive and emotional functioning increases.

(continued)

TABLE 12.2 (CONTINUED)

Study	Inclusion/Exclusion Criteria	Description of Interventions	Number and Description of Participants	Outcomes	Findings
Subramaniam & Woods (2012) 5 studies Systematic review	RCTs Individual intervention. Individuals with dementia.	Two types of reminiscence: life story book approach ($n = 3$) and general reminiscence ($n = 2$). Session length = 30 minutes to 1 hour. Treatment duration = 6–12 weeks with one session per week.	258 participants; 101 participants were involved in reminiscence interventions. Mean age = 84 years. Sites = nursing homes and personal care facilities.	Outcomes were well-being, quality of life, depression, and memory performance.	Three of the studies reported positive, beneficial effects of reminiscence. Outcomes = increased well-being, social engagement, enhanced autobiographical memory and decreased depression.
Woods, Spector, Jones, Orrell, & Davies (2005) 5 studies Systematic review	RCTs. Persons with dementia. Interventions = > 3 wks, sessions = > 5. Led by a professional facilitator.	Group format = 3; individual format = 2. Modal duration = 30 minutes. 1–2 sessions per week. Treatment duration = 4–18 weeks.	185 participants. Personal care home residents = 2 studies; nursing home residents = 1 study; Community dwelling = 1 study (one no report). Mean age = 81.4 years.	Cognitive functioning orientation, depression, social engagement, autobiographical memory, caregiver burden.	Improvements for caregiver burden, behavioral functioning, mood. Slight improvements were found on cognitive functioning and depression.

The meta-analysis reviewed RCTs of reminiscence therapy for four outcomes with dementia patients (Kwon, Cho, & Lee, 2013). Inclusion criteria included the following: (1) sample of > 60 years; (2) a diagnosis of dementia by a mental health doctor or neurologist; (3) study used a reminiscence therapy approach with two or more groups in an RCT design; and (4) study included statistical values in reporting results. The criteria yielded 10 studies that were included in the analysis, but neither participant demographics nor intervention designs were included.

Positive findings were reported for three of the four outcomes. Reminiscence was statistically significant, with a strong effect size for enhanced cognitive functioning, decreased depression, and enhanced quality of life for participants. However, the therapy did not improve behavioral outcomes for the participants. As a result, the researchers conclude that reminiscence therapy has overall effectiveness when intervening in cognitive and emotional domains. Evidence does not exist that this approach decreases behavioral outcomes in dementia.

Two of systematic reviews focused on cognitive functioning as an outcome. Cotelli, Manetti, and Zanetti (2012) included research that focused on the effects of reminiscence interventions on cognitive functions and/or mood for individuals with dementia. Studies compared reminiscence interventions to comparison conditions (e.g., social support, reality orientation) or no treatment. Session duration ranged from 30 minutes to 1 hour. Length of treatment ranged from 1 to 5 weeks. A total of 209 participants were included; 98 persons with dementia were in reminiscence interventions, with 111 in controls/comparison conditions.

Positive outcomes were found on cognitive functioning after reminiscence interventions. Other significant changes included decrease in agitation, and increase in autobiographical memory. Reminiscence interventions increased abilities and functioning in cognitive and emotional functioning. Most positive outcomes were found when reality orientation and reminiscence were combined in an intervention.

A second systematic review also focused on cognitive functioning (Woods, Spector, Jones, Orrell, & Davies, 2005). Five studies were included, with a total of 185 participants with an average age across studies of 81.4 years. Inclusion criteria were the following: interventions had to (1) last at least 4 weeks, (2) have a minimum of six sessions, and (3) be led by a professional facilitator. Three interventions were run in group formats; two were individually administered. The modal duration of sessions was 30 minutes. One administration offered five sessions per week, but the rest had one to two sessions per week. The treatment duration was between 4 and 18 weeks. Two studies were focused on personal care home residents, one on nursing home residents, and one on community-dwelling older adults (one study did not indicate population).

In addition to cognitive functioning and orientation, outcomes included depression, social engagement, autobiographical memory, and caregiver burden. The authors reported improvements on caregiver burden, behavioral functioning of the care recipient, and recipient mood. Only slight improvements were reported for cognitive functioning and depression.

The third systematic review also included depression as an outcome, as well as memory performance, quality of life, and well-being (Subramaniam & Woods, 2012). This review included five studies with a total of 258 participants with 101 participants involved in reminiscence interventions. The inclusion criteria were (1) original research, and (2) reminiscence provided as an individual intervention for people with dementia. The studies represented two reminiscence structures: life story book approach ($n = 3$) and general reminiscence ($n = 2$). Session lengths ranged from 30 minutes to 1 hour, with treatment duration of 6–12 weeks of one session per week. When age was reported, the average across studies was 84 years. Two intervention sites were nursing homes and three were personal care facilities.

The authors reported positive, beneficial effects of reminiscence in three studies that used the life story book approach. These outcomes were increased well-being, social engagement, enhanced autobiographical memory, and decreased depression. However, the generalized reminiscence studies did not lead to significant treatment effects.

CONCLUSIONS

By all accounts, life review and reminiscence interventions are effective during later life. While not the same, both of these approaches involve the use of past experiences to enhance well-being or decrease difficulties such as depression or anxiety. A positive outcome of these interventions is to promote interactions among older adults and facilitate a sense of connection to their past experiences. In addition, there is evidence that these interventions are helpful with preparing for end of life.

The studies in this chapter provide interesting conclusions about whether there is greater effectiveness of life review versus reminiscence. For mental health and well-being outcomes, there is inconclusive evidence that life review is more effective than simple reminiscence. While Pinquart and Forstmeier (2012) and Bohlmeijer et al. (2007) reported a greater effect for life review, Bohlmeijer et al. (2003) concluded that there were no differences in outcomes by either type. The mixed conclusions could be a result of several factors. Although different conceptually, the practice of life review and reminiscence may have more similarity than difference. Additionally, the length and/or duration of the intervention might also be a factor. There are some indications that longer duration of interventions lead to better results for these two outcomes, which might be the case regardless of whether a reminiscence or life review protocol is administered. Additional comparison of life review and reminiscence would resolve this question, including studies that provided similar session and duration structures.

A second issue is the effectiveness of these interventions for depression versus well-being outcomes. The greatest positive changes were in the reduction of geriatric depression, as this outcome was evaluated in the largest number of reviews. While the results are again inconclusive, there is greater evidence that these interventions are more effective with depression than elements of well-being, such as life satisfaction or self-esteem. Since well-being is connected to present-day functioning and experiences, reminiscence and life review interventions that do not make a strong connection to current experiences may not be effective in these areas. Linking past with present, as in the case example of Mrs. Jewell in Chapter 11, provides individuals with an opportunity for exploring options in current life situations.

While there is consistent evidence related to depression, well-being outcomes are less clear. In some studies, these outcomes did improve after reminiscence; however, in other studies, these outcomes were no different as compared to control or comparison conditions. Some studies suggest that the intervention approach (e.g., individual versus group) is critical, as well-being outcomes may include a more social component that increases in the context of interventions with other individuals. This conclusion merits further empirical investigation, especially as studied across the diversity of populations of older adults.

In the subpopulation with dementia, however, positive changes are reported in both mental health functioning and quality of life outcomes. Decreased depression occurred for the individual with dementia and decreased burden for the care providers. In addition, Kwon et al. (2013) reported that quality of life outcomes were more positive after reminiscence.

Additionally, reminiscence seems to have other positive outcomes for individuals with dementia. In the area of cognitive functioning, Woods et al. (2005) reported slight improvements. Cotelli et al. (2012) reported more significant gains in cognitive functioning and slight improvement in autobiographic memory as well.

There are mixed results on the ability of reminiscence that result in behavioral changes in patients with dementia. Woods et al. (2005) reported positive behavioral gains, such as decreased agitation, enhanced communication, and increased social engagement. However, Kwon et al.'s (2013) meta-analysis reported that there was no support for behavioral changes as a result of reminiscence. However, this second analysis did not specify the types of behavioral changes that were included in the individual studies. As a result, it is impossible to determine which behavioral outcomes were targeted in these studies. Clearly, additional research is needed on the outcomes for behavioral functioning.

There is some evidence that the structure of the life review or reminiscence intervention may produce different effects. Two articles determined that interventions for caregivers that produced a legacy outcome (e.g., life story, audiotape) had a significant outcome for caregivers (Keall et al., 2015; Subramaniam & Woods, 2012). Both sets of caregivers were providing care for populations with significant and deteriorating conditions—either dementia or patients receiving palliative care. In these circumstances, life review or reminiscence work that results in a tangible remembrance of the care recipient and his or her experience appears to be especially significant.

In spite the optimistic findings overall, there are some limitations in the state of the outcome research. The variation in administration across different studies is remarkable and makes interpretation difficult. As both Tables 12.1 and 12.2 indicate, the duration and length of the intervention sessions are vastly different, which translates into different dosage rates in the various studies. In order to address the effectiveness of the interventions, questions about length of sessions, duration of treatment, and titration (e.g., length between intervention administration) need to be considered and evaluated.

Issues related to samples also are critical in evaluating the effectiveness of the interventions. For the most part, the reviews report age, gender, and residential context of the participants. Additionally, there was specific focus on the population with dementia. Beyond those sociodemographic descriptions, little is known about the study populations. Critical questions about intervention effectiveness with various populations, including diversity in race, ethnicity, immigration experiences, educational attainments, and sexual/gender identities, need to be considered.

A second sample issue relates to sizes. While several meta-analyses and systematic reviews are available, many contain small numbers of studies. Based upon the criteria for inclusion, numerous studies were excluded due to small sample sizes, insufficient specificity about the intervention, lack of description of participants, or lack of comparison or control groups. Additionally, many studies did not determine if outcomes were sustained after the conclusion of the program. As a result, there continues to be a need for rigorous research in this area.

Going forward, there are several areas of potential research in this area. First, ongoing research on sustainability of the intervention will help determine whether inoculation needs to take place at regular intervals after conclusion of the program. Continued evaluation of different administrative protocols (e.g., groups, individual activities, technology based) will provide an array of options based upon participate preference, program resources, and so on. In addition, there is promising work with programs that have tailored interventions to particular client experiences, such as behavioral or physical health challenges. Interventions that synthesize these experiences into a reminiscence or life review structure should continue to be evaluated.

The results that both group and individual interventions are effective is good news for practitioners. Depending on context and circumstances, interventions can be delivered in either administration structure, which provides options. The flexibility in these approaches makes them adaptable across several different settings, including the community, as well as long-term care.

However, trying to make a case for these interventions can be limited by the homogeneity of samples that were part of the studies. Participants were very similar in age and gender, which makes generalization to different segments of the population difficult. Most individuals were in their mid-70s, and the majority of all participants were female. Additional research that targets diverse subpopulations is necessary.

REFERENCES

Bohlmeijer, E., Roemer, M., Cuijpers, P., & Smit, F. (2007). The effects of reminiscence on psychological well-being in older adults: a meta-analysis. *Aging & Mental Health, 11*(3), 291–300.

Bohlmeijer, E., Smit, F., & Cuijpers, P. (2003). Effects of reminiscence and life review on late-life depression: a meta-analysis. *International Journal of Geriatric Psychiatry, 18*(12), 1088–1094.

Chin, A. M. (2007). Clinical effects of reminiscence therapy in older adults: a meta-analysis of controlled trials. *Hong Kong Journal of Occupational Therapy, 17*, 10–22. doi:10.1016/S1569-1861(07)70003-7.

Cotelli, M., Manenti, R., & Zanetti, O. (2012). Reminiscence therapy in dementia: a review. *Maturitas, 72*, 203–205. doi:10.1016/j.maturitas.2012.04.008.

Keall, R. M., Clayton, J. M., & Butow, P. N. (2015). Therapeutic life review in palliative care: a systematic review of quantitative evaluations. *Journal of Pain and Sympton Management, 49*(4), 747–761.

Kwon, M. H., Cho, B. H., & Lee, J. S. (2013). Reminiscence therapy for dementia: meta analysis. *Healthcare and Nursing Science and Technology Letters, 40*, 10–15.

Lin, Y., Dai, Y., & Hwang, S. (2003). Effect of reminiscence on the elderly population: a systematic review. *Public Health Nursing, 20*(4), 297–306.

Pinquart, M., & Forstmeier, S. (2012). Effects of reminiscence interventions on psychosocial outcomes: a meta-analysis. *Aging & Mental Health, 16*(5), 541–558. doi:10.1080/13607863.2011.651434.

Subramaniam, P., & Woods, B. (2012). The impact of individual reminiscence therapy for people with dementia: systematic review. *Expert Review of Neurotherapeutics, 12*(5), 545–555. doi:10.1586/ern.12.35.

Woods, B. Spector, A. E., Jones, C. A., Orrell, M., & Davies, S. P. (2005). Reminiscence therapy for dementia. *Cochrane Database of Systematic Reviews*, Issue 2, Art. No. CD001120. doi: 10.1002/14651858. CD001120.pub 2.

III

CHALLENGES IN IMPLEMENTATING EVIDENCE-BASED TREATMENT

13

IMPLEMENTATION ISSUES

Throughout the previous chapters, five intervention approaches with the older population have been described, applied to case examples, evaluated, and critiqued. Clearly,
practitioners with older adults and their families have a body of literature that can serve
as a resource in evaluating whether a practice approach has a demonstrated level of effectiveness. This is a heartening conclusion since attention to the needs and experiences of
older clients is crucial, with the increased number and diversity of the older population.

In spite of progress, there is much work to be done in geriatric practice. Questions and
limitations remain about the implementation of interventions. Critical questions about
treatment fidelity exist, and require attention and evaluation in the evidence based literature. These include the following:

- What is meant by treatment fidelity, and how is it assessed and measured?
- What protocols increase treatment fidelity, and how are they integrated into research
  and practice?
- How are interventions evaluated to determine whether they are comparable across dif-
  ferent treatments or applications?
- How does the context or treatment setting influence the administration of treatment?

These important questions need to be addressed, as conducting interventions within
real-world settings is a dynamic experience. As practitioners, part of the professional role
is to address the effectiveness of interventions with clients. The question about whether
an intervention has helped is a research question. Did the intervention result in clinically
significant outcomes with the clients? An additional question is whether the intervention
as implemented is the same as what *was intended*. A related question is whether the intervention is consistent across multiple administrations. These are also research questions

that shape how practitioners evaluate existing studies, as well as how interventions are implemented within their own practice.

Unfortunately, questions about implementation and consistency of interventions are often neglected. The lack of discussion about intervention administration creates confusion about what actually constitutes treatment (Kropf & Cummings, 2008). As Naleppa and Cagle (2010) state, "there has been considerable focus on measuring outcomes (i.e., dependent variables) . . . [while] less attention is given to the independent variable and the mechanisms of change in the intervention process" (p. 2).

This chapter discusses the implementation of interventions. Initially, principles that have been developed to guide evidence-based practice are presented. Additionally, the practice literature is evaluated to determine adherence to these guiding principles, with specific application to interventions with older adults. Finally, challenges to conducting evidence-based research within real-world-settings are discussed.

TREATMENT FIDELITY

Treatment fidelity is a fairly recent concept in intervention research. This section presents a brief history of the concept, along with current definitions. In addition, strategies to increase treatment fidelity within psychosocial research are presented.

HISTORY AND DEFINITIONS

Although the term "fidelity" appeared earlier in a small group of studies, the formal definition emerged in the early 1990s (Bellg et al., 2004). Moncher and Prinz (1991) formally introduced this concept in their evaluation of outcome studies and treatment effectiveness. This early article promoted two different aspects of fidelity. *Treatment integrity* is the determination of whether the intervention is delivered as intended. A good example of establishing a protocol to assess treatment integrity is presented by Hidebrand et al. (2013). This research team developed a data-driven model that compares interventionist adherence and competence to the clinical model. In this way, the team could oversee the execution of the treatment across interventionists and administration sites and determine whether the treatment was delivered as intended. A second aspect, *treatment differentiation*, concerns the uniqueness of an intervention; that is, is the treatment condition different enough from non-treatment conditions (either no treatment or another type of treatment approach) to differentiate and compare these experiences?

Since the term was initially defined, multiple definitions of treatment fidelity have emerged. *Fidelity* refers to the extent to which the essential components of the intervention are delivered as intended by established treatment protocols (Cohen et al., 2008; Gearing et al., 2011; Naleppa & Cagle, 2010; Tucker & Blythe, 2008). A more extensive definition has been promulgated by the Behavioral Change Consortium (BCC), which is a group of researchers funded by the National Institutes of Health (NIH), investigating treatments for behavioral change. This group states that "an intervention can be said to satisfy treatment fidelity requirements if it can be shown that the treatment provided was given consistently to all participants randomized to treatment, there was no evidence of non-treatment-related effects, and the intervention was true to the theory and goals underlying the research" (Resnick et al., 2005, p. 46).

STATUS OF FIDELITY ASSESSMENT

In spite of the importance of assessing treatment fidelity in research, studies often do not report this information. Evaluations of intervention research indicate that implementation of the intervention (the independent variable) is often neglected entirely or given scant attention (Corley & Kim, 2016; Naleppa & Cagle, 2010; Tucker & Blythe, 2008). Examined empirically, only about 45%–55% of intervention studies include fidelity assessment in their findings (Borrelli et al., 2005; Frank, Coviak, Healh, Belza, & Casado, 2008; Moncher & Prinz, 1991).

To assess how fidelity was considered in the research contained in this book, the meta-analyses and systematic reviews were examined to determine if an inclusionary criterion was established about having a control or comparison condition as part of the research studies. This would provide evidence that there was treatment differentiation in the studies contained in the reviews. Unfortunately, only 30% of the meta-analyses or systematic reviews included a criterion that selected studies including control or comparison conditions. This level indicates that the majority of studies were not required to have a non-treatment condition. As with other intervention studies, studies of the effectiveness of interventions with older adults need to include content on how those completing treatment compare to those who did not participate, or those who participated in other treatment forms (e.g., usual care).

What are some of the reasons that fidelity remains such an elusive concept in psychosocial intervention research? In their analysis of the literature, Tucker and Blythe (2008) discuss two reasons that few studies assess treatment fidelity. Relatively few methods are available to assess fidelity, which leads researchers to abandon this endeavor entirely. Second, training in this area may be neglected. As the various studies on treatment fidelity indicate, intervention research does not constitute a large segment of the social work and related research literature (e.g., Corley & Kim, 2016; Thyer, 2001). "Given the lack of feasible methods for assessing treatment fidelity and the very small number of published examples, research training may offer limited coverage of the topic" (Tucker & Blythe, 2008, p. 189).

While ensuring that treatment is consistent across participants and sites, the reality of intervention in real-world settings means that modifications and adaptations are necessary. However, significant changes can decrease the effectiveness of the treatment (Jenson & Bender, 2014), so an important question is how much the intervention can be modified and retain effectiveness. Additionally, what are the reasons that an intervention should be modified from the original form? As Washington et al. (2014) state, "Finding the balance between fidelity and flexibility can be challenging" (p. 159).

Importantly, dignity and respect for the participants are crucial, and this may result in needed changes in the established protocol of the intervention. As Naleppa and Cagle (2010) state, "treatment implementation . . . should never be mechanical or conducted without regard to client diversity. Thus, deviation from treatment protocols may, and in some cases should, occur when testing an intervention. In other words, researchers and practitioners should refrain from using so-called cookie-cutter approaches" (p. 6). These authors call for an openness in adapting interventions, with a willingness to act in innovative and creative ways to introduce treatments as necessary.

STRATEGIES TO ENHANCE TREATMENT FIDELITY

The BCC Working Group has developed a set of recommendations that can be used to enhance treatment fidelity in both research and practice (Bellg et al., 2004). Within research, these standards provide the framework to implement a study and structure for reporting the critical components that were part of the study. However, these also are useful principles for practice and creating a new program or intervention approach. The five stages of the process consist of the design, training, treatment delivery, receipt of treatment by participants, and enactment of treatment skills. In each of these stages, there are particular issues that must be addressed to enhance treatment fidelity.

The initial stage is the *design*, which involves how treatment will be introduced to the clients or participants. A critical determination involves treatment dosage, and ensuring that the same dose occurs within the various conditions; that is, how much of the treatment will each client or participant receive? For example, a reminiscence program may be established within several nursing homes, and there is a desire for comparability across sites. Decisions about design include how often these sessions will be offered (e.g., 2 times per week), the length of the sessions (30 minutes each), and the duration (6-week program). In addition, these standards need to be implemented in a consistent manner across sites. This is an important initial step in establishing an intervention approach and determining that the participants in the reminiscence approach receive comparable treatment.

The second phase is assuring that the providers of the intervention are *trained* to deliver the treatment adequately and systematically. To accomplish this goal, training protocols need to be standardized, with competency or performance criteria established. While standard training is critical, there also should be enough flexibility to take into account variation in treatment provider background and expertise. Methods to enhance treatment provider performance include employing a structured practice in training, measuring provider adherence to training by a standard checklist of performance criteria, minimizing performance decay by offering booster training sessions and supervision, and conducting a sample of participant exit interviews to ascertain the delivery of treatment components.

Additionally, *treatment delivery* considers how the intervention is provided to participants. In this area, fidelity is assessed by monitoring how the treatment is carried out, as practice or clinical circumstances arise that require changes in the implementation of the intervention. For example, the facilitators of the reminiscence intervention within the nursing home settings may have a script that is used at the beginning of each session. In this way, standard instructions and introductory content are given to all participants, regardless of the site or facilitator. As an evaluation tool, a sample of sessions can be videotaped and assessed by treatment experts (e.g., supervisors or advanced clinicians) to determine the performance of the facilitator in real-world applications. Facilitators who are evaluated to deliver the intervention as designed 80%–100% of the time are considered to have high integrity in delivery. Low integrity is considered to be 50% or less (Gearing et al., 2011; Perepletchikova & Kazdin, 2005).

In monitoring the *receipt of treatment*, determination is made about whether the participants are able to improve as a result of the intervention. A typical way to determine that change has resulted from the treatment is including pre–post test measures within the design. However, other methods can be used. One is to include the use of hypothetical examples that provide participants with the opportunity to employ skills within the context of the intervention itself to demonstrate performance. In a nutrition-based psychoeducational group, for example, participants are taught how to prepare healthy meals to manage their diabetes. An assessment of their ability to choose the healthier foods from an array of options might be one indicator of how they have mastered the course material.

Finally, *enactment of treatment skills* indicates the level to which participants are able to employ knowledge and skills within the larger environment. Assessment methods include evaluating how well participants can employ skills or information that is part of treatment by self-monitoring or reporting. For example, participants in a caregiving social support group may be asked to keep a journal about managing stress. As a result of participating in the group, situations that might have previously created stress may be managed more effectively, which results in lower stress thresholds.

INTERVENTIONS WITH OLDER ADULTS

Within the older population, the heterogeneity of functional and cognitive abilities creates challenges in ensuring fidelity in implementing interventions. Differences in hearing, sight, recall, and processing can factor into how the intervention is delivered and also how the participant engages in and receives it. Challenges to, and strategies for, implementation of interventions specific to the older population are highlighted in this section.

CHALLENGES IN IMPLEMENTATION

Delivering interventions has challenges, regardless of context or client population. In treatment approaches with older adults, however, complication can arise as a result of multiple factors. These involve the setting or context for the intervention, the characteristics or abilities of the participants, and staffing and personnel matters.

A major issue in aging-related research and practice is the difficulty associated with treatments delivered within residential settings such as assisted living or nursing homes. Within residential contexts, non-participants may be exposed to the intervention by virtue of being in a shared space. In that situation, it is difficult to determine who actually benefited from the intervention. For example, in treatment programs that are delivered in long-term care settings, it may be difficult to control who is included (and who is not). Kolanwski, Buettner, and Moeller (2006) offer suggestions about how to minimize these internal threats. One suggestion is to select or randomize *sites*, not individuals within sites; for example, participants for treatment are selected from one nursing home, while a control group is from a second site. If this strategy is not possible, then identifying space for the intervention within the facility is critical. An activity intervention could be delivered in a separate room of the facility, with only the participants present. This change would reduce the possibility of dispersing the treatment beyond the participant sample.

Even with these cautious approaches, interventions often occur in environments that experience rapid and significant change, which can compromise treatment effectiveness or complicate results. This is particularly difficult if staff are tracking outcomes for participants in an intervention. Buckwalter et al. (2009) defines highly unstable environments as those that have "high rates of attrition/turnover of staff, students, or patients, or that are subject to unpredictable external forces, such as regulatory change" (p. 111). For example, a study of quality indicators to assess nursing home residents' abilities and function indicated a high level of instability within the facilities (Rantz et al., 2004); that is, the rates of factors such as falls, resident weight loss, or activity level vary due to organizational factors such as quality of care. As a result, changes in outcomes may reflect changes from the interventions *or* from the quality of staffing within the facility. These authors suggest that two 6-month evaluation periods be analyzed to determine variability in quality indicators prior to introducing an intervention.

To deal with the factors that can compromise treatment fidelity, modifications of the treatment may be necessary. In an examination of modifications in health-care interventions, Cohen et al. (2008) identified three sets of factors that created the need for modification of treatment. While this list was constructed for health-care interventions, the findings have utility for other intervention types as well.

Accommodations to practice circumstances may be required to implement the intervention. For example, an evidence-based practice model may include specific ways of recruiting participants or collecting assessment data, yet these protocols may not fit with established routines within agency workflow processes. While agencies or organizations may be able to make a certain level of change, extensive changes are often impossible. Implementation barriers may include variations in workflow or organizational culture, which create a new set of responsibilities or tasks for the staff. For example, staff in a senior center may be asked to track interactions between participants to determine if they are more socially engaged after an intervention is implemented. If this request does not fit well with the staff's other responsibilities, there is a real danger that incomplete or poor quality data will be provided. Unfortunately, this might be a point where "many new practices are abandoned, because the power of the status quo is strong" (Nichols, Martindale-Adams, Burns, Zuber, & Graney, 2016, p. 138).

As a result, modifications in the intervention structure must be considered. Some of the common changes that occur are reassigning responsibilities or changing data recording structures to be more accommodating of staff. Another possibility is altering intervention delivery methods, such as structuring when intervention sessions are offered, to fit with agency program schedules. These types of modifications promote integration of the intervention within the real-world contexts of health and social service provision.

A second area is *accommodating participants' circumstances*. With older adults, changes may be necessary based upon participants' health and functioning levels. Some changes that are instituted include methods of transmitting information (e.g., how written material is prepared, supplementing oral content with written materials). In the interventions in the previous chapters, several interventions were developed to be delivered in a technology format (e.g., web-based or videophone). These alternate delivery formats were developed so that older participants who were homebound or lacked transportation could participate. In addition, participant preferences also need to be taken into account, such as providing handouts, or shortening the duration of sessions. These changes promote adherence to interventions and reduce dropout rates.

A third type of change is associated with *intervention costs*. Personnel costs are a concern in many programs, as hiring individuals to administer the intervention can quickly escalate overall costs. This is especially the case when special skills or knowledge are required, such as certifications or licenses (e.g., a LCSW is needed to teach classes). Instead, less qualified individuals can be supervised or trained by master teachers or clinicians. A second modification is the cost of delivery format. Instead of individual sessions, the intervention may be modified to hold group sessions with participants, which minimizes time and costs and fits better within organizations' budgets.

EXAMPLES OF FIDELITY ASSESSMENT

The areas just discussed provide a framework for understanding why modifications may be necessary within interventions. Realistically, every point in the intervention design and implementation involves decisions that impact treatment fidelity. Since the majority of interventions are developed and tested outside of the care system, problems occur in implementation within real-world settings (Gitlin, Marx, Stanley, & Hodgson, 2015). "Hence, a translational phase is necessary to modify complex protocols and interventionist training to derive a better fit with service environments and identify environmental supports and barriers to implementation" (Gitlin et al., 2015, p. 212). Two examples of intervention programs with older adults and their families are provided to demonstrate how treatment was modified in the context of real-world situations.

The first program, Families Matter in Long Term Care, was a multi-site intervention for care providers to enhance involvement with their family members and facilitate communication with staff within the setting (Washington et al., 2014). Several issues emerged that required changes within the treatment protocol and assessment of fidelity. As these authors stress, flexibility is key in overcoming challenges and barriers. Some of the challenges experienced include care providers being unable to attend in-service workshops, variation in treatment plan adherence across the family caregivers, and staff inability to participate as initially determined. As a result, the intervention team faced numerous decisions that had an impact on the original protocol. Based upon the five areas articulated in the recommendations by the BCC, Table 13.1 is a summary of the original fidelity strategy and modifications to the protocol that were implemented as a result of the challenges encountered.

A second example of assessing fidelity of interventions for older adults included four health-promotion programs. These interventions were examined to determine how fidelity was tracked, as well as modifications in protocols to deal with real-world circumstances in implementation (Frank et al., 2008). The four behavior-change programs targeted increased activity, falls prevention, depression management, and self-management of diseases.

The BCC Working Group standards were also used to assess fidelity in this analysis. Similar to the family caregiver example preceding section, the five areas of the BCC framework were examined to ascertain how the intervention programs addressed fidelity. In addition, modifications to the original protocols are articulated as a result of implementing the intervention within agency settings (see Table 13.2). Changes stemmed from several factors that the projects had to face in implementing the intervention within these real-world contexts. Some examples of issues that the teams faced were the following:

- Using master trainers who were certified in certain areas to train and supervise leaders of the intervention. This was done instead of having certified trainers deliver the intervention to the participants.
- Gathering data about outcomes from case managers instead of directly from participants themselves. This change was derived from delivering the program within participants' homes, which made data collection more difficult.

Fidelity Category	Original Fidelity Strategy	Modification
Study Design: Plan for implementation setbacks; establish fixed doses	Participants attend the full version of a workshop about the intervention.	Shortened version of the workshop was created to accommodate participants' schedules.
	Participants created a service plan about the intervention in person with a staff member at the residential facility.	A shortened version of the workshop and service plan creation was conducted with those who couldn't attend in person.
	Fixed doses based upon workshop attendance and creation of service plan.	Varied doses of the intervention based upon the workshop attendance of the participants, the extent to which they adhered to their service plan, and service plan reinforcement.
Provider Training: Assess the training of treatment providers	Implementation by LTC staff	Interventionist assumed full role for training.
	Caregivers create individualized service plans with the input of staff.	Interventionist helped develop individualized service plans if staff members were unavailable to do so.
Treatment Delivery: Deliver the intervention as intended	Staff members undergo rigid training on intervention delivery.	Interventionist completed rigid training due to change in implementation of intervention.
Treatment Receipt: Establish a method to verify that participants understood and could perform the behavioral skills prescribed in the intervention	Observe staff delivery.	Observe interventionists' delivery.
	Direct observation of caregivers' behavioral skills	Follow-up calls to caregivers to address barriers to treatment receipt
Treatment Enactment: Establish a method to monitor and improve the ability of patients to perform treatment-related behavioral skills in real-life settings	Follow-up calls to assess adherence to service plans at months 1, 3, and 5.	Follow-up calls reduced to months 1 and 3.
	Postcard reminders mailed at months 2 and 4 to enforce adherence.	Postcards mailed at 1 month.

Adapted from: Washington et al. (2014).

Fidelity Category	Methods of Assessment Modifications in Interventions	Examples of Modifications
Study Design: Plan for implementation setbacks; establish fixed doses	Consult with designers of original program to consult about possible changes, consult with experts in subject matter, consult with community agency providers.	Changed method of instruction (e.g., participants were seated instead of standing), peers led classes instead of professionals, extended durations of sessions, included visit by health professional to review intervention.
Provider Training: Assess the training of treatment providers	Use instructor, participant, and master training manuals, implement workshops and listservs for technical assistance, survey master trainers about outcome of training, offer booster training sessions.	Shorten training from original length for greater participation of trainers, use videos to demonstrate activities for trainers, increased frequency of booster sessions, assign "coaches" to help with technical assistance issues of trainers.
Treatment Delivery: Deliver the intervention as intended	Master trainer performed observations of intervention, program evaluated by external consultants, mentor system for volunteer coaches, surveys from participants or master instructors.	Recruited facilitators who were not affiliated with sponsoring organizations to deliver intervention; program was embedded in programs already offered at an agency site.
Treatment Receipt: Establish a method to verify that participants understood and could perform the behavioral skills prescribed in the intervention	Self-reports of health status, attendance records, focus groups with participants	Changed time of survey administration to participants to better coincide with content in the intervention, intervention given in either English or Spanish, provided written materials to compliment oral presentation/instructions.
Treatment Enactment: Establish a method to monitor and improve the ability of patients to perform treatment-related behavioral skills in real-life settings	Record health status results of participants, included follow-up performance measures at 6 and 12 months, compared outcome data to baseline, follow-up telephone survey of participants.	Changed times of follow-up calls, included a participant newsletter in follow-up design, compared outcomes to baseline of participants instead of using a control group, promoted post-program classes to graduates who wanted to participate.

Adapted from: Frank et al. (2008).

- Including qualitative comments as well as quantitative outcome data. These additional data provided insight into changes in participants' functioning abilities, and added a context for some of the outcomes.

These two examples illustrate how the implementation of interventions is a dynamic process that involves adaptations from the original model. While the programs that are showcased had to initiate significant modifications, the use of a framework such as the one drafted by the BCC Working Group provides a process for cataloging and assessing the impacts of modifications on the fidelity of the interventions. In intervention research, an assumption should be that modifications are a usual part of adapting evidence-based practice models into diverse settings with different participant populations. As Cohen et al. (2008) state, "The need to adapt does not indicate a poor intervention or an inexperienced research team; it is a common part of the research process. It is the journey of translating evidence based research into practice" (p. S387).

For the five approaches presented in this book, each chapter contained a summary of how interventions were modified for older clients. Typical changes included shortening the duration of sessions, holding fewer sessions, providing material in multiple forms (e.g., oral and written material), and making the treatment accessible for older individuals (e.g., in-home or technology-based). In some of the studies, these changes were empirically evaluated to determine if these modifications resulted in different outcomes. Additional work in this area is necessary as a greater breadth of treatment approaches are employed with older clients.

In summary, evidence-based practice requires that interventions be introduced into diverse settings and with different participant populations. In order to implement interventions, modifications are typically required that impact the effectiveness and fidelity of the treatment. Although vitally important, research often lacks information about the translation of treatment *models* into treatment *practices* that occur in real-world settings. All of these factors need to be integrated into the plans to introduce, implement, and evaluate interventions with older adults.

REFERENCES

Bellg, A. J., Borrelli, B., Resnick, B., Hecht, J., Minicucci, D. S., Ory, M., . . . Czajkowski, S. (2004). Enhancing treatment fidelity in health behavior change studies: best practices and recommendations from the NIH Behavior Change Consortium. *Health Psychology, 23*(5), 443.

Borrelli, B., Sepinwall, D., Ernst, D., Bellg, A. J., Czajkowski, S., Breger, R., . . . Orwig, D. (2005). A new tool to assess treatment fidelity and evaluation of treatment fidelity across 10 years of health behavior research. *Journal of Consulting and Clinical Psychology, 73*(5), 852–860.

Buckwalter, K. C., Grey, M., Bowers, B., McCarthy, A. M., Gross, D., Funk, M., & Beck, C. (2009). Intervention research in highly unstable environments. *Research in Nursing & Health, 32*(1), 110–121.

Cohen, D. J., Crabtree, B. F., Etz, R. S., Balasubramanian, B. A., Donahue, K. E., Leviton, L. C., . . . Green, L. W. (2008). Fidelity versus flexibility: translating evidence based research into practice. *American Journal of Preventive Medicine*, 35(5), S381–S389.

Corley, N. A., & Kim, I. (2016). An assessment of intervention fidelity in published social work intervention research studies. *Research on Social Work Practice*, 26(1), 53–60.

Frank, J. C., Coviak, C. P., Healy, T. C., Belza, B., & Casado, B. L. (2008). Addressing fidelity in evidence based health promotion programs for older adults. *Journal of Applied Gerontology*, 27(1), 4–33.

Gearing, R. E., El-Bassel, N., Ghesquiere, A., Baldwin, S., Gillies, J., & Ngeow, E. (2011). Major ingredients of fidelity: a review and scientific guide to improving quality of intervention research implementation. *Clinical Psychology Review*, 31(1), 79–88.

Gitlin, L. N., Marx, K., Stanley, I. H., & Hodgson, N. (2015). Translating evidence based dementia caregiving interventions into practice: state-of-the-science and next steps. *The Gerontologist*, 55, 210–226.

Jenson, J. F., & Bender, K. A. (2014). *Preventing child and adolescent problem behavior: evidence-based strategies in schools, families, and communities*. New York: Oxford University Press.

Kolanowski, A., Buettner, L., & Moeller, J. (2006). Treatment fidelity plan for an activity intervention designed for persons with dementia. *American Journal of Alzheimer's Disease and Other Dementias*, 21(5), 326–332.

Kropf, N. P., & Cummings, S. M. (2008). Effective practice with older adults: concluding thoughts. In S. M. Cummings & N.P. Kropf (Eds.), *Handbook of psychosocial interventions with older adults: evidence based treatment* (pp. 345–355). London: Routledge.

Moncher, F. J., & Prinz, R. J. (1991). Treatment fidelity in outcome studies. *Clinical Psychology Review*, 11(3), 247–266.

Naleppa, M. J., & Cagle, J. G. (2010). Treatment fidelity in social work intervention research: a review of published studies. *Research on Social Work Practice*, 20(6), 674–681.

Nichols, L. O., Martindale-Adams, J., Burns, R., Zuber, J., & Graney, M. J. (2016). REACH VA: moving from translation to system implementation. *The Gerontologist*, 56(1), 135–144.

Perepletchikova, F., & Kazdin, A. E. (2005). Treatment integrity and therapeutic change: issues and research recommendations. *Clinical Psychology: Science and Practice*, 12(4), 365–383.

Rantz, M. J., Hicks, L., Petroski, G. F., Madsen, R. W., Mehr, D. R., Conn, V., . . . Maas, M. (2004). Stability and sensitivity of nursing home quality indicators. *The Journals of Gerontology Series A: Biological Sciences and Medical Sciences*, 59(1), M79–M82.

Resnick, B., Bellg, A. J., Borrelli, B., De Francesco, C., Breger, R., Hecht, J., & Czajkowski, S. (2005). Examples of implementation and evaluation of treatment fidelity in the BCC studies: where we are and where we need to go. *Annals of Behavioral Medicine*, 29(2), 46–54.

Thyer, B. A. (2001). What is the role of theory in research on social work practice? *Journal of Social Work Education*, 37(1), 9–25.

Tucker, A., & Blythe, B. (2008). Attention to treatment fidelity in social work outcomes: a review of the literature from the 1990s. *Social Work Research*, 32(3), 185–190.

Washington, T., Zimmerman, S., Cagle, J., Reed, D., Cohen, L., Beeber, A. S., & Gwyther, L. P. (2014). Fidelity decision making in social and behavioral research: alternative measures of dose and other considerations. *Social Work Research*, 38, 154–162.

14

FUTURE DIRECTIONS IN INTERVENTIONS WITH OLDER ADULTS

The purpose of this book is to provide a summary of evidence-based interventions for individuals in later life. As the initial chapters highlight, aging individuals are a diverse group more different from each other than any other age cohort. This is a result of their individual life trajectories combined with social experiences which results in unique life courses. In addition, older adults have a range of functional abilities and health and social statuses. As a result, their residential circumstances vary from living with family or alone in the community, to residing in a long-term care facility. This scenario makes practice with older adults an exciting and challenging venture.

At the beginning of this book, the quote by Betty Friedan reminds us that society's image of older adults is quite different from how older adults view and experience themselves. For practitioners who are working with older clients, this message is an important one to "take to heart," spending time to understand *this older individual* as a unique person. In addition, Friedan reminds us that moving forward, we also must be ready to do things differently, for example, for practitioners, to look for new ways to assist clients with overcoming the challenges of later life, and to explore different methods and interventions with the older population. Her words have marked meaning as we prepare for the number of baby boomers who bring different life experiences and expectations to their later years.

PROMISING INTERVENTION APPROACHES

While the previous chapters have explored intervention approaches that have an evidence base with the older population, this chapter will present some promising practice approaches. These interventions have been effective in work with other populations, but have not been well established with older clients. Two approaches will be described, including their method of intervention, client populations, and resulting outcomes. Modifications or adaptations for practice with older adults will also be explored. To heed Friedan's words, these may be the "surprising new possibilities" in treatment approaches in coming years (1993, p. 31).

MINDFULNESS-BASED STRESS REDUCTION

Mindfulness-based stress reduction (MBSR) is a mind-body intervention that has had wide usage with clinical (e.g., health-care patients and mental health clients), and non-clinical populations. This intervention emphasizes a mind-body connection, and a non-judgmental awareness of the present, rather than worry and anxiety about the future, or re-experiencing the past (Lenze et al., 2014). Within the intervention approach, individuals become aware of sensations in their body, the soundscape, and their mind states.

Intervention Approach

MBSR was founded by Jon Kabot-Zinn, who started out as a molecular biologist. After earning a PhD at MIT, Dr. Kabot-Zinn became focused on the mind-body interaction, especially for healing and management of chronic pain. Although initially connected to Buddhist principles, MBSR has evolved into practice that has a scientific and empirical foundation. In 1979, Dr. Kabot-Zinn founded the Center for Mindfulness at the University of Massachusetts Medical School. Over the ensuing years, a literature on MBSR outcomes has developed, with effectiveness in several areas including a "moderate and persistent" effect on mental health, as well as chronic health conditions, across a variety of populations (De Vibe, Bjørndal, Tipton, Hammerstrøm, Kowalski, 2012, p. 8).

MBSR uses a structured approach to intervention. The standard approach is 26 hours of session time, which is spread across an 8-week class of 2.5 hours, and includes one 6-hour class, which typically occurs on a weekend during the sixth week (Kabat-Zinn, 1990). Session content includes gentle yoga, body awareness meditations (e.g., body scan), and concentration meditations. Besides the sessions, participants are expected to commit to daily practices of meditation and yoga exercises that last 45–60 minutes. During class sessions, participants' experiences with these assignments are discussed and processed with the facilitators. MBSR courses are offered in a variety of settings and contexts within community and health-care settings. In addition, worksite environments are also becoming more common places for MBSR courses to deal with work demands and to foster innovation and creativity (Hensen, 2012). A typical MBSR group size is 10–40 participants.

Outcomes

Although initially developed to help those who suffer from chronic pain, MBSR continues to be an intervention employed with individuals who face significant health challenges. However, MBSR is now also used in a variety of populations to deal with mental health and health issues. In addition, non-patient populations are also participating in MBSR classes to enhance well-being and decrease stress levels.

A number of meta-analyses and systematic reviews have been conducted on MBSR groups. Outcomes of these studies are presented to determine effectiveness for various conditions. While these have analyses are not specific for older adults, several yield positive results that have relevance for the issues that challenge the older population.

Health-Related Outcomes Five meta-analyses or systematic reviews report outcomes of MBSR for health-related conditions. Three of these included varied chronic health conditions, such as diabetes, cardiovascular conditions, arthritis, headache/migraines, fibromyalgia, irritable bowel syndrome, asthma and respiratory illness, chronic fatigue, and back and spine issues. Two studies specifically focused on outcomes for cancer patients.

A review by Merkes (2010) reported outcomes of this intervention for adults with chronic conditions in 15 studies. The median number of participants in the studies was 27, and the majority of participants were female. The average age of participants in these studies ranged from 44 to 70, with the majority in the mid- to late forties. For mental health outcomes, six studies reported significant reductions in anxiety, and an additional six reported reduced depression rates. Other mental health outcomes included positive changes in mood, global mental health, reduced psychological distress, and reduced obsessiveness, psychosis, and paranoid ideation. Positive physical health outcomes included reduction in pain, increased global health functioning, and reductions in fatigue and sleep disruptions.

Bohlemeijer, Prenger, Taal, and Cuijpers (2010) also reported on outcomes for patients across varied diagnoses. Eight RCTs were included, with outcomes reported for depression, anxiety, and psychological distress. Overall, the majority of participants in these studies ranged in age from 45–55 years, with the majority being female. The number of participants included in the various studies ranged from 37 to 200. For all three outcomes, small to moderate positive effects were reported, with anxiety having the greatest reduction overall.

In a review by Crowe et al. (2016), intervention studies for community-based adults with long-term health symptoms or conditions were included. Fifteen studies were part of the systematic review; 11 were RCTs, and the remaining four were pre–post test designs. The mean age of the participants ranged from 38 to 75, and most studies were majority female. Differing from most of the studies, however, two included in this review had majority male participants (Gans et al., 2014; Mularski et al., 2009). Studies were evaluated on physical outcomes related to the long-term health issue. Improvements were found for sleep, symptoms related to irritable bowel symptoms, asthma, fibromyalgia, and tinnitus.

MBSR has been used with individuals diagnosed with cancer. In a meta-analysis on mental health outcomes for patients with breast cancer, Zainal, Booth, and Huppert (2013) included nine studies on the impact of MBSR on depression and anxiety. All participants in the studies were women, with the majority having completed cancer treatment. The mean age of participants was 45.4 to 61.6 years, with 90% being White. Seven of the studies included measures of depression, with MBSR having a significant moderate impact on this outcome. Four studies included anxiety with a large significant impact on this outcome. Overall, this intervention was effective in the reduction of negative psychosocial outcomes associated with breast cancer.

A second meta-analysis on patients with cancer included participants with various diagnoses (Ledesma & Kumano, 2009). These included breast, gastrointestinal, prostate, neurological, hematologic, and gynecologic cancers. Ten studies were included, with outcomes related to both physical and mental health factors. The majority of study participants were female (79%), with Stage II being the modal stage in the disease. The average age across studies was 54.75 years. For mental health outcomes, MBSR was found to improve quality of life, relieve anxiety and stress, reduce sleep disturbance, and help overall mood. Small effects were found for physical health outcomes, including body mass changes, blood cell counts, or other health indicators. As a result, the conclusion of the authors is that MBSR has a greater impact on mental health than the physical correlates of cancer.

Depression and Anxiety Four meta-analyses focused on the reduction of depression and anxiety as a result of MBSR practice. Goyal et al. (2014) included 47 RCTs that focused on stress-related outcomes in adult populations. The average number in the studies was 74.79 (range 18–186), with no additional information about study participants. Mindfulness moderately improved outcomes for anxiety, depression, and the experience of pain. Limited or no evidence was found for impact on positive mood, sleep, or weight. This analysis also reviewed any harmful outcomes of meditation on participants, and none was reported within the studies.

A meta-analysis on stress reduction and health benefits was conducted across a variety of participant populations (Grossman, Niemann, Schmidt, & Walach, 2004). Twenty studies were included, with both clinical populations (e.g., pain, cancer, cardiac disease, depression, anxiety) as well as non-clinical groups who were experiencing stress. Both mental and physical health outcomes produced moderate positive effects at intervention outcome. As a result, these authors conclude that "mindfulness training might enhance general features of coping with distress and disability in everyday life, as well as under more extraordinary conditions of serious disorder or stress." (p. 39).

Khoury, Sharma, Rush, and Fournier (2015) specifically analyzed studies of healthy (non-clinical) participants. The outcomes of stress and anxiety were reviewed, with a total of 29 studies included within the analysis. Study participants included students ($n = 10$), health-care professionals ($n = 9$), the general population ($n = 4$), MBSR groups ($n = 3$), and pregnant women ($n = 1$). Moderate effects were found for stress reduction, depression, anxiety, and increased quality of life. The target population that had the greatest overall change from MBSR was health-care professionals.

Given the positive findings, a fourth analysis focused on the process of MBSR and the method to reduce stress, and improve mental health and well-being (Gu, Strauss, Bond, & Cavanagh, 2015). The twenty studies included 15 RCTs and five quasi-experimental designs. Sample sizes ranged from 27 to 205 participants; eight for those with depression, four with cancer patients or survivors, three with non-clinical samples, two with anxiety disorders, two with distress-relates symptoms, and one unspecified sample. The majority of outcomes were mental health conditions (e.g., depression, anxiety, distress, negative affect). Mindfulness (e.g., the experience of being in the present moment) was the process that had the greatest impact on outcomes. Other processes that produced changes were self-compassion and reduction of repetitive negative thinking.

The meta-analyses and systematic reviews on MBSR yield positive results in several outcomes. Although the research consisted of heterogeneous populations, many of the conditions are also experienced by older adults. In particular, depression and anxiety decrease upon completion of an MBSR intervention with consistency across studies. These are the most frequent mental health issues of later life, and MBSR holds promise in decreasing the severity and experience with the older population.

MBSR and Older Adults

Although in its beginning stages, a literature is starting to develop for MBSR treatment with older adults. In particular, MBSR has been used with older clients or care providers who are depressed, anxious, or in pain. In addition, this approach has been implemented to increase the quality of life for those who are isolated or who live in residential settings. Individual studies that have been conducted with older adults will be summarized and highlighted.

Depression In one study, community-based older adults were randomly assigned to an MBSR ($n = 100$) or wait-list group ($n = 100$) (Gallegos, Hoerger, Talbot, Moynihan, & Duberstein, 2013; Gallegos, Hoerger, Talbot, Krasner, Knight, Moynihan, & Duberstein, 2013). The sample consisted primarily of women (62%), with an average age of about 73 years. The group was highly educated, with about 88% having attended college. An average of two health conditions was reported by the participants.

The MBSR intervention took place within a university setting, and the groups were held with 15–20 members in each. Seven sessions lasted 2 hours, with a mid-treatment session of 7 hours. The MBSR protocol included yoga, sitting meditation, informal meditation (e.g., walking meditation, other activities), and body scan (mindful attention to sensations within the body). Outcomes were measured for positive affect, depressive symptomotology, and immune functioning through blood assays. Findings indicated that MBSR had greater efficacy for improving positive affect for participants who had lower baseline depression scores. Those with higher levels of depression reported less improvement at the conclusion of the intervention. The authors suggest that older adults who are experiencing depression may benefit from more emphasis on the MBSR principles of non-striving and acceptance, such as recognizing and tolerating limitations that result from the aging process. In addition, blood assay analysis indicated that MBSR—particularly yoga—had the greatest positive impact on physiologic functioning.

A study in Bangalore, India, evaluated the impact of MBSR on older adults who resided in residential facilities (Kumar, Adiga, & George, 2014). A total of 60 participants were randomly assigned to a treatment or control group. The majority of participants in both groups were between the ages of 60–64 years (n = 73% treatment; n = 57% control). The majority of both groups were male (57%), and all were married. Most had lived in the residential facility for 2 years or less. The intervention consisted of 5 weeks of five MBSR sessions. Each session lasted for 20–30 minutes, and consisted of mindful breathing, body scan, mindfulness of thoughts, sounds, and feelings. The outcomes that were measured were depression and mindfulness, operationalized as "the awareness that emerges through paying attention in purpose, in the present moment, and non-judgmental to unfolding of experience moment to moment" (p. 6). The outcomes indicated that the MBSR participants had both lower depression scores and higher mindfulness scores at post-test and compared to the control group.

MBSR has also been used to help care providers of older adults. In a study in Hong Kong, caregivers of persons with chronic health conditions and who experienced caregiver strain were randomly assigned to a treatment (n = 70) or control group (n = 71) (Hou et al., 2014). The overall sample had an average age of 58 years, and 83% were female. The majority of care providers were either spouses or children of the care recipient, and typically assisted with 5–6 ADLs daily. The intervention consisted of eight weekly 2-hour sessions, but no day-long retreat was included. The various components of MBSR were the body scan, sitting meditation, yoga, and mindfulness in daily activities (e.g., walking, eating). Each class consisted of 12–15 participants. Results indicated that the intervention participants had significantly lowered depression scores at post-test and 3 months post-intervention. Although these caregivers had considerable time constraints, the majority were able to attend six or more of the sessions. Additionally, over half of the participants continued to practice mindfulness meditation at the 3-month follow-up period.

Quality of Life Factors Several quality of life indicators have also been studied in older MBSR participants. In one study, older adults who complained of worrying and memory were included in an MBSR intervention (Lenze et al., 2014). Thirty-four participants in two sites participated in either the traditional (8-week) or modified (12-week) intervention. The average age of the participants was about 71 years, about 73% were female, the majority were White, and most had some post-secondary education. Two intervention types were compared as part of the study. The traditional intervention consisted of an 8-week, 2.5-hour session protocol and included a day-long retreat. The modified intervention was extended to 12 weeks, with a reduction to 2.5 hours for the retreat. Outcomes included functioning of participants, as well as their subjective assessment of the intervention. From pre-to post-test, participants in both the traditional and modified intervention showed a trend toward improvement of cognitive functioning, including memory and recall. In addition, improvements in severity of worrying were found in both conditions, and extended to the 6-month follow-up. Again, there was no difference in change between the two treatment conditions, which suggests that extending the length of the intervention does not increase treatment effects. In the subjective outcomes, older participants evaluated the experience. Overall, the most preferred practices were meditation (40%) and yoga (32%). The most disliked component was the body scan, but this was only reported by a minority of participants (12%). At the 6-month follow-up, a significant percentage reported that they continued to practice mindful breathing (83%), meditation (59%), and mindful eating (59%) a few times per month or more.

A community-based study researched the impact of MBSR on loneliness, measured through both subjective appraisal and pro-inflammatory gene expression (Creswell et al., 2012). Loneliness was measured by participant responses, and participants also had 10 ml of blood drawn at pre- and post-treatment. Forty older adults were randomly assigned to a treatment or control condition. The average age of the sample was 65 years, was mainly White (64%), female (80%), and educated beyond high school (98%). The MBSR intervention consisted of an 8-week intervention of weekly 120-minute sessions and one midpoint day-long retreat. Sessions included mindfulness meditation, yoga, group discussions to bring awareness to moment-to-moment experiences. Those in the intervention completed an average of 7.2 sessions. Results indicate that intervention participants reported significantly less loneliness from baseline, as compared to the control that had a slight increase in scores. In addition, the intervention group also had lowered physiologic levels that correlate with loneliness. As a result of these combined results, the authors conclude that MBSR is an effective intervention for loneliness that enhances both the mental and physical health of participants.

Some older adults suffer from insomnia, which can negatively impact mental and physical health and functioning. In a randomized controlled trial of Chinese adults 75 years and older, 60 participants were assigned to either an MBSR or control group (Zhang et al., 2015). The average age in the study was 77 years, and 58% were male. The MBSR intervention was conducted at a hospital in a modified format. Two-hour sessions were held for an 8-week time frame, with a 2-hour silent retreat between the sixth and seventh weeks. The sessions consisted of the body scan and sitting, walking, and standing meditations. Due to the age of the participants, the yoga component was omitted in the structure. Results indicated that MBSR decreased the incidence and experience of insomnia, as well as depression scores. However, measures of anxiety did not change within the treatment group from pre- to post-test.

Two additional studies examined quality of life issues in older adults who resided in long-term care settings. In one study, MBSR was introduced in a continuing care community (Moss et al., 2015). Thirty-nine older adults were randomized to an MBSR ($n = 20$) or control ($n = 19$) group. The average age of the sample was 82 years, all were White, 64% had post-secondary education, and 82% were female. Participants had an average of

4.2 medical conditions, including arthritis, sleep problems, hypertension, cardiac issues, and chronic pain. The MBSR program consisted of 8 weeks of 2-hour sessions held one time per week. The intervention did not include a retreat. The intervention consisted of a body scan, sitting meditation, mindful walking, loving kindness meditation, and yoga, which was conducted in chairs instead of on the floor. Outcomes were measured on health-related quality of life, acceptance and psychological flexibility, mindfulness, self-compassion, and distress. At post-test, those in the MBSR intervention had increased scores on two outcomes of psychological flexibility, and increased quality of life related to physical limitations. These two significant outcomes related to participants' ability to demonstrate greater acceptance of the challenging conditions experienced and perception of lower levels of physical barriers in functioning.

Finally, one study measured the experience of chronic pain, anxiety, and distress for nursing home residents (McBee, Westreich, & Likourezos, 2004). The sample size was small ($n = 14$), but the population had significant health issues (minimum of 20 health conditions for each resident). Many of these conditions are accompanied by severe levels of pain, such as osteoarthritis, fractures, and cancer. The goal of the intervention was to reduce pain and increase positive feelings for the participants. The majority (92%) were women, mainly Jewish (86%), and were 85 years of age. The intervention was a 10-week modified MBSR structure. The sessions consisted of deep breathing, quiet sitting, mindful eating, body scan, gentle chair yoga, visualization and communication exercises, and loving kindness meditation. Sessions were held weekly for 1 hour each, and a retreat was not included. Pre-and post-treatment analysis indicated that the participants were less sad, and showed a downward trend in experiencing pain.

The Promise of MBSR with Older Adults Although few studies have been conducted on MBSR with the older population, there is a significant literature in general. The outcomes targeted, such as decreased depression, anxiety, and physical symptomology, are issues that threaten older adults' functioning and abilities. In addition, the positive outcomes achieved with non-clinical populations also make MBSR an appealing approach for preventive work as well.

The few studies that have targeted the older population have indicated that this approach has utility in decreasing geriatric depression and enhancing quality of life. Since MBSR can be introduced into diverse contexts, such as senior center programs and residential settings, it is easily integrated into sites where older adults congregate. Although not empirically evaluated yet, those studies that do report compliance rates suggest that older adults who take MBSR complete the majority of sessions.

One study specifically targeted care providers, and this is an area to explore further. The mindfulness component has the potential of decreasing caregivers' stress levels, and also helping them stay present to experience the joys and rewards that exist. Although care provision is a demanding role, the research with care providers reported that the majority continued to practice mindfulness after completion of the formal course.

Several of the studies that employed MBSR with older adults modified the structure in certain ways. If necessary, the yoga was modified for gentler poses, with shorter durations, or was omitted totally. In addition, many courses omitted or shortened the retreat, which was traditionally held at the midpoint for an entire day. If a retreat was included, the duration was shortened to a half-day or less. In addition, the session durations were also shortened from the traditional 2.5 hours. Modified session times were typically 1 hour or less. In spite of the shortened duration, positive outcomes were achieved, which is consistent with evaluations of other MBSR studies that have adjusted class time (Carmody & Baer, 2009). These results are encouraging, and invite additional research on outcomes with diverse populations of older adults.

BEHAVIORAL ACTIVATION

Behavioral Activation (BA) is an approach that originated within the cognitive-behavioral orientation to treatment. However, BA has become an independent intervention approach that has demonstrated efficacy in working with depressed clients. The approach differentiates depressed persons' internal state (e.g., mood, outlook) from their behavior (e.g., isolation, dysregulation). The goal of BA is to intervene within the behavioral realm, with the subsequent positive change in individuals' mood state. Because results are achieved without the corresponding therapeutic attention to clients' cognitions, BA has been promoted as a more parsimonious approach to relieving depression than cognitive-based therapy (Dimidjian et al., 2006).

Intervention Approach

BA has origins in the work of Ferster (1973), who identified the role of avoidance, isolation, and inertia in depressed individuals. While these avoidance coping mechanisms may alleviate short-term discomforts, the longer outcomes include an inability to derive pleasurable experiences within the environment and disruption of routines. Clinicians work with depressed clients to establish *social zietgebers*, or "social regulators of biological rhythms, our dependence on social/environmental routes to maintain emotional stability" (Jacobson, Martell, & Dimidjian, 2001, p. 259). Using a more environmental (vs. medical) paradigm, BA seeks to increase access to pleasurable and antidepressive experiences and to establish functional routines that promote steadiness and stability for the individual.

The course of the intervention is focused on behavioral change of the client and typically lasts 12–16 sessions. Jacobson et al. (2001) provide a summary of the various stages of this intervention approach (see Box 14.1). Typically, the process begins with an assessment of life domains (e.g., family, work, health, hobbies/recreation, spirituality) of the client to determine areas that the individual wants to target within therapy (Lejuez, Hopko, & Hopko, 2001). Strategies employed within BA interventions are numerous and include activity logs where clients monitor activities and their level of pleasurable

BOX 14.1 COURSE OF TREATMENT IN BEHAVIORAL ACTIVATION

The following is a general guideline for the progress of BA.

1. *Establishing a good therapeutic relationship and presenting the model to the client.* BA emphasizes the understanding of the client in this approach, and the treatment process begins with an overview of BA. As part of this initial phase, a summary of depression (e.g., symptoms, experience, hopefulness of being helped) is included. Additionally, the myth that changes in mood need to be achieved prior to behavior is dispelled.

2. *Developing treatment goals.* This process is a collaborative one between the clinician and client. Treatment goals are discussed and are divided into both short- and longer-term goals, identification of which is a priority for the work together. During this phase, the two work together to identify those situations that are secondary problems/behaviors that may be at work to maintain depression, for example, ways that a client is using avoidance or escape to avoid a situation. Likewise, ways that the client's routine is dysregulated (e.g., don't get out of bed, miss school) are also identified.

3. *Conducting a functional analysis.* In this phase, contextual issues are identified that trigger depressive experiences. These types of questions help guide work at this level (Jacobson et al., p. 261).
   a. What particular set of depressive symptoms is the client experiencing?
   b. How is the client responding to or trying to cope with the depression?
   c. To what extent are avoidance patterns exacerbating the depression?
   d. What routines have been disrupted?

4. *Employing activation strategies.* Through the use of various strategies such as monitoring logs and activity reports, clinicians and clients review their experiences. As part of this process, these experiences are appraised (e.g., "Attending mass on Sunday—coffee hour afterward. Spoke with 5 individuals. Was enjoyable.").

5. *Modifying avoidance.* Clients are helped to identify the functioning of avoidance and to choose alternative coping behaviors. Two acronyms are used:
   a. *TRAP*—decoded as
      i. *Trigger*
      ii. *Depressive response*
      iii. *Avoidance pattern*
   b. *TRAC*—which is
      i. *Trigger*
      ii. *Response*
      iii. *Alternative coping.*

The movement from TRAP to TRAC might include modifying the client's environment, such as choosing to spend time with different sets of individuals or bringing home work every night, or changing behavioral experiences, such as doing a 5-minute meditation prior to engaging in demanding caregiving tasks.

6. *Attending to routines*. Routines and structure provide a degree of mood elevation and accomplishment. By mastering tasks (e.g., rising, taking a shower, making coffee), the client can regain energy to undertake more novel experiences. The following acronym provides the steps in this process for a client:

   a. *A*—Assess whether what I am doing will add to my depression. Am I avoiding?

   b. *C*—Choose to behave in a way that will increase the chances that my life situation and mood will better.

   c. *T*—Try the behavior that I chose.

   d. *I*—Integrate the new behavior into my routine.

   e. *O*—Observe the result. Do I feel better or worse as a result of this new activity?

   f. *N*—Never give up! If something doesn't work—try again!

7. *Attending to experience*. In depressed individuals, negative thoughts become part of their experience. Instead of reinforcing, the clinician continues to focus on ways to activate the client. For example, what activities will block these thoughts? Through observation of times when the client is not engaged in negativity, the clinician seeks to increase the experience of positive experiences and interactions.

responses; goal setting, where the client determines the level of change that is acceptable or desired; and rewarding progress, which involves positive reinforcement for goal-related attainment (e.g., getting a massage).

Although derived from cognitive and behavioral therapies, BA offers a unique perspective on overcoming depression (Jacobson et al., 2001). So, what is different or new about BA? First, this approach helps clients modify their environment, and does not focus on the internal world such as emotions and cognitions. Second, the social withdrawal that is symptomatic of depression is viewed as the interaction of negative or painful life circumstances and the individual's challenge in changing these conditions. Finally, there is not an emphasis on skill development, as in other therapies. Instead, a clinician works to identify natural contingencies or reinforcements that the client is not enacting and enables the client to link to these potential sources of pleasure and positive reward.

BA and Depression

BA has specific effectiveness in treating depressed patients. A randomized control trial compared BA, cognitive therapy, and antidepressant medication in adult depressed patients ($n = 241$) (Dimidjian et al., 2006). Results indicate that BA was as efficacious as antidepressants and outperformed cognitive therapy. This finding is significant, as BA is the most parsimonious and easy-to-implement intervention among the three approaches evaluated.

Two meta-analyses have reviewed studies on BA. Cuijpers, van Straten, & Warmerdam (2007) included 16 studies that totaled 780 individuals. Ten studies recruited samples from the community, four from clinical settings, and two were unspecified. The majority ($n = 10$) compared BA to some type of cognitive therapy outcome. Results indicated that activity scheduling, a major component of BA, is effective in treating depression in adults. When compared to cognitive therapy, findings indicate that these two approaches yield similar positive outcomes that last up to 6 months post-intervention.

In a second meta-analysis, 34 RCTs were included ($n = 2,055$ participants) (Mazzucchelli, Kane, & Rees, 2009). Sixteen studies compared BA to control conditions such as waiting lists or usual treatments. The effectiveness of BA compared to control conditions was large and significant, with more positive outcomes achieved. A second analysis compared BA to other treatment conditions ($n = 23$ studies). Fifteen studies compared cognitive therapies to BA, with a result of no difference between these two treatment conditions. In an additional 17 studies, BA was compared to other psychotherapies or interventions (e.g., behavioral interventions, problem-solving therapies). Results favored BA as the most effect intervention within this subgroup of studies.

BA with Older Adults

Studies that evaluated BA with the older population have included individuals suffering from geriatric depression and complicated bereavement. In addition, BA has been implemented with dementia caregivers. In a study with those experiencing geriatric depression, BA was implemented as an in-home intervention (Yon & Scogin, 2009). Using a multiple baseline design, 14 older adults (mean age = 75 years) completed an average of 14.67 individual BA sessions. Overall, geriatric depression scores decreased significantly from pre- to post-test. In addition, 71% of those who experienced major depression no longer scored in this range at the end of the intervention. Overall, 56% of the sample experienced clinically significant improvement at post-test scores.

A second study evaluated BA treatment as applied through a bibliotherapy structure (Moss, Scogin, Di Napoli, & Presnell, 2012). Twenty-six participants were randomized into a 4-week intervention or wait-list group. Those in the intervention group received a copy of the book *Overcoming Depression One Step at a Time* (Addis & Martell, 2004), which includes both narrative and exercises to complete. Each week, intervention participants received a phone call to check for questions, monitor symptoms, and check progress on readings and assignments. At the conclusion of the intervention, treatment participants had decreased scores on a clinician-rated measure of depression. However, self-reported symptoms were not significant at post-test, but these scores decreased significantly at 1 month post-intervention. Interestingly, a finding suggested that the greater the amount of bibliotherapy received by a participant, the greater the improvements in depressive symptoms.

Two studies applied BA interventions to care providers of individuals with dementia. Losada, Márquez-González, and Romero-Moreno (2010) evaluated a group intervention to train caregivers to identify dysfunctional thoughts and barriers that block seeking positive and pleasant activities. The groups met for 12 weeks, with a maximum of eight participants in each group. Results indicted that at post-test, caregivers were less depressed, experienced fewer dysfunctional thoughts, and had higher scores on pursuing leisure activities.

A final study evaluated a telephone-based intervention to support Chinese caregivers (Au, 2015). Two groups of caregivers (n = 93) participated in a treatment group for 4 weeks. Both groups started by receiving a psychoeducational intervention that helped increase caregiver knowledge on dementia, stress, and community resources. After 4 weeks, the BA group received weekly phone calls to increase the pleasant activities that they experienced and facilitated communication with the care recipient and others. The second group received weekly phone calls that reinforced content that was originally presented within the 4-week psychoeducational sessions. At baseline and after the initial 4 weeks, there were no differences between the two groups. After the additional 4-week intervention, the BA group experienced a significant decrease in depression scores. In addition, the BA treatment group had a significant increase in positive communication and coping skills.

Promise of BA with Older Adults As with MBSR, BA interventions hold promise as effective interventions with the older population. There are several features that make this treatment approach appealing as a intervention strategy. First, geriatric depression is a significant mental health issue in later life and occurs as a result of health and social transitions, relocations, and other events that might decrease pleasurable activities for individuals. These changes may lead to major lifestyle alterations—such as a person who has to dramatically change a diet because of a medical condition. In attempting to cope, the person may abandon several pleasurable activities, such as cooking or eating out with friends. This all-or-nothing strategy can lead to feelings of deprivation, disconnection, and isolation. BA strategies can assist the individual to integrate new approaches, such as trying different restaurants, or taking a cooking class on healthy food preparation.

Second, the implementation of BA is very flexible, which allows integration into multiple settings. Studies have been conducted in group and individual formats, using technology and web-based applications, and within a home-based, residential, and community environment. In addition, training to deliver BA is relatively easy and can be incorporated into settings where there are scarce mental health resources (e.g., nursing homes).

Since BA focuses on integrating pleasurable experiences and activities, the approach may be viewed as less stigmatizing for older cohorts who are not drawn to insight-oriented treatments. In addition, the course of BA treatment can be brief, which provides positive outcomes and symptom relief quickly. These outcomes are encouraging since evidence exists that treatment effects continue post-intervention.

These two treatment approaches, MBSR and BA, are examples of emerging therapies that hold promise for older adults. While neither one has an extensive literature base with older clients yet, the emerging literature indicates that both approaches yield positive results. In addition, both approaches are flexible enough to be administered within different contexts. Moving forward, evaluations of other promising interventions need to be undertaken to expand the array of treatment approaches with older adults and their families.

NEXT STEPS IN EVIDENCE-BASED PRACTICE WITH OLDER ADULTS

To expand the evidence base of treatment approaches, there are several next steps that need to be taken. Some of these are expanding existing approaches that are effective in practice with older adults into new populations, using innovative approaches within diverse contexts. In addition, research on emerging therapies with the older population require additional evaluation to increase understanding of effective practice.

EXPANDING EXISTING EVIDENCE-BASED PRACTICE APPROACHES

A major question in intervention research is whether an intervention or treatment model will yield significant results within practice settings. This topic was addressed as part of the issue in implementation fidelity (see Chapter 13), with examples of modifications that were necessary to ensure that the intervention was feasible and had achievable outcomes. Besides intervention fidelity, however, there are other factors that impact whether an intervention can be carried out as intended.

An intervention may have significant, positive impacts when using one type of administration, yet performs poorly if offered in a different format. An example is an intervention that was created by one of the authors of this book, titled Let's Talk about Raising Grandchildren. Using an audio-based format, this was a psychoeducational intervention constructed for grandparents who were raising grandchildren. In an effort to reach frail or isolated care providers, the intervention contained eight modules on caregiving topics that grandparents could listen to individually. A workbook accompanied the audio component so grandparents had the opportunity to apply the practice concepts within their life. As an individually focused intervention, this approach had success in helping grandparents with care-related tasks (Kropf & Wilks, 2003).

Due to the initial effectiveness with custodial grandparents, the intervention was introduced as a curriculum for a group intervention with these care providers. Unlike the individually based administration, it did not go well in a group format. In fact, the grandparents asked that it be discontinued after the third week! What was the reason? They stated that they wanted the chance to talk about *their* experiences, and not be bound to the topic that was introduced from the intervention. That is, the *supportive* aspect of the group intervention was the most valuable for the participants. This (very humbling) example demonstrates the importance of considering the context for a new intervention, as well as empirically evaluating efficacy using different treatment administrations.

When evidence exists, this knowledge needs to reach practitioners to advance their understanding of what interventions work to achieve which outcomes. Evidence-based models need to be integrated into the curricula of programs that educate the next generation of clinicians (cf., Gibbs & Gambrill, 2002; Rubin 2011). Practice-based classes, as well as internships and externships, need to include those approaches that are founded on empirical outcomes. This can be exciting for students who can become researchers themselves as they evaluate methods of practice in their assignments and field work experiences. These topics also need to be inserted into continuing education modules, as existing practitioners may not have been exposed to this content during their own studies.

Researchers need to also bolster the evidence base within intervention studies. Within research, operationalizing the independent variable is crucial and, unfortunately, is given little or no attention (Corley & Kim, 2015; Naleppa & Cagle, 2010; Tucker & Blythe, 2008). Crucial information includes duration, length of treatment, administration protocol, fidelity issues of treatment, and sequence of content. In order to determine comparability of interventions, more detailed summaries and descriptions must appear within the literature.

EVALUATING PROMISING INTERVENTION APPROACHES

In addition, evidence on the effectiveness of new and innovative approaches needs to be generated and evaluated. With the increasing complexity issues brought by aging clients into practice, clinicians need to draw from a variety of practice approaches. Consider some of the issues presented within the case examples of the chapters—older adults with addictions, those who are in care provider roles (versus being a care recipient themselves), or older adults with lifelong psychiatric issues. Do we have enough clinical data to make good decisions about effective practice approaches with these clients?

As new treatments are introduced with the older population, a critical question is whether they will produce the same level of effectiveness as with younger cohorts. Clearly, the chapters on evidence-based practice stress the importance of adapting and modifying approaches to be congruent with changes and preferences within the older population. In fact, there is not one set of necessary modifications, as the "older population" is often multiple decades of older individuals. Careful analyses of functional abilities and sociocultural aspects (e.g., lower education level in the oldest cohorts) need to be taken into account within intervention approaches. As evaluated in Chapter 13, modifications in approaches need to be empirically evaluated.

In summary, practice and treatment with older adults and their families is in an exciting place! As the population grows, health and social service professionals will increasingly address practice issues of later life. As evidence-based practitioners, clinicians have greater resources as more attention to the older population has been integrated into health and mental health research and practice. Additionally, there are numerous opportunities to evaluate whether practice approaches that are effective with other populations have utility with older clients.

These are some of the "new possibilities and new directions" that Betty Friedan suggested in her book *The Fountain of Age*, which was quoted at the beginning of Chapter 1. Moving forward, all health, mental health, and social service practitioners will experience these possibilities and challenges of aging in their professional work. As authors of this book, we hope that the contents provide a resource for practice—and open avenues to consider how to effectively intervene within the lives of older adults.

REFERENCES

Addis, M. E., & Martell, C. R. (2004). *Overcoming depression one step at a time: the new behavioral activation approach to getting your life back*. Oakland, CA: New Harbinger Publishing.

Au, A. (2015). Developing volunteer-assisted behavioral activation teleprograms to meet the needs of Chinese dementia caregivers. *Clinical Gerontologist, 38*(3), 190–202.

Bohlmeijer, E., Prenger, R., Taal, E., & Cuijpers, P. (2010). The effects of mindfulness-based stress reduction therapy on mental health of adults with a chronic medical disease: a meta-analysis. *Journal of Psychosomatic Research, 68*(6), 539–544.

Carmody, J., & Baer, R. A. (2009). How long does a mindfulness-based stress reduction program need to be? A review of class contact hours and effect sizes for psychological distress. *Journal of Clinical Psychology, 65*(6), 627–638.

Corley, N. A., & Kim, I. (2015). An assessment of intervention fidelity in published social work intervention research studies. *Research on Social Work Practice, 26*(1), 53–60.

Creswell, J. D., Irwin, M. R., Burklund, L. J., Lieberman, M. D., Arevalo, J. M., Ma, J., . . . Cole, S. W. (2012). Mindfulness-based stress reduction training reduces loneliness and pro-inflammatory gene expression in older adults: a small randomized controlled trial. *Brain, Behavior, and Immunity, 26*(7), 1095–1101.

Crowe, M., Jordan, J., Burrell, B., Jones, V., Gillon, D., & Harris, S. (2016). Mindfulness-based stress reduction for long-term physical conditions: a systematic review. *Australian and New Zealand Journal of Psychiatry, 50*(1), 21–32.

Cuijpers, P., Van Straten, A., & Warmerdam, L. (2007). Behavioral activation treatments of depression: a meta-analysis. *Clinical Psychology Review, 27*(3), 318–326.

De Vibe, M., Bjørndal, A., Tipton, E., Hammerstrøm, K. T., & Kowalski, K. (2012). Mindfulness based stress reduction (MBSR) for improving health, quality of life, and social functioning in adults. *Campbell Systematic Reviews*, 8(3). DOI:10.4073/csr.2012.3.

Dimidjian, S., Hollon, S. D., Dobson, K. S., Schmaling, K. B., Kohlenberg, R. J., Addis, M. E., . . . Atkins, D. C. (2006). Randomized trial of behavioral activation, cognitive therapy, and antidepressant medication in the acute treatment of adults with major depression. *Journal of Consulting and Clinical Psychology*, 74(4), 658–670.

Ferster, C. B. (1973). A functional analysis of depression. *American Psychologist*, 28(10), 857.

Gallegos, A. M., Hoerger, M., Talbot, N. L., Krasner, M. S., Knight, J. M., Moynihan, J. A., & Duberstein, P. R. (2013). Toward identifying the effects of the specific components of mindfulness-based stress reduction on biologic and emotional outcomes among older adults. *The Journal of Alternative and Complementary Medicine*, 19(10), 787–792.

Gallegos, A. M., Hoerger, M., Talbot, N. L., Moynihan, J. A., & Duberstein, P. R. (2013). Emotional benefits of mindfulness-based stress reduction in older adults: the moderating roles of age and depressive symptom severity. *Aging & Mental Health*, 17(7), 823–829.

Gans, J. J., O'Sullivan, P., & Bircheff, V. (2014). Mindfulness based tinnitus stress reduction pilot study. *Mindfulness*, 5(3), 322–333.

Gibbs, L., & Gambrill, E. (2002). Evidence-based practice: counterarguments to objections. *Research on Social Work Practice*, 12(3), 452–476.

Goyal, M., Singh, S., Sibinga, E. M., Gould, N. F., Rowland-Seymour, A., Sharma, R., . . . Ranasinghe, P. D. (2014). Meditation programs for psychological stress and well-being: a systematic review and meta-analysis. *JAMA Internal Medicine*, 174(3), 357–368.

Grossman, P., Niemann, L., Schmidt, S., & Walach, H. (2004). Mindfulness-based stress reduction and health benefits: a meta-analysis. *Journal of Psychosomatic Research*, 57(1), 35–43.

Gu, J., Strauss, C., Bond, R., & Cavanagh, K. (2015). How do mindfulness-based cognitive therapy and mindfulness-based stress reduction improve mental health and wellbeing? A systematic review and meta-analysis of mediation studies. *Clinical Psychology Review*, 37, 1–12.

Hensen, D. (2012) A guide to mindfulness at work. *Forbes* (October 31). http://www.forbes.com/sites/drewhansen/2012/10/31/a-guide-to-mindfulness-at-work/

Hou, R. J., Wong, S. S., Yip, B. K., Hung, A. T., Lo, H. M., Chan, P. H., . . . Mercer, S. W. (2014). The effects of mindfulness-based stress reduction program on the mental health of family caregivers: a randomized controlled trial. *Psychotherapy and Psychosomatics*, 83(1), 45–53.

Jacobson, N. S., Martell, C. R., & Dimidjian, S. (2001). Behavioral activation treatment for depression: returning to contextual roots. *Clinical Psychology: Science and Practice*, 8(3), 255–270.

Kabat-Zinn, J. (1990). *Full catastrophe living: using the wisdom of your body and mind to face stress, pain and illness*. New York: Delacorte.

Khoury, B., Sharma, M., Rush, S. E., & Fournier, C. (2015). Mindfulness-based stress reduction for healthy individuals: a meta-analysis. *Journal of Psychosomatic Research*, 78(6), 519–528.

Kropf, N. P., & Wilks, S. (2003). Grandparents raising grandchildren. In B. Berkman & L. Harootyan (Eds.), *Social work and health care in an aging society* (pp. 177–200). New York: Springer.

Kumar, S., Adiga, K. R., & George, A. (2014). Effectiveness of mindfulness based stress reduction (MBSR) on stress and anxiety among elderly residing in residential homes. *International Journal of Nursing Care*, 2(2), 81–85.

Ledesma, D., & Kumano, H. (2009). Mindfulness-based stress reduction and cancer: a meta-analysis. *Psycho-Oncology*, 18(6), 571–579.

Lejuez, C. W., Hopko, D. R & Hopko, S. D. (2001). A brief behavioral activation treatment for depression treatment manual. *Behavior Modification, 25*(2), 255–286.

Lenze, E. J., Hickman, S., Hershey, T., Wendleton, L., Ly, K., Dixon, D., . . . Wetherell, J. L. (2014). Mindfulness-based stress reduction for older adults with worry symptoms and co-occurring cognitive dysfunction. *International Journal of Geriatric Psychiatry, 29*(10), 991–1000.

Losada, A., Márquez-González, M., & Romero-Moreno, R. (2010). Mechanisms of action of a psychological intervention for dementia caregivers: effects of behavioral activation and modification of dysfunctional thoughts. *International Journal of Geriatric Psychiatry, 26*(11), 1119–1127.

Mazzucchelli, T., Kane, R., & Rees, C. (2009). Behavioral activation treatments for depression in adults: a meta-analysis and review. *Clinical Psychology: Science and Practice, 16*(4), 383–411.

McBee, L., Westreich, L., & Likourezos, A. (2004). A psychoeducational relaxation group for pain and stress management in the nursing home. *Journal of Social Work in Long-Term Care, 3*(1), 15–28.

Merkes, M. (2010). Mindfulness-based stress reduction for people with chronic diseases. *Australian Journal of Primary Health, 16*(3), 200–210.

Moss, A. S., Reibel, D. K., Greeson, J. M., Thapar, A., Bubb, R., Salmon, J., & Newberg, A. B. (2015). An adapted mindfulness-based stress reduction program for elders in a continuing care retirement community quantitative and qualitative results from a pilot randomized controlled trial. *Journal of Applied Gerontology, 34*(4), 518–538.

Moss, K., Scogin, F., Di Napoli, E., & Presnell, A. (2012). A self-help behavioral activation treatment for geriatric depressive symptoms. *Aging & Mental Health, 16*(5), 625–635.

Mularski, R. A., Munjas, B. A., Lorenz, K. A., Sun, S., Robertson, S. J., Schmelzer, W., . . . Shekelle, P. G. (2009). Randomized controlled trial of mindfulness-based therapy for dyspnea in chronic obstructive lung disease. *The Journal of Alternative and Complementary Medicine, 15*(10), 1083–1090.

Naleppa, M. J., & Cagle, J. G. (2010). Treatment fidelity in social work intervention research: a review of published studies. *Research on Social Work Practice, 20*(6), 674–681.

Rubin, A. (2011). Teaching EBP in social work: retrospective and prospective. *Journal of Social Work, 11*(1), 64–79.

Tucker, A., & Blythe, B. (2008). Attention to treatment fidelity in social work outcomes: a review of the literature from the 1990s. *Social Work Research, 32*(3), 185–190.

Yon, A., & Scogin, F. (2009). Behavioral activation as a treatment for geriatric depression. *Clinical Gerontologist, 32*(1), 91–103.

Zainal, N. Z., Booth, S., & Huppert, F. A. (2013). The efficacy of mindfulness-based stress reduction on mental health of breast cancer patients: a meta-analysis. *Psycho-Oncology, 22*(7), 1457–1465.

Zhang, J. X., Liu, X. H., Xie, X. H., Zhao, D., Shan, M. S., Zhang, X. L., . . . Cui, H. (2015). Mindfulness-based stress reduction for chronic insomnia in adults older than 75 years: a randomized, controlled, single-blind clinical trial. *EXPLORE: The Journal of Science and Healing, 11*(3), 180–185.

INDEX

CPSIA information can be obtained
at www.ICGtesting.com
Printed in the USA
BVHW040100210919
559038BV00001B/1/P